LIVING IN A WORLD TRANSFORMED

Perceptual and Performatory Adaptation to Visual Distortion

LIVING IN A WORLD TRANSFORMED

Perceptual and Performatory Adaptation to Visual Distortion

Hubert Dolezal

Department of Psychology
Northeastern Illinois University
Chicago, Illinois

THE BLACKBURN PRESS

Reprint of the 1982 Edition, by Academic Press, Inc.

Living in a World Transformed
Perceptual and Performatory Adaptation to Visual Distortion

ISBN-10 1-932846-02-6
ISBN-13: 978-1-932846-02-7

Library of Congress Control Number: 2004110239

THE BLACKBURN PRESS
P. O. Box 287
Caldwell, New Jersey 07006 U.S.A.
973-228-7077
www.BlackburnPress.com

To Nick, Renée, and Christopher

Contents

11

Theoretical Foci and Paradigms: Products and Processes of Adaptation 261

12

Practical Applications: Sleep and Space Travel 303

A

Appendix: Long-Term Adaptation to Up-Down Reversal: Observer's Direct Reports 315

Preface

This book, a waystation, inspects an ancient puzzle: How are the real world and its truths preserved in visual perception? In my boyhood I watched with amazement as a broomhandle bent as it was lowered into a water tank and then straightened again as it was withdrawn. It was then that I first wondered whether visual realities could be trusted. As a graduate student at Cornell, I became acquainted with the enterprising experiments of George Stratton and Ivo Kohler. Both had attached to their heads prismatic spectacles that inverted or reversed the light that entered their eyes. For extended periods, they then tried to go about their everyday business. Was adaptation to this radical optical transformation possible, and how did it work?

The reports of their experiences contained seemingly contradictory observations and interpretations. Ambiguities and outright contradictions were apparent in the textbooks that related their findings (e.g., Boring, 1950, p. 678). All in all, I and many others were left fascinated, bewildered, and unsatisfied. I simply had to find out first-hand what it was like to live in such an ostensibly different world; here was my chance to turn back the clock and step through Alice's looking glass, into the transformed world of Walter Mitty.

The plan of my project, then, was to wear reversing prisms for an extended period, collect the facts, and describe them accurately without linguistic ambiguity. One specific task was to describe how the visual system must work with the motor system when the optical information incorrectly specifies the location of places, objects, people, events, and visible parts of the self. Accomplishments in the areas of cognition, memory, and aesthetic judgment were also covered. I tried to heed Leonardo Da Vinci's advice that science comes by observation, not authority; getting accurate facts is the most basic task and precious commodity of science—its flywheel of change.

This book also aims to provide a paradigm case for future long-term adaptation experiments. Thus, rather than featuring a broad survey of the vast literature of related research—excellent ones by Howard and Templeton (1966), Rock (1966), and Welch (1978) are already available—this book aims at an in-depth description and analysis of a carefully controlled 5-week study during which I wore up–down reversing prisms affixed to a football helmet and lived as normally as possible in an outdoor environment, a mountainous coastal village in Greece. The book also provides an in-depth analysis of selected issues of concern to several major researchers and theorists in the field: Hermann von Helmholtz, George Stratton, Ivo Kohler, Richard Held, Irwin Rock, Charles Harris, and Ian Howard.

My treatment of the subject matter differs in several other respects. The method followed was in the phenomenological tradition as taught me by Robert MacLeod. Analysis of the observations is Gibsonian. Understanding perceptual and performatory adaptations to optical transformation in the full interactive complexity of everyday life calls for this emphasis: to describe the nature of the information that at first confuses and misleads the spectacle-wearer, yet eventually enables him or her to see meaning in what he or she perceives and to act competently. Thus, the study is a primary source of raw data for perceptual theory, which will, I hope, enhance methodological rigor, help dispel misconceptions, encourage models that represent reality more accurately, and lead to new areas of research. As the title of this book implies, the perceiver is transformed no less that the visible world.

I hope the book will be useful to undergraduates, graduate students, and researchers in psychology who want access to original source material and an in-depth analysis of a paradigmatic study. Those studying human perception and performance skills, especially as related to the development and modification of these skills here on earth and in weightless environments, should also find the book helpful.

Acknowledgments

This book is in your hands today because of the good will of many people and the continuous support of my university.

There are those to whom special recognition belongs: Paul Hauptly constructed the helmet system and mounted the two prism units; Rebecca Moskowitz typed several drafts superbly and flawlessly with good cheer, sound advice, and unbelievable patience; Mitchell Beales organized figures and references, and replenished my desk with books and articles; Carol Podraza did excellent typing. A good combination of support and leeway came from the staff of Academic Press, who understand the pertubations of authorship, and series editor E. C. Carterette made valuable suggestions for pruning the manuscript.

Looking over my shoulders, especially during the early phases of this project, were my honored Cornell teachers: Robert MacLeod, James J. Gibson, Eric Lenneberg, and Ulric Neisser. I also thank loyal friends and family for being there: Tom Toleno, Anthony Barrand, Sam Boyian, James Lackner, Ann Graybiel-Lackner, Bea MacLeod, James Mancuso, Leslie Schneider, Patrick Cabe, my brother Herman, his wife Diane, and my mother.

Two scholarly souls, Larry Benowitz and Randy Easton, critically appraised the manuscript and made suggestions for improvements and revisions of most of it. How often they saved me from folly!

The central place in my dedication belongs to my wife, Renée, who gave her time to me willingly and lovingly. She edited every draft, acting as a persistent and candid critic, and encouraged me to see this book through. The other two dedications are for Nick, my father for 23 years, and for my loving son Christopher.

LIVING IN A WORLD TRANSFORMED

Perceptual and Performatory Adaptation to Visual Distortion

Introduction

The sun falls slowly out of the water. I watch it as it descends into the Grecian sky, brightening the world into day. Towering Mount Pelion hangs from the water's surface, a cheap pasteup, stuck there carelessly. Suddenly I visually perceive that I am geographically down there, below me, standing on my head, looking up at the sky. Somehow my head is dissociated from my body or hanging upside down. I make these seemingly bizarre observations from a balcony overlooking the coast of St. John's. My world and I have been transformed: I have just begun to wear up–down reversing prisms. In the days to come I will try to ride a bike, hike on steep mountain trails, water ski, drive a car, read, play chess and soccer, and go on with the banalities of daily life, all in my world transformed.

Descriptive data like these are presented and analyzed throughout this book and directed toward exploring basic questions about perception. How dependent is knowing and doing on perceiving? How are humans able to get around successfully in the real world? How do we perceive and represent mentally what there is to know about ourselves, especially in relation to the world, and how do we put this knowledge to work in action?

The method for my exploration suggested itself after I read Stratton. He applied a unique test to learn how the human perceiver and performer copes with misinformation created by transforming spectacles. Would the spectacle-wearer come to know again the real attributes of the self and of the world? Could he or she rediscover truth? Here was the tool par excellence I had sought to investigate how humans acquire knowledge and how successful we are at reacquiring consistent perception and competent action when the conventional visual information to do is perturbed. In donning spectacles, I, too, was to discover how resourceful people are under unique conditions of survival. All in all, this book is but a link in the exploration of perception.

PLAN OF THE BOOK

My first goal is to provide a reasonably full description and explanation of adaptation phenomena—of the perceptual experiences and actions produced when a person lives in a natural environment with optically transforming spectacles. To that end, Chapter 2 outlines several experimenter requirements for describing and measuring adaptation, including a brief discussion of the variables that have been found to be influential. Chapter 3 then details the optical conditions that spectacles impose on an observer and the consequent unique adapting requirements for perceiving and acting. A widely neglected and important factor in adaptation research is treated in Chapter 4: the restricted field of view (FV). All spectacle-adaptation experiments limit the normal FV and thus produce effects that have been confounded with, and attributed to, the optical transformation. Results of a 1-week study, the Tube Study, in which I limited my field of vision to 12° by placing plain paper tubes over my eyes, explored the relationship between central and peripheral vision and documented the importance of peripheral visual information for body position knowledge and for all forms of action.

In keeping with my second goal, to provide a paradigm case for long-term adaptation experiments, Chapters 5–10 emphasize an in-depth description and analysis of such an investigation, the Prism Study: a 5-week experiment during which I wore up–down reversing prisms affixed to a football helmet and lived as normally as possible in an outdoor environment. Chapter 5 features the method and Chapter 6 describes the control stages and baseline adaptations to the increased weight, size, and restricted FV of the helmet system. The immediate effects, gradual modifications, and final accomplishments to reversing the FV are discussed in three further chapters; visual stability during head and body movements (Chapter 7); visually guided actions (Chapter 8); and the perception of the self and of events (Chapter 9). Chapter 10 considers the aftereffects (*a*) of adaptation to reversing the FV; (*b*) of restricting it; and (*c*) of having increased the size and weight of the observer's functional head with the helmet. The nature of the information that is responsible for the observed effects, adaptations, and aftereffects is emphasized in Chapters 7–10. Chapter 11 is devoted to an analysis of the main descriptive, experimental, and theoretical contributions of seven influential researchers and theorists: Stratton, Kohler, Rock, Harris, Helmholtz, Held, and Howard. My views are also juxtaposed and summarized. Finally, Chapter 12 offers a brief discussion of future implications, especially for sleep research and for adaptation to the weightlessness sickness experienced by space travelers. Appendix A contains some of my direct observations from the Prism Study that are relevant to Chapters 7–10. Appendix B is a description of the prisms, the construction of the helmet, and the time course of the Prism Study. As it turns out, this book is a treatise in defense of *visual knowledge.*

CHECKING UP ON THE AUTHOR: HOW TO BUILD A DO-IT-YOURSELF REVERSING SPECTACLE

I recommend that you make a simple and inexpensive device that up–down reverses the light available to your visual system and approximates the apparatus I used. Such observations are fascinating and will make this book more comprehensible since the relationships of the geometrical optics of light can be hard to grasp.

First, get a pair of round welder's goggles that fit snugly over the eyes. Next, tape both sides of the lower three-quarters of each glass with black electrician's tape, leaving free a narrow slit at the top. Now, get a rectangular, highly reflecting metal sheet or a mirror (not safe), the length of which matches the width of your forehead. Place the reflector's edge against your forehead as if it were a visor cap. You can free your hand by attaching the reflector to a light plastic (welder's helmet) harness that can be placed on the head and adjusted to fit snugly. Use tape to make *absolutely* sure that no light other than light bouncing off the surface of the reflector enters your eyes. Any nonreversed light will invalidate any "pure" observation. Note that to see anything your eyes must always remain cast up toward the reflector, a problem faced by Kohler and his observers. In my Prism Study, I used prisms instead of mirrors, and this allowed me to move my eyes freely. Extreme care should be taken if you wish to do more than sit and point, read, or write with this apparatus; have someone near to prevent a fall if you plan to move about.

THE EXPERIMENTER AS SUBJECT: BENEFITS AND PROBLEMS

Scientific discovery initially depends on the direct observations and private experiences of individuals. Firsthand observations may be communicated more accurately because the data need not go through an additional translation from subject to experimenter. Also, the broader and more focused knowledge of the prepared Experimenter makes more likely the discovery of evidence that the normal subject might purposefully ignore (i.e., because of instructions from the experimenter that focus the subject's attention elsewhere). Thus, the researcher doubling as observer, is freer to supersede her–his original intentions and pursue data in support of divergent hypotheses. Chances are also that the trained experimenter can better distinguish fact from inference and thus collect more clean, theory-free data (Dolezal & Toleno, 1975; MacLeod, 1949, 1975). The following discoveries in the psychological phenomenology of human perception confirm these advantages: Goethe's, Purkinje's, and Hering's work on the perception of color; Stumpf, on tone; Katz, on touch; Max Wertheimer, on apparent motion; Rubin, on figure-ground; Michotte, on causality; and James, on consciousness (Dolezal, 1975, p. 225; Mac Leod, 1968, p. 69, 1970, p. 250; Spiegelberg, 1965; Thinès, 1977, Chapter 2).

Yet, the misgivings and suspicions about single-observer research have not been stilled. When only one observer collects data, their reliability is thought to be in serious jeopardy. The uniqueness of the individual is considered a hazard to reliability. Drawing conclusions from single-observer studies that imply a general principle is seen as a particularly dangerous practice, and so it can be. However, these reservations have not stood in the way of reliable, valid, and significant measurement and generalizations. Thus, substantial agreement exists that single-observer, or small-N, research has yielded major breakthroughs due to intensive observation and reflection upon a few cases (Carini, 1975). Piaget's fruitful conceptualizations serve as prime examples. Part of the reason for increased precision is the improved possibility for determining the sources of variability (Kratochwill, 1978, Chapter 1; Hersen & Barlow, 1976, Chapter 2). Single-observer studies have an honored history because of their remarkable track record of fertile methodological, factual, and conceptual groundwork, all of which turned out to be essentially accurate upon parametric repetition with many observers. Weber's work on the psychophysics of thresholds, that of Fechner on afterimages, that of Ebbinghaus on human memory, and that of Mach on the role of the semicircular canals in the perception of movement of the body are further examples of this viable tradition (Thinès, 1977). Studies of adaptation to transformations (especially the observations of Helmholtz and Stratton, who served as both experimenter and observer have proven themselves repeatable and heuristic goldmines.

Indeed, as we venture into highly uncommon environments such as outer space where a few wander for relatively short periods, our development of single-observer methodology becomes increasingly important. No doubt, data collected under the complex and uncontrolled conditions of everyday life should be rechecked under exacting laboratory conditions. By encouraging the dual mode of scientific investigations in life and in the laboratory, flexibility of inquiry will be preserved. I hope that others will choose to continue the tradition of single-observer investigation and that this book will aid them to do so.

1

Historical Perspective

PHILOSOPHICAL ORIGINS

The need to understand the unknown, including the very process of knowing, distinguishes humans from other species. Sustained discourse on the question, "What is the nature of human knowledge?" can be found in Plato's *Cratylus, Phaedrus,* and *Republic.* Broad questions of this kind generate two false expectations: that a single answer is possible and that it might suffice. Neither is true. The thinking of philosophers most concerned with the problem of human knowledge over the last 23 centuries[1] is characterized by a process of observing, noting distinctions, and following up with more detailed questions. The enterprise is powered by curiosity. Unwieldy problems posed by philosophers thus have

[1]Plato, *Phaedrus,* Vol. 7, 115-141; Aristotle, *Physics,* Vol. 8, 259-355; Augustine, *The Confessions,* Vol. 18, 1-125; Aquinas, *The Summa Theologica,* Vols. 19 & 20; Descartes, *Rules for the Direction of the Mind,* Vol. 31, 1-40; Spinoza, *Ethics,* Vol. 31, 355-463; Locke, *An Essay Concerning Human Understanding,* Vol. 35, 85-400; Berkeley, *The Principles of Human Knowledge,* Vol. 35, 403-444; Hume, An Inquiry Concerning Human Understanding, Vol. 35, 451-509; Kant, *The Critique of Pure Reason,* Vol. 42, 1-250; Hegel, *The Philosophy of Right,* Vol. 46, 1-150; and James, *The Principles of Psychology,* Vol. 53. (All volumes published by Encyclopaedia Britannica, Chicago, 1952, as part of the Great Books of the Western World series.)

been reformulated and refined until they eventually became the factual inquiry of psychologists.

The concern of this book, adaptation to visual transformation, is a contemporary representative of several ancient but persistent questions about the validity and reliability of knowing activities: How accurately does perception represent reality; how stable an index of reality is perception? These broad questions remain partly unanswered because they still contain meanings that reach beyond the factual details accumulated by modern methods and theories and are, ultimately, the thrust of this book.

DISCOVERY: THE RETINAL IMAGE IS INVERTED[2,3]

The central role of light in the study of perception was explicitly recognized by the ancient Hellenes. The cycle, making plain observations and then asking questions about them, eventually yielded the realization that light arriving at the retina is inverted and reversed with respect to light before it enters the eyeball. When light reflected from an external object passes through a small hole punched in a sheet of thin material making up one wall of a room, an inverted and reversed image is cast on the opposite wall. Such a room is known as a *camera obscura* (dark chamber), and its miniature is a pinhole camera (Figure 1.1). Although its invention is often attributed to Porta (e.g., Helmholtz, 1962, Vol. I, p. 116; Southall, 1964, p. 5), the *camera obscura* was long used by Arab astronomers to safely view solar and lunar eclipses, and the Arabian scholar Alhazen (Ibu al-Haytham, 965–1039 or 1040) compared the *camera obscura* to the structure of the eye and its inverted image to that formed in the eyeball (Polyak, 1957, p. 20). Indeed, Alhazen's elaborate, seven-volume treatment of vision and optics in his *Optics* foreshadowed many modern developments but was almost totally neglected (cf. Sabra, 1978, Chapter 6).

[2]Inversion refers to the optical reversal of up for down *and* right for left.

[3]We need to distinguish between two kinds of images: *optical* and *retinal-physiological*. An optical image consists of structured light and is either static or fluid, representing immobile or moving distal sources, that is, an object or event. The retina is either relatively stationary during fixation or moves with respect to the optical images of the ambient array during saccadic and pursuit movements. The retina "samples" optical images; it is a light-sensitive surface that moves "behind" a sea of shafts of light—behind optical images. A retinal image is a portion of the ambient array containing optical images that have impinged on the searching retina. Most importantly, it is the structural characteristics of the optical image, not the supposedly "visible," or pictorial characteristics of the retinal "image," that constitute the proximal stimulation for vision.

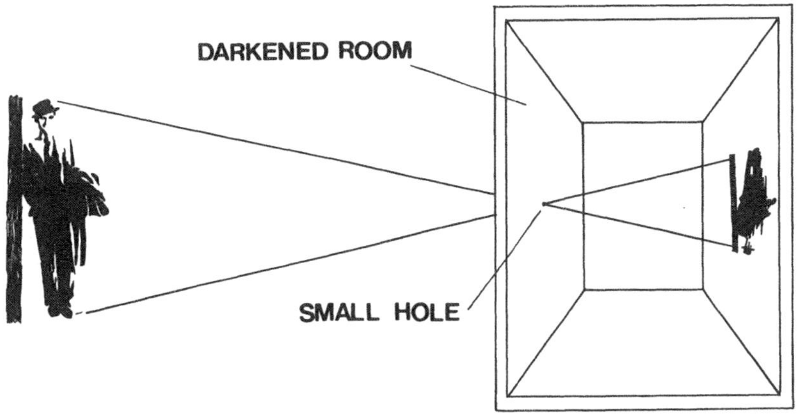

FIGURE 1.1. The camera obscura. The optical image is inverted (right–left and up–down reversed) when passed through a pinhole, analogous to entering the eye through the pupil.

Although it is possible that Leonardo Da Vinci (1452–1519) also invented the *camera obscura,* it is more likely that he knew of Alhazen's eleventh century (1038) description, which was translated into Latin in the late twelfth or early thirteenth century by an unknown person (Sabra, 1978, p. 179). Da Vinci did more than describe the analogical relationship between the pinhole and the pupil and the common image-inversion effect within a chambered enclosure. He was clearly the first to ponder the apparent incongruity of humans seeing objects as being normally oriented while they are evidently unaware of the inverted image within the eyeball. To Da Vinci, this discrepancy required a solution. Although his descriptions are fragmented, they contain clear evidence that he assumed that the inverted image must be reinverted to make vision possible. His knowledge of the fact that light is refracted at an interface of air with a denser medium such as water or a lens may well have helped mislead him (Leonardo Da Vinci's *Notebooks,* 1958, pp. 225–226). Indeed, he erroneously postulated that the lens reinverts the inverted image, supporting his argument by three diagrams (Polyak, 1941, Figure 24). Da Vinci said, "no image of however small a body enters within the eye without being turned upside down, and as it penetrates the crystalline sphere it is turned again upside down, and so the image within the eye becomes upright as was the object outside the eye [1958, p. 259]."

Aranzi, an Italian writing in the then customary Latin, was the first to demonstrate experimentally that the retinal image is inverted in the animal eye. Removal of part of the opaque coats (sclera and choroid) in the back of the eyeball allowed the image formed on the retina or a plate behind it to become directly visible.[4] The experiment itself predates 1586, yet his contribution, published in 1595, remained without influence (Polyak, 1957, pp. 38, 97). Two further donations to understanding the behavior of light—one, theoretical and the other, empirical—were required before the inverted retinal image could become a generally accepted fact and thence, a tenaciously cherished puzzle. First, based on his knowledge of the behavior of light when passed through positive lenses, Kepler had, by 1611, drawn an accurate representation of the formation of an optical image "on" the retina (Polyak, 1957, pp. 36–37; Walls, 1951, p. 4). Second, in 1625, Jesuit friar Christopher Scheiner demonstrated convincingly that an inverted and minified image was projected on the human retina (Helmholtz, 1962, Vol. I, p. 91). In this instance, Scheiner was more successful than even Da Vinci in satisfying Da Vinci's credo that science comes by observation, not authority. Leonardo's riddle became the bewilderment of many, including Descartes, Molyneux, and Berkely. Consequently, it could hardly escape becoming a full-sized puzzlement with which even twentieth-century experimental psychologists grappled: How can we accurately perceive the location and orientation of objects in the environment if the light from them is inverted and reversed inside the eye? Who or what "turns it around again" inside the perceiver? Somehow, somewhere, the inverted retinal image had to be restored to harmony with its external object before vision could be understood.

A new authority had thus been invited into scientific thought, namely, the unquestioned assumption that the inverted image must be erected to allow for veridical vision. That assumption had two other assumptions tucked under its wings: (*a*) That visible, pictorial characteristics of the retinal image are somehow "looked at" by some part of the brain during visual perception; (*b*) That accurate perception necessitates a *correspondence* of orientation, location, shape, size, etc. of object and retinal image characteristics. The first assumption requires a Cartesian homunculus who "sees" the retinal image and inverts it again in so doing; it promises an indefinite regress. The second has given rise to

[4]It is important to recognize that the so-called *inversion* of the retinal "image" *cannot* in principle be directly demonstrated unless we can get a *retina* to report on what a retinal "image" looks like. Thus, it should not be said that the retinal "image" is inverted by any of the devices that have been utilized in the sort of experiments we will be considering. Rather, the structure of the optical image that has passed through an inverting lens or prisms may be described as inverted with reference to the light that has not yet passed through.

many postulates about perceptual "constancies" and to isomorphism between characteristics of stimulation and brain processes. All notions of isomorphism that rely on a literal correspondence have failed. Both suppositions deserve to be rethought carefully.

The history of psychology is replete with memorable experiments generated by unsound assumptions. Such experiments remain memorable not because they anwer their intended question but because either the method employed or the facts unearthed supplant the original false puzzle. The most notable example in the area of adaptation to visual transformation is Stratton's first (1896) experiment in which he sought an empirical answer to the question: "*Is* the inverted image a necessary condition of our seeing things in an upright position [Stratton, 1896, p. 611]?" Motivated by the results from his first experiment, as well as by two critical essays by Hyslop (1897a, b), Stratton shifted his main theoretical aim to clarifying the relationship between vision and touch.

IMPORTANT DEVELOPMENTS

Claim: Touch Supplies Vision with Spatial Values

Stratton thus found himself unwitting heir to a second puzzle: Is sight or touch the more dominant and reliable guide to an object's real direction and distance? Ever since a simplified version of this question had been explicitly posed by Molyneux in a now famous letter to Locke (James, 1890/1950, p. 210), it had seemed settled. Molyneux posited the case of an adult, blind from birth, who could distinguish between a sphere and a cube by touch and who was suddenly given sight. Could he, without touching, distinguish the two by his new-found sight? Both Molyneux and Locke answered this thought-experiment with a resounding "no," and later empiricists found no fault with their answer. It would be almost 300 years before factual evidence forced a reassessment.

The question of the relationship between the two avenues of gaining knowledge, sight and touch, was taken up by Berkeley in his *An Essay Towards a New Theory of Vision* of 1709. His view led him to the conclusion that concurrent tactual experience provides vision with the appreciation of *distance* as well as *orientation*. Berkeley believed that distance or depth cannot be perceived directly if only one point of light is projected in the line of sight and if the object is viewed monocularly and without eye or head movement because no difference in the retinal image would result under these conditions (Berkeley, 1969, Section 2 ff).

Surprisingly, Berkeley was right, provided this point of light appears in an optically homogeneous or "empty" environment. The distance-from-self of the light would be judged "indeterminate." Unfortunately, Berkeley considered this static and highly contrived case as the prototypic representative of "distance" judgments. The solution to the puzzle of the perception of distance-from-self lies in disclaiming Berkeley's premise that "distance [is] a line turned endwise to the eye" and that a line in that situation cannot project more than one single point to the eye (Berkeley, *Alciphron,* IV, 8: III, 150–151, cited by Donagan, 1978, Chapter 11). Berkeley may be read to imply that if visible objects were represented by more than one line or point, then a basis for perceiving different distances would exist.

The answer to Berkeley's falsely cast puzzle indeed lies here. In modern translation I would say that the array of light, reflected from the environment and oneself, contains many such "distance lines" that, by their relational nature, provide the observer with direct optical information for the distance-from-self of any visible thing. Given that people do make accurate judgments and do not usually knock over their tea cup, Berkeley had to cast about for an explanation. He firmly believed that both the objects and ideas of sight and touch are distinct things (Berkeley, 1969, Sections 49 and 79, respectively) and that we attribute to sight what touch conveys because of the "customary and close connection" between the ideas of sight and touch, which are "blended and confounded together [1969, Section 79]." Tactile experience, implied Berkeley, supplies sight with spatial value. Thus, Berkeley asserted that "a man born blind, being made to see, would, at first, have no idea of distance by sight [1969, Section 41]."

Berkeley, fully aware of the inverted retinal image, remained consistent in his discussion of the relationship between seen and felt *orientation.* He insisted that the confusion over explaining erect vision arose from a failure to distinguish between touch and sight (Berkeley, 1969, Section 91). The sense of touch, and touch experience, determines and distinguishes unequivocally geographical down (the surface of support) and up (1969, Sections 93, 94). Consequently, a man born blind, when first given sight, would not be able to make judgments about, or be able to apply, the terms *up* or *down, erect* or *inverted;* only by tactual experiences would he come to do so by and by (1969, Sections 95, 102).

Controversy: Nature versus Nurture in Spatial Orientation

Berkeley's conclusions were widely accepted. His claim that touch educates vision in the perception of the distance and orientation of objects faced no serious theoretical challenge until the introduction of the "local sign" concepts of Lotze and Hering and until Helmholtz's analysis of the problem of visual direction.[5] Berkeley's claim faced no empirical defiance until the now famous demonstration by Helmholtz of eye-hand adaptation to visual displacement by wedge prisms, which seemed to show that accurate reaching is directed by the visual system. Claim aroused controversy. The touch-vision controversy, still alive today, gathered significant momentum when Stratton's results became known. (See Chapter 11 for a detailed discussion.)

The discovery that the retinal image is inverted, coupled with the claim that touch educates vision, generated a false dichotomy that has haunted and occupied psychologists since they began to seek to understand human perception: Our capacities for spatial orientation are presumed either to originate in innate mechanisms that provide perceptual knowledge (e.g., of direction) and do not depend on environmental learning opportunities (nativism) or they are thought to depend on the perceiver's environmental learning history for their appearance, maintenance, and termination (empiricism). Opponents of these two assumptions, myself included, regard them as a false dichotomy because, in its extreme, neither position can be made even linguistically intelligible, let alone be formulated as a mutually exclusive and empirically confirmable or disconfirmable proposition. Behavior is mutually dependent on the relationships between anatomical structures and their functions and their complex systemic products. Biological foundations and environmental events and their necessarily experiential product influence one another. Last but not least, behavior depends on the generative capacity of the nervous system for novel thought and action.

MODERN CONCERNS

Not until the nineteenth century was there an explicit realization that the retinal and postretinal neural transformations of information reaching the brain were more important by far in understanding the basic phenomena of perception, learning, remembering, cognition, and language than the transformation of the optical image by the lens system of the eye. Both Helmholtz and Stratton supplied us with facts and hypotheses that rendered Da Vinci's false paradox of the inverted image innocuous and the nature-nurture controversy in its original form meaningless. The modern concerns that may be traced to the retinal image problem are all manageable research topics. Sperry's (1943) and Arora

[5]For a splendid historical account of the problem of visual direction see Walls (1951).

and Sperry's (1963) *anatomical disarrangement* studies are representative.

The modern trend of reformulating philosophical or dichotomous problems into empirically testable issues has yielded the following questions concerned with visual transformation: "How, and to what extent, can perception and competent action, once established, be modified? Under what conditions can such competences be abolished and then reestablished to high levels of competence? What is the relative contribution of genetic, anatomical, functional, environmental, and experiential factors in modifying perceptual-performatory competences?"

Studying adaptation to *natural or experimental deprivation* has become a favorite twentieth-century method. Though the idea is traceable to antiquity, Itard's (1962) report of the feral boy of Aveyron stirred up much speculation. Experimental studies more directly concerned with the touch–vision issue gathered momentum after von Senden's (1960) monumental analysis of cases of the blind restored to sight, Schlodtmann's (1902) pressure phosphene study in blind children, and Gregory and Wallace's (1963) investigation of a 50-year-old blind man, restored to sight by binocular grafting of donated corneas. Held and Bauer's (1974) experiments with infant monkeys reared with a ruff around their neck to prevent sight of the hands is a more recent application of the deprivation technique to the nature–nurture/touch–vision issues. (The work of Hubel and Wiesel (1959) and Riesen (1961) quickened the vigor of related investigations.) The aim of these studies is to determine the degree of built-in competence (i.e., reaching accuracy, its robustness to resist a nonnurturing environment, and the necessary and sufficient conditions to maintain and perfect the earliest available abilities).

Imposing an external optical tranformation onto a young or adult creature became another popular method of studying the nature–nurture controversy. These so-called *rearrangement* or *recombination* experiments followed Sperry's cue but without interfering with anatomy. Early representative animal studies that attached right–left displacing prisms to the head of chicks were reported by Hess (1956), Pfister (1955), and Rossi (1968). Representative inversion experiments were conducted with kittens by Bishop (1959) and with a rhesus monkey by Foley (1940).

Experiments with human observers are most numerous. Many (e.g., Kohler, Wallach, Held, Taylor) seem to subscribe to the at least implicit assumption that one way to learn about perceptuomotor development in (child) development is to study these adaptation processes in the adult (cf. Kohler's dictum, "Der Umbau macht den Aufbau klar" i.e., Modification illuminates development [e.g., 1964, p. 148]). The most important reason why this assumption is troublesome is this: The adult comes to the prismatic adaptation situation with a vast repertoire of well-learned and overlearned abilities that are abruptly disrupted; infants developing normally do not. Therefore, the adult probably will have to do some unlearning and ignoring of information as well as relearning in the face of competing information, attention, and competences (cf. Gibson, 1969, p. 209). Not so the infant: Mostly new discriminations and new learning are his or her context for change. Nevertheless, even though very different reasons for achieving visually guided competences are likely to be at work, the difficulties experienced by the adult shortly after donning transforming spectacles are strikingly similar to the bumblings of the young, normally developing child (cf. Chapter 8 and Appendix A, Table A8.2).[6]

The proliferation of research topics and trends is both encouraging and disconcertingly hard to keep up with, even though most are derived from a few fundamental concerns. A conference on "recombination procedure as a tool for the study of visual perception" occupies an entire issue of *Perception* (Welch, 1974) and attests to the liveliness of the field. Examples of recent and future trends are the interest in adaptation to optical transformations under water (see Welch, 1978, Chapter 12 for a summary of this work), during sleep (cf. my Chapters 7 and 12), and prior and during space travel (cf. my Chapter 12).

In summary, two great nineteenth-century pioneers, Herman von Helmholtz and George Stratton, launched the current era of factual inquiry into the problem of adaptation to visual transformation. Numerous twentieth-century studies were motivated by the methods, results, and interpretations of their experiments. Helmholtz and Stratton inherited, and grappled with, three historical developments that emerged from the background of centuries of philosophical disputation about the makeup of human knowledge. These three origins of adaptation studies are first, the discovery that the retinal image is inverted with respect to external objects; second, the empiricist claim that touch educates vision about the direction and orientation of objects; and third, the pseudocontroversy about whether spatial orientation is innate or learned.

[6]Both experience disorientation and loss of balance and engage in awkward movements in dressing, catching a ball, handling a spoon, eye-head tracking of fast moving animals like birds, in sitting on a chair, getting into slippers, and walking down stairs. Groping, repeated experimenting, clumsy effort, poor timing, and frustration are exhibited by both a normal 16–22-month-old and by an adult (the author) adapting to the wearing of reversing prisms. Both appear to have serious difficulty in understanding the spatial relationships between body parts and visible objects in the environment as well as between actions and their consequences.

2

Describing and Measuring Adaptation Phenomena

In 1865, Aubert, while writing on the physiology of retinal adaptation, introduced the term *Umstimmung*. *Umstimmung* literally means "tuning," as in tuning an instrument to a new key—an apt metaphor because it suitably describes the phenomenon of adjustment experienced by wearers of transforming spectacles.

The first recorded attempt to measure the adaptation of action came in 1866. Helmholtz conducted a seemingly simple experiment in which he compared the accuracy of pointing at an object during and after gazing briefly through laterally displacing prisms (1867, Vol. I, pp. 601–602; 1962, Vol. III, pp. 246–247). Hundreds of short-term studies, using light-displacing wedge prisms, may be traced to Helmholtz's demonstration. Stratton ushered in a rather different trend 30 years later: the long-term experiment primarily concerned with the description of phenomenal experiences and gross motor actions during the course of spectacle wearing (1896, 1897b). He spent 21.5 hours in 1896 and 87 hours in 1897 wearing a monocular lens system that optically inverted his field of view (FV).[1]

[1]The normal field of view of the human observer is approximately 180° horizontal × 150° vertical (Gibson, 1950, pp. 27, 46). It is bounded by the cheeks, eyebrows, and nose.

In describing and measuring adaptation phenomena, the experimenter examines changes in the observer's *visual perception,* overt *actions,* and *verbal descriptions* of both. Thus, the experimenter seeks to describe the observer's vast array of confusing and unfamiliar, yet unrelenting, present perceptions and how he or she manages to reconcile these with past perceptual memories and past visual imagery. The experimenter must also describe the subject's actions, how his or her visual experiences affect past skills, and how he or she comes to perform competently. Finally, the experimenter has to note the spectacle-wearer's ability to describe his or her own perceptions and actions.

One important goal of researchers who study adaptation is to answer the question, "To what does the observer who wears spectacles adapt?" One preliminary answer is that the subject adapts to the incongruous appearance of everything within his or her FV as well as to his or her inability to direct any body part competently under visual guidance. Another answer is that the observer adapts to the special characteristics of the spectacles. Consequently, the experimenter must become familiar with the effects of various transforming spectacles.

Spectacles that displace, invert, reverse, or tilt the incoming light introduce a discrepancy between the actual and apparent (phenomenal) *location* of all seen places, objects, people, events, and the observer's body parts (see Figure 2.1). Inverting, reversing, and tilting spectacles also produce a change in the apparent *orientation* of everything represented in the observer's FV.[2]

REQUIREMENTS FOR DESCRIBING AND MEASURING ADAPTATION PHENOMENA

On the empirical front, the scientist seeks to move from the domain of private experience and observation to the domain of publicly confirm-

---

When both eyes are pointed toward the environment, they command a horizontal arc of 180° or more, particularly when the eyes are mobile (Helmholtz, 1962, Vol. I, pp. 93–94). A subject's FV invariably contains optical information about the location and orientation of his or her body parts, about places, objects, events, and often about other creatures. The FV may consist of one of several kinds of vistas that remain fixed during every fixation of the eyes: it moves with every eye movement (*the FV of the eyes*), with every eye-head or head-eye movement (*the FV of the head*), and with every eye-head-body movement (*the locomotion FV*). The binocular FV of fixation is shown in Figure 4.1.

[2]I define the *location* of a body part (e.g., of the head) as the place occupied by the head relative to the other body parts (e.g., the shoulders). The *orientation* of a body part (e.g., the head) is defined as the manner in which the head is placed or arranged relative to other parts (e.g., the shoulders). Thus, the head may be perceived to be located between the knees and up-down reversed, (i.e., the observer may perceive that the top of the head is closer to the ground than the chin is).

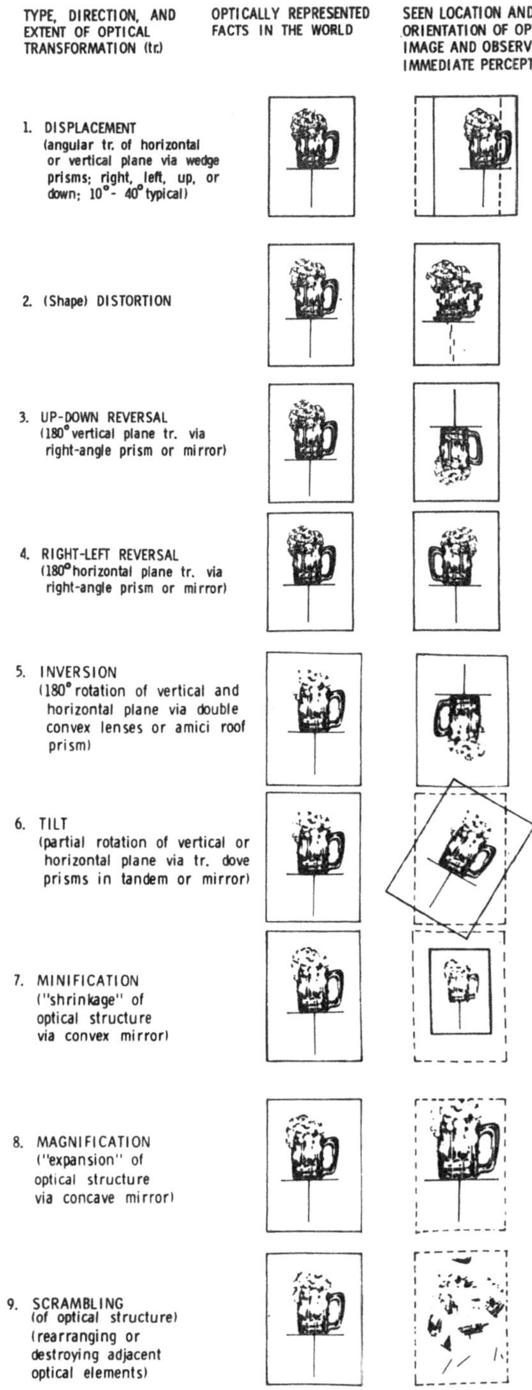

FIGURE 2.1. Various types of optical transformations. The actual and perceived location and orientation of objects in the observer's field of view (FV) is represented by the mug. Solid lines represent the seen edges of the observer's restricted FV before and after the transformation is introduced. Broken lines indicate the place in the world represented in the FV. Shape distortions and color fringes that are introduced by displacing prisms are not shown (see Kohler, 1964, and Ogle, 1968, for examples). In any study care is taken that only light that has passed through the transforming system reaches the observer's eyes. The idea for this illustration came from seeing Hochberg's Figure 13.34 (1971, p. 532).

able fact, demonstrating the existence of adaptation as a phenomenon, measuring its magnitude, and describing how and why it occurs.

On the analytic front, the researcher who aims at an exhaustive description and explanation of adaptation phenomena must do the following:

1. Distinguish between two classes of adaptation: perceptual and performatory (Chapter 2).
2. Distinguish between adaptation and the immediate effects of looking through transforming spectacles (Chapter 2).
3. Distinguish among three basic ways of describing and measuring adaptation: (*a*) The gradual modifications; (*b*) the final accomplishments after a given period of wearing spectacles; and (*c*) the aftereffects once the spectacles are removed (Chapter 2).
4. Describe the differences between looking and acting with and without spectacles (Chapters 3 and 4).
5. Describe the information that makes adaptation possible.[3] More

[3]I regard *information* as the primary and sustaining source of knowledge and *perception* as the fundamental means of gaining it. Information *about* the varied characteristics of the environment and about the self are postulated to be "contained in" and "carried by" the spatial and temporal characteristics of every form of energy. The relatively persistent structural characteristics of energy are the variables discriminable by an observer's perceptual system and constitute either potential or effective information for places, objects, events, people, and the self (cf. Gibson, 1966, p. 245). Hence, a tree can be a source of varied forms of *potential* information for many centuries. Its very presence constitutes information for all organisms who might come in bodily contact with it, who explore it as a kind of obstacle, who live in it as a source of shelter, and who ingest its leaves as a source of sustenance. Given ambient light, the structural characteristics of thc light reflected from the tree specify its shape, size, location, and other characteristicts. Hence light, as any other form of energy, is the carrier, and thus revealer, of information. Given a surrounding medium in which chemicals diffuse, the odor of its buds and bark are contained in that medium. When an observer perceives an environmental fact directly, he or she gains *effective* information. Information is thus the vehicle that potentially conveys meaning and knowledge about oneself and the environment. Information contained in the structure of ambient energy is postulated to be meaningful because it *specifies* spatiotemporal *consistencies* about the characteristics of observer–environmental objects and events. Thus, the branches of a tree are perceived to be attached to its trunk rather than floating in midair because this *spatial relationship* is preserved, regardless of nature of the energy that carries that information. Similarly, the sound of the falling tree is not perceived to precede the event because this *temporal relationship* is preserved in whatever energy specifies that event. This is one sense in which meaning can be said to be "carried by" or "contained in" ambient energy. The *perception* of the meaning *in* information is enhanced when the observer notices consistencies and the relationship among consistencies (and occasional inconsistencies) among facts and among events. Information, by its very nature, is embedded in a broader, nonarbitrary matrix of more information. This "overlap" is spatial as well as temporal and is postulated to be the precondition for the orderly appreciation of

precisely, describe the information that accounts for the immediate effects that occur, the gradual modifications, the final accomplishments, and for the aftereffects experienced and performed by the observer who has been exposed to gazing through the transforming goggles, and further, describe how, in adapting, the spectacle-wearer actually utilizes the potential information available to him or her (Chapters 7–10).

Requirement 1. Distinguishing and Measuring Perceptual and Performatory Adaptation

To validly measure adaptation one must distinguish between two main types: the adaptation of perception and that of action. The changes the observer notices in the appearance of what he or she perceives while gazing through transforming spectacles is a different phenomenon from the changes in actions in which the observer engages. This difference is underscored by the very different verbal descriptions that delineate changes in phenomenal experience and action. Moreover, perceptual and performatory adaptation can be experimentally dissociated. (Irving Rock [1966, 1973, 1975] has been the clearest and most persistent champion of this distinction.) The distinction is, of course, not a denial that perceiving depends on actions such as eye, head, or limb movements; it also does not ignore the concomitant, synchronous, and reciprocal relationship between perceiving and performing (cf. Chapter 8).

The experimenter has the basis for inferring either an effect or a rapid adaptation of visual perception rather than of visually guided action if the observer reports differences in the appearance of the visual world immediately after he or she begins looking through spectacles. The experimenter can tell that perceptual adaptation has occurred if, after a period of time, the observer makes visual judgments that reflect a

---

events and causality, of object "constancy," in short, of a perceptually stable and relatively permanent world. Most importantly, the notions of context and meaning may be used interchangeably, in that context is informative and hence meaningful. Indeed, when this context is artifically reduced, restricted, or disturbed, meaning is lost or compromised. Although I will be most concerned in this book with the direct perception of information as discriminable structure and with information that specifies the meaningful visuomotor relations of the observer in the natural ecology, the known facts also seem to demand a further meaning of information: Direct perception is greatly supported by what may be termed *knowledge-based information* (cf. Chapter 8). The perceiver–performer can draw from this rich fund of perceptuocognitive meanings and understanding that likely consists of memorially stored and cognitively manipulated perceptual input–output relations and schemas.

reliable change in this original appearance. The experimenter can also infer perceptual adaptation if the subject simply describes changes in how things appear. Thus, perceptual adaptation does not only exist separately from the adaptation of action in the beginning, but can be distinguished throughout the adapting process. For example, in the first hour of the first day of wearing up–down reversing spectacles,[4,5] in the Prism Study, I reported:

> *I'm sitting on a chair, head stationary. Here I am again, sitting, but standing on my head. This is the feel of the situation now. It's not just visually true. I am, in truth, in some strange way, standing on my head without feeling the weight of my body suspended on it, gazing at the scene . . . I am seated on a balcony 100 feet above the beach and sea. Whatever I view has an aspect of entire irreality. I am surprised that the sea does not float toward the sky. The sea has become the sky. The waves are behaving oddly. The progress of swimmers is irreal; it is hard for me to say whether they are coming toward the shore or going out to sea. A man or boy walking—I cannot be sure which—appears to be a two-legged crab moving in strange fashion.*

Change in the original perception or appearance was reported 118 waking hours later on the ninth day of wearing the spectacles and still 170 hours later on the thirteenth day.

> *During inactivity, perceptual consistency is the rule: As I'm sitting up here on the balcony, without moving my head, observing the scene, people walking up and down stairs, washed clothes hung on the line, ball on the ground, the only difference really, between the first days of Stage 2 [prespectacle baseline observations] and today is that clearly I'm visually with the [top of the] head toward the ground. All else seems to be going on quite comfortably and "normally." There is consistency in what I see. I am not confused about whether people are walking up or down stairs as I initially was; I am aware, however, that somehow I'm looking at the world from a different point of observation—from just a foot or two off the ground.*

The experimenter–observer of this experiment has been able to describe the immediate effects and changes in the initial appearances, and there-

[4]Whenever the terms *up* or *down* are employed, they mean geographically up or down, that is, parallel to the imaginary line of the pull of gravity. Thus, raising the eyes, head, or arm always means moving skyward, whereas lowering means moving groundward—toward the surface of support. Gravity entails an up–down polarity that remains a constant, quite independent of any optical transformation imposed upon an observer's FV and quite independent of any process of perceiving one's surface of support.

[5]Unless otherwise indicated, all observations cited in examples throughout the book are based on the protocol of a long-term (5-week) experiment in which I served as both experimenter and observer and wore up–down reversing spectacles attached to the head (discussed in detail in Chapters 5–10): the Prism Study.

fore the experience of adaptation can be classified as perceptual in nature.

Visually guided *actions* are invalid as an indicator of visual adaptation. When a spectacled observer moves his or her eyes but keeps the head, body, and limbs stationary, only visual adaptation can be measured, and hence, only conclusions about perceptual adaptation are appropriate (unless we are measuring changes in eye movements per se). Thus, exposure and test conditions must be identical to allow valid inferences. If the observer points incorrectly, the experimenter may not conclude that perceptual adaptation has not occurred because such a conclusion assumes that perceptual adaptation is equivalent to or necessarily leads to performatory competence; performatory competence only may be lacking. Note that such an invalid conclusion implies that perceptual adaptations cannot occur independently of a performatory criterion. On the other hand, if the subject reaches competently in a postexposure test, the researcher is on safer ground with his–her inference that visual adaptation has taken place as well (on the still-debated assumptions that some form of visual adaptation constitutes either a necessary or sufficient condition for the control of competent action).

Perceptual Consistency

The experimenter must be able to tell when perceptual adaptation has occurred in order to measure it. I maintain that the observer achieves perceptual adaptation when he or she consistently perceives the novel information available. The observer has adapted if (*a*) his or her phenomenal (visual) experiences cease to be characterized by unfamiliarity, discrepancies, incongruence, and phenomenal contradictions; (*b*) his or her verbal descriptions of phenomenal experiences cease to contain contradictions; and (*c*) his or her looking (eye–head) movements become errorless. Thus, achieving perceptual consistency is tantamount to having adapted.

Phenomenal Experiences Become Consistent

To adapt perceptually, observers must gradually comprehend what they perceive and what they perceive themselves to be doing. Linguistic and conceptual ambiguity and confusions riddle the description of phenomenal experiences of the observers and the experimenters who have worn inverting and reversing spectacles (cf. Chapter 11). The initial visual experiences of these researchers have been characterized by perceptual confusions, discrepancies, phenomenal contradictions, and unfamiliarity in appearance of symbols, objects, events, and people. To illustrate, Kohler reported this observation of one of his observers who wore up-down reversing goggles: ". . . two adjacent heads, one upright, the other [actually] inverted, were *both* perceived as upright. Gradually, more and more objects appeared right side up [1964 p. 32; originally 1951, p. 17]." How both the experimenter and the observer can avoid such ambiguity of description is discussed on pages 265 and 269–271.

Particularly apparent in the observer's experiences and descriptions are confusions about his or her own actions and the seen relationships of body parts to one another and to the environment (e.g., observers Kundratitz, Marte, Scheffler, Fjelstadt [up-down reversal]; Grill [right-left reversal]; observer and experimenter Kohler [right-left reversal]; all detailed in Kottenhoff (1961)[6] and, in part, in Kohler (1951; 1964). A new perceptual consistency is established as the experienced discrepancies cease. I postulate that the observer experiences changes in what events signify, what his or her own actions phenomenally signify, and what the subject perceives that he or she can now accomplish with many actions.

The observer must gain and establish new perceptual meanings rather than regain and reestablish previous perceptual meanings because I postulate that, throughout perceptual adaptation, the observer is aware of the visual differences in what he or she perceives with spectacles and what he or she remembers before donning them. Operationally, no matter how long the observer adapts, he or she should continue to be able to make factually correct same-different judgments about phenomenal experiences with and without spectacles.

Verbal Descriptions Become Consistent

During perceptual adaptation, descriptions of the following kinds of experiences cease to contain verbal contradictions: the appearance, recognizability, and familiarity of objects, faces, print, and events; their apparent location and orientation relative to the location and orientation of the observer's own body parts; the appearance of the observer's own movements. For the most part, these phenomenal experiences concern discrepancies within the FV. However, verbal descriptions are also influenced by discrepancies and by the lack of equivalent information among different perceptual systems. In particular, the experience of the observer's own performance is partly made up of the awareness of the acoustic, nosmic, but especially, haptic-kinesthetic components of visually guided action. (*Haptic* awareness refers to the felt position of unmoving body parts; during their movement *kinesthetic* awareness is

[6]This work, unfortunately only available in German, is probably both the least read and, overall, the best *monograph* on the subject of adaptation to optical reversal. It is rich in history, in data from little-known long-term experiments, and in interpretation. It deserves to be read and will reward its readers richly.

possible.) Not incidentally, the existing discrepancies between visual information and haptic information must also be resolved to achieve verbal consistency. The process of achieving consistency in verbally expressed phenomenal experience is gradual and, I hypothesize, partly dependent on looking behavior becoming less error prone.

Looking Behavior Becomes Errorless

"Looking" includes three levels of scanning (movement) activities performed by the visual system: (*a*) *Eye scanning* consists of movements of the eyes within a stationary head; (*b*) *head scanning* includes movements of the head (with compensatory eye movements) and movements of the eyes followed by a head movement (e.g., eye-head pursuit); and (*c*) *locomotion scanning*, which includes head–eye, or eye–head movements during locomotion.

In experiments in which the observer is free to move, errors in the *direction* of head movements are expected to occur, especially during attempted eye-head pursuit, while wearing inverting and reversing spectacles. Errors in the *extent* of head movements are expected to occur while wearing displacing, tilting, minifying, and magnifying spectacles. Finally, errors in the normal *rate* of head movements are expected with all types of transforming spectacles.

The following observations from the Prism Study illustrate how errors in looking can foster errors of judgment and verbal contradictions during the course of perceptual (as well as performatory) adaptation. The point that perceiving inevitably entails performing and vice versa also is made. At first, I lost knowledge of head posture immediately upon donning the spectacles. I continued to be confused about the posture of my head even after some 10 days (182 hours) of wearing spectacles, particularly after I had tilted my head toward either shoulder. Also, I committed errors in attempting eye-head pursuit of a moving object–event.

In the first hour of the first day of looking through the reversing prisms, I reported:

> *On numerous occasions today I have been unable to say in what position my head was, that is, whether it was slightly tilted to the right, below, or above the primary position,*[7] *and so on. This was particularly true after keeping my head in the chin-to-chest position, which causes general disorientation. I remained uninformed*

[7]An observer's head is in the primary position when he or she holds it normally erect, not inclined or turned toward either shoulder and not tilted forward or backward. The observer's eyes are in the primary position when the lines of sight, the imaginary lines through the center of each pupil, are horizontal and perpendicular to the line of gravity as he or she stands erect on a flat plane with a normally erect head.

as to my head posture until I head-scanned and found the horizon line or some known or identifiable visual frame of reference, say the street, a telephone pole, or a house.

On the fourteenth day (or 182 waking hours later) I reported:

I often do not know the exact or even approximate posture of my head during onto-the-shoulder tilt head movements: Though I know that I have moved *my head during such head movements, I do* not *know how much or how far I have moved it and what position my head is in upon completion of the head movement (either relative to the primary position or relative to either shoulder).*

On the same day in the evening (after 192 hours of wearing reversing spectacles) I concluded that the information for head posture is primarily visual:

If called upon, I can give an account of what posture my head is in relative to some standard, say the primary position. That is, after any given head movement, I can say whether my head is above or below the primary position, whether and to what approximate degree my head is tilted to the right or left, and so on. I can do this provided I simultaneously have visual information as to symmetrical objects or places in the FV. These may consist of the horizon line, a building, a fence, etc. Otherwise, as I have noticed, my head may be tilted quite a bit, and I may not be aware of it at that time.

Errors in the direction of head movement while following a moving object or event were also reported during the first hour:

I intended to keep my son's head in my FV as someone else lifted him off the ground. Instead of moving my head geographically upward I moved it downward the instant my son began to be lifted. Thus, I came to see his feet rather than his head.

On the second day (13.5 hours later) I noted:

I made several errors in the direction of head movement in following the flight of birds. On four occasions I moved my head toward the ground rather than skyward, as required to visually pursue the birds. Upon noticing my error I made a conscious attempt to throw my head backward to visually intercept the flying doves. This attempt at conscious intervention was successful.

I gained the distinct impression that my head was (somehow) visually controlled, guided in much the same way that my arms (and limbs) are during a reaching or grasping movement. I perceived my head as just another appendage that followed the "commands" of the visual system—the movements of the eyes.

Errorless looking, whether it entails a new control of eye, or eye-head movement combinations, may still be a necessary condition for achieving perceptual adaptation of event perception and the perception of the self. To be sure, the most convincing measurement of perceptual adaptation requires an observer with a fixed head and body and as little of his or her body visible as possible. Ideally, the perceptual test should involve only the same kind of eye movements executed during exposure to the spectacles. Curiously, an experiment meeting these rigorous requirements to measure perceptual adaptation has not been reported.[8]

Performatory Competence

Acting competently is tantamount to achieving performatory adaptation. The main criterion that enables the experimenter to judge whether or not performatory adaptation has occurred is whether or not the observer has come to act competently. Regardless of how the observer perceives himself–herself and the environment, he or she must act according to the facts of the ecological condition in order to survive. Though obvious, this fact has frequently been ignored, particularly when adaptation is operationally defined as *mispointing* after the spectacles have been removed.

It must be noted that performatory *consistency* cannot be accepted as the sufficient criterion of performatory adaptation because the observer could simply be consistently incompetent. As is the case with perceptual adaptation, gaining performatory competence is a gradual process with a measurable product rather than a finite state that is attained suddenly and fully. Unlike perceptual adaptation, however, the emphasis in performatory adaptation is on regaining and reestablishing performatory competence because, ultimately, the tasks the observer must perform to get about in the environment cannot depend only on the phenomenal appearances within his or her FV.

Consistent Perception Necessary for Competent Action

I propose that consistency of phenomenal (visual) experiences, consistency of their verbal descriptions, and especially errorless looking are all requisite to competent action. Inaccurate, discrepant, and contradictory visual perceptions direct incompetent action. Thus, if the observer

[8]Gibson's (1933) and some subsequent experiments (e.g., Coren & Festinger, 1967; Koehler & Wallach, 1944; and Rausch, 1952), concerned with the "normalization" and with "figural aftereffects" of the curvature of line drawings viewed through prisms, may be exceptions; however, the severely limited extent of negative and figural aftereffects (approximately 2°), as compared with the 10–15° shifts that are routinely observed with laterally displacing prisms, suggests that we are dealing with two different phenomena.

is phenomenally wrong or unsure about the location of a cup relative to himself–herself, he or she should misreach it. Similarly, if the observer commits errors in head movements while localizing an object, incorrect reaching is likely. The interpretation that perceptual consistency leads to performatory competence has important implications for the hotly debated issue of whether active movement by the observer during exposure to transforming spectacles is required for achieving performatory adaptation or whether, indeed, passive movement of the observer during exposure is a sufficient condition. This controversy is taken up in Chapter 11.

Requirement 2. Distinguishing Immediate Effects and Adaptation

The experimenter must separate what happens immediately after the observer starts looking through transforming goggles and what he or she experiences and does later. The experimenter needs to know how accurately and how reliably the observer can carry out the task(s) assigned before exposure to the transformation (pretest). The conditions under which the preexposure tests are taken must remain the same for the entire study; the exception is the introduction of the optical transformation and any other independent variable, of course. The measures the researcher takes of perceptual judgments and–or performatory activities constitute a baseline of normal behavior and serve as a basis of comparison for all subsequent measures he or she collects (Figure 2.2).

Next, immediately upon exposing the observer to the transforming spectacles, the experimenter should determine again the observer's performance on all preexposure measures. The immediate perceptual and performatory effects constitute yet another baseline with respect to which the experimenter can compare future changes in perception and action (see Figure 2.2). Measurements must be carried out as soon as possible after exposure to avoid confounding the immediate effects with rapid adaptations. Immediate effects are a rich source of data and of empirical hypotheses about both the nature of the imposed transformation and about future changes that can be expected; even so, adaptation can be inferred without this step.

Requirement 3. Distinguishing Three Methods of Measuring Adaptation

The most complete description of adaptation phenomena requires measuring the gradual changes, the final level of accomplishment just before the goggles are removed, and the aftereffects.

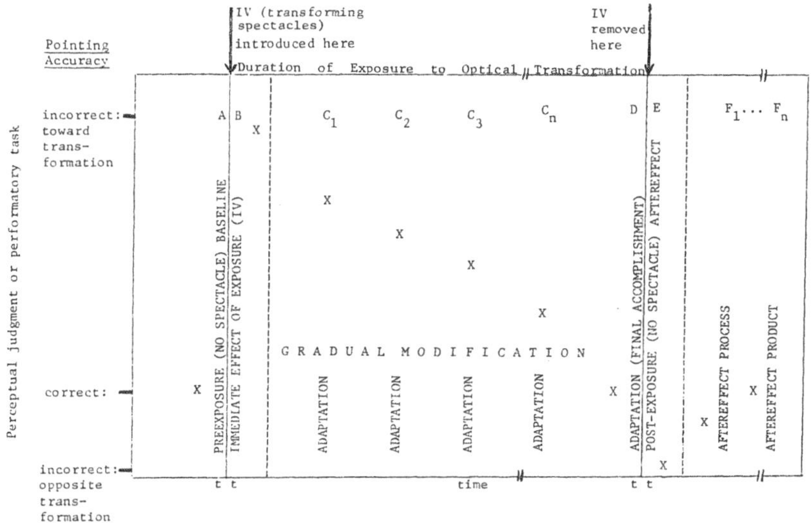

FIGURE 2.2. Measurement options in studies of adaptation to transforming spectacles (t indicates optimal time of measurement). Points are plotted (Xs) for a hypothetical case in which maximum pointing error occurs immediately after donning spectacles. Error gradually decreases until pointing is correct at D. On removal of prisms error occurs in the opposite direction with a gradual return to correct pointing.

Gradual Modification: Process

The experimenter monitors the course of adaptation by repeatedly measuring the observer's performance on the tasks assigned (see Figure 2.2). A comparison (e.g., by time-trend analysis) of these multiple measures during the period of exposure to transforming spectacles enables the researcher to provide a description of the process of adaptation. He or she must also account for how much the very act of repeated measurement influences (speeds, slows, or otherwise alters) the course of various forms of adaptation. A process description is indispensable for finding out how different perceptual capabilities and performatory skills adapt at different rates and in different ways. Another advantage of this approach is that it is extremely informative about the relationship of adaptation to other phenomena that have exhibited similar parameters in their "history" (e.g., learning). Moreover, a process description is uniquely suited to providing hints about what information the observer uses to adapt and what brain mechanisms may be at work. Knowing only that adaptation *has occurred,* but not the parameters of change except the end-product, leaves largely unanswered the questions of *how* and *why* adaptation occurs.

Final Accomplishment: Product

The experimenter measures the product of the cumulative spectacle-wearing exposure relative to a baseline level, ideally against the data on immediate effects (see Figure 2.2). The main benefit of this measurement is that it tells the experimenter the flexibility limits of the adapting observer. Moreover, it is the method of choice for finding out if and to what extent different perceiving activities and performance skills can become perfected under conditions of transformation. Such differentiated information clearly has value in the quest for an understanding of the mechanisms underlying adaptation phenomena.

Aftereffects of Adaptation

The experimenter measures any disturbance that lingers in the perceptual or perceptuomotor systems following removal of the spectacles (see Figure 2.2). Two main measurement routines are employed. With the first, the researcher notes the differences in perception and action between the aftereffects of wearing spectacles and the final product of wearing them. The second and most popular procedure is used mostly in short-term, displacing prism studies and measures adaptation by subtracting the first postexposure score from the last preexposure score. The main advantage of these methods is their simplicity. Aftereffect data may suffice to infer that adaptation *did* take place, though not necessarily (cf. Chapter 10). An aftereffect measure does save the labor of monitoring the immediate effects, the gradual changes, or the end-product of adaptation. Its virtue is that the measurement process is isolated from, and cannot interfere with, the process of adaptation. Yet, it is also intrinsically unsatisfying because it chooses to disregard almost all of the available information about adaptation phenomena as they exist in all their richness. Perceptual adaptation, especially, simply cannot be monitored with the aftereffect technique. Finally, describing the aftereffect process and product itself may also yield useful information, especially about the "readaptation" to the original, pretransformation conditions (see Figure 2.2).

VARIABLES IN ADAPTATION TO TRANSFORMATION STUDIES[9]

To predict the behavior of an observer exposed to transforming spectacles and to understand how adaptation works requires knowing

[9]For an analysis of the stimulus, response, and task variables in displacement experiments, see Howard (1968).

under what environmental, organismic, and task conditions he or she is required or allowed to function. Some of the important variables that should be considered in conducting any adaptation study are listed in Table 2.1. Discussion of these parameters is most meaningful in the context of an empirical problem and within the theories that give them special attention (see Chapter 11).

TABLE 2.1
Variables in Studies of Adaptation to Optical Transformation

I. Independent variables (IVs)

A. *Characteristics of spectacles:*

1. Type of optical transformation: displacement, reversal, inversion, tilt, minification, magnification, distortion, destruction ("scrambling") of optical structure
2. Direction of optical transformation
3. Extent of optical transformation
4. Location of spectacle relative to the observer: Attached to the observer's head; to eyes; external to the observers. Binocular disparity created by two optical elements, one in front of each eye
5. Size of the restricted field of view (FV)
6. Shape of the restricted FV
7. Weight of the spectacles (if attached to the observer, eyes, or head); size of the goggle housing the transforming elements, i.e., how far it extends from the observer's head or eyes

B. *Characteristics of the stimulation-information display available to the observer:*

8. Structural complexity of the optic array (FV): during exposure to the optical transformation and during the test for adaptation: Observer views stationary scene; observer views events; observer views self stationary; observer views self moving, e.g., observer looks at his or her moving arm through spectacles either while aiming at a target (method of Harris) or while moving randomly (method of Held); observer views others moving, e.g., a surrogate arm
9. Target characteristics (for pointing tasks): true location; orientation; and distance from the observer's point of observation; true size; intensity; and on-duration
10. Error information available to the observer during exposure
11. Suddenness with which the optical transformation is introduced
12. Duration of exposure
13. Continuous or intermittent exposure
14. Photopic or scotopic viewing condition

C. *Characteristics of the task environment:*

15. Distance and orientation of spectacles relative to eyes: constant; variable
16. Monocular or binocular exposure
17. Foveal and/or peripheral viewing of scene/target
18. Instructions to the observer
19. Knowledge of results, e.g., error-corrective feedback following having pointed at a target
20. Body parts moved by the observer (allowed or necessary) before, during, and after exposure: eyes; head; shoulders; body; arms; hands; fingers; legs; feet

(continued)

TABLE 2.1 (*Continued*)

21. Position assumed by the observer (allowed or necessary) before, during, and after exposure, i.e., while baseline-, process-, product-, and aftereffect-measures of adaptation are collected (all body parts as in 20)
22. Movement type: Active movements by the observer; being moved passively by the experimenter
23. Kind of practice: massed; spaced
24. Amount of practice, e.g., number of pre-exposure target pointings
25. Time delay between target presentation and responding
26. Sleep (rapid eye movement sleep (REM) or non-REM sleep) duration; duration of presleep exposure to optical transformation

D. *Combination IVs:* Linked to the direction and extent of the optical transformation and the task environment

27. Type of eye posture and movement the observer assumes/must assume for a task
28. Type of eye movement–head movement combination necessary to execute task
29. Type of eye-, head-, body-, limb-movement combination necessary to execute task

E. *Characteristics of the observer:*

30. Focused attention the observer pays to the available information during exposure

II. Dependent variables (DVs)

A. *Nature of the task:* (spatial, temporal, complexity characteristics)

1. Type and complexity of positioning and movements before, during, and after exposure of the observer's eyes, head, neck, shoulders, body, arm, finger, and legs allowed the observer and required of the observer
2. Relationship of these movements to one another
3. Characteristics of these positionings of movements: frequency; rate of speed; duration; accuracy (or number, frequency, or rate of error)
4. The observer moves actively, passively, or not at all (only perceptual judgments are required)

B. *Nature of the test:*

5. Location of target (e.g., pointing accuracy) using any body part (eyes, nose, fingers, toes, etc.); "target" may be another body part (test is typically conducted without sight of the pointing body part)
6. Production (e.g., drawing); exposure and test conditions must be identical
7. Reproduction (e.g., geometric figures)
8. Intermanual transfer
9. Interocular transfer
10. Phenomenal description: memory comparison; successive matching; simultaneous comparison

C. *Perceptual-performatory system(s) stimulated and/or tested:* visual; haptic; vestibular (orienting); auditory; nosmic; gustatory

D. *DVs indicating perceptual adaptation:* (verbal-perceptual reports implying adaptation). Question: Does the novel condition (appearance) of the transformed visual world become the normal quality (appearance) of the phenomenal world? If yes, perceptual adaptation took place

(*continued*)

TABLE 2.1 (*Continued*)

E. *DVs indicating performatory adaptation:* (performatory criteria implying adaptation). Question: Did performance improve toward greater competence when compared to performance immediately after exposure? If yes, performatory adaptation took place

III. Organismic variables (OVs)

1. Visual acuity
2. Strabismus
3. Astigmatism
4. Field defects, e.g., tunnel vision
5. Proneness to motion sickness
6. Attention the observer pays to available information
7. State of motivation–emotion: e.g., anxiety vis-à-vis the experimental task
8. Characteristics of prior exposure to optical transformations of same or specified other type: duration; extent; degree of adaptation achieved; time elapsed since last adaptation
9. Age

IV. Relevant secondary variables (SVs)

A. *Characteristics of the spectacles:*
   1. Light absorption characteristics of lens, mirror, or prism used
   2. Percentage light reflected by mirror used, e.g., is it a front surface mirror

B. *Characteristics of the stimulation–information display:* Error information available to the observer about the direction and/or extent of the transformation during exposure and testing

C. *Characteristics of the task environment:* Temperature; humidity; noise level; etc.

D. *Characteristics of the observer:*
   1. Special competence the observer may have, e.g., champion archer used in a pointing task
   2. Effects of unknown magnitude: response set; handedness; sex; intelligence; knowledge; etc.
   3. The observer's familiarity with the testing environment

E. *Characteristics of the experimenter:* Experimenter effects (bias)

SUMMARY

This chapter outlines what the perception researcher must do to fully describe and accurately measure the adapting behavior of observers who are exposed to prismatically transformed light. The subject perceives himself–herself and his or her visual world as different than they are. This is also the reason why the observer performs unskillfully immediately after donning spectacles. The experimenter seeks to measure these immediate effects of unique appearances and actions. The gradual modification of these effects is a measurable process, which yields a measurable product. The final accomplishments of adaptation, I contend, consist of the observer coming to perceive consistently and act competently: (*a*) The adapted observer is skillful once again. When he or she achieves perceptual consistency, unfamiliar and disturbing sights appear familiar and aesthetically pleasing again; (*b*) he or she is well oriented and understands the visual meanings of body movements; (*c*) errors in the performance components of looking (e.g., head movements in the wrong direction) drop out; (*d*) the observer's verbal descriptions of all these perceptual and performatory accomplishments cease to be confusing and contradictory. Achieving visual consistency is a prerequisite for performing complex actions skillfully once more; yet, skillful action is not tantamount to perceptual adaptation. After the observer adapts to his or her world transformed and removes the spectacles, the experimenter's challenge is to measure whether the subject has suffered any aftereffects of this adaptation.

The final section lists the most potent experimental variables the experimenter is likely to encounter in the laboratory or in real life. They are (*a*) the type, direction and extent of the light transformation imposed on the observer; (*b*) where the spectacles are attached (i.e., to the subject's eyes, head, or to a table top); (*c*) how severely the observer's field of view is limited by the optical device; (*d*) the duration of exposure; (*e*) the type of eye-, head-, body-, and limb-movement combination necessary to carry out any desired task; (*f*) whether he or she moves voluntarily or is passively transported; and (*g*) whether the subject pays attention to the information available to him or her.

3

Light and Its Demands

Only if we know the behavior of light as it passes through the transforming spectacle can we begin to understand what unique demands spectacle-wearing imposes on our observer, what obstacles to adapting he or she faces, and what information may be available to him or her. This information at first confuses and misleads the subject, yet provides enough consistency to make eventual adaptation possible.

In this chapter I seek to answer three questions in order to describe to what the spectacle-wearer adapts. First, how is light transformed when passed through a prism or lens? Briefly, the observer adapts to the new direction of light that creates a discrepancy between the visually perceived and actual location and orientation of everything in his or her field of view (FV). Second, what is transformed with spectacles? The observer adapts to the features of the visual world that become altered once spectacles are donned. Specifically, the observer's entire FV—including all objects, events, and body parts—changes in appearance. Third, what are the unique *adapting requirements* (invariants) for successful looking and competent action that every optical transformation imposes upon the subject? For example, an observer looking through displacing prisms must point the eyes to one side to regard an object dead ahead of the nose. Figure 3.1 illustrates this unique adapting require-

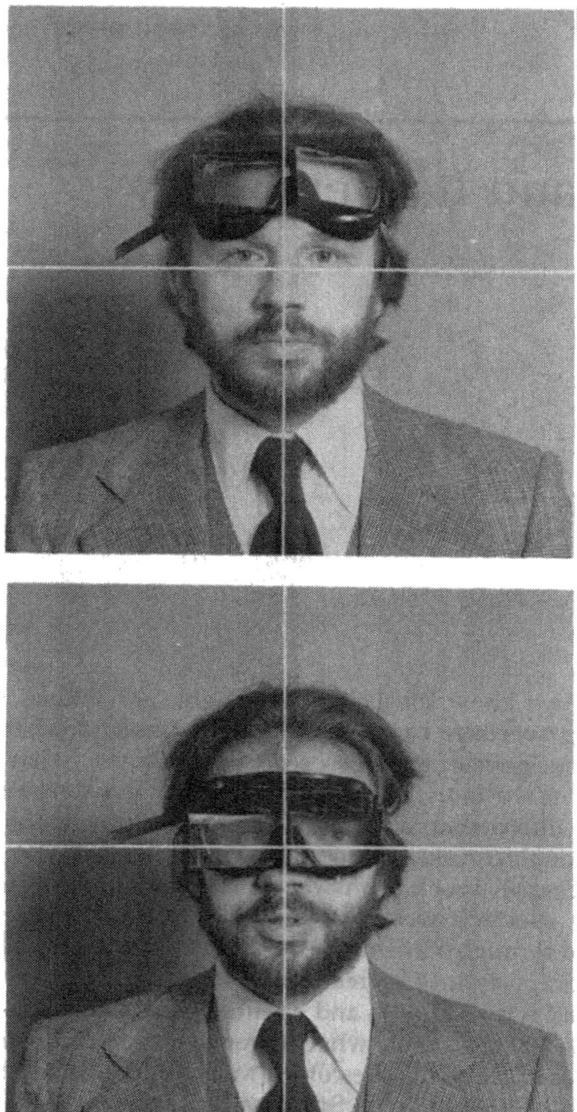

a

b

FIGURE 3.1. Unique adapting requirement for the observer looking through base right displacing prisms. The apex (thin portion of the wedge) points toward the observer's left and the apparent displacement of everything seen through the prisms is in that direction: (*a*) The observer is fixating crosshairs directly in front of the nose without the prisms; (*b*) to foveate (see clearly) the crosshair while maintaining the head in the primary position, the observer must point the eyes (fixate) in the direction of the optical displacement: to his left (see Figure 3.4.); *(continued)*

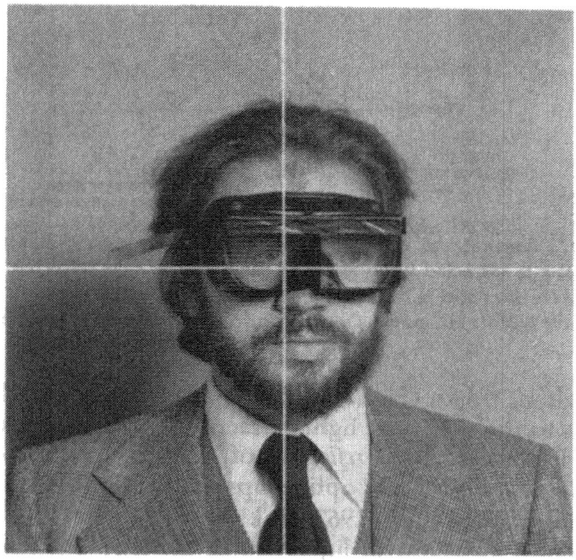

c

FIGURE 3.1. (*continued*) **(c) eye and head position when the observer *visually judges* that the head is straight ahead as in *b*—in the primary position—and the crosshairs dead ahead. 21° prism. Eye-cross hair distance 125 cm (50"). (Photos made 3/79.)**

ment. Or, take the case of an observer wearing right–left reversing prisms who wants to regard and point successfully at a horse emerging from the starting gate on his or her left and moving up the track to the observer's right. The eyes must move *right* to *left* while the head and hand move in the opposite direction!

The following analysis will focus on the problems of adaptation to up–down reversal of the FV in which the spectacles are assumed to be attached to the observer's head. Nonetheless, its principles are directly transferable to other forms of optical transformation.

PASSING LIGHT THROUGH REVERSING PRISMS[1]

Helmholtz (1962, Vol. III, p. 60) was the first experimenter to diagram what happens to light as it passes through a reversing (right-angle

[1]Since a great number of experiments use laterally displacing prisms, a reference to some notable descriptions of their geometrical optics may be useful. The optical distortions produced by laterally displacing plano prisms were given general quantitative expression by Ogle (1951, 1952). (A plano prism is plane [flat] on one side and concave or convex on the other.) He demonstrated that the apparent distortion of the image seen through an ophthalmic prism depends upon the physical dimensions of the prism (prism power,

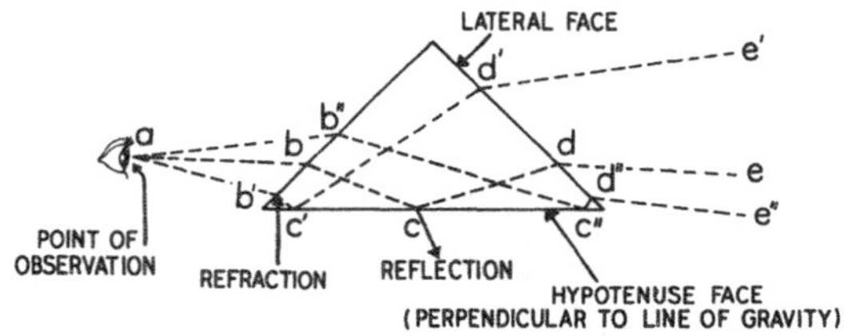

FIGURE 3.2. Geometrical optics of light passing through a reversing prism. Light originating at *e* is refracted upon entering the prism at *d,* is reflected from the mirrored hypotenuse face at *c,* and is refracted again upon leaving the prism at *b.* (Adapted from Helmholtz, 1962, Vol. III, p. 60. Dover Publications. Used by permission.)

isosceles glass) prism (Figure 3.2). He also gave general mathematical expression to the theory of light refraction in a prism (1962, Vol. II, pp. 92–101). He showed how *reflection* of light from the internal face of a right-angle prism produces optical up–down or right–left reversal of the structure of incident light (1962, Vol. II, p. 110). Helmholtz furthermore discussed how *refraction* of light within the medium of glass produces apparent displacement of a viewed object relative to a fixed point of observation (1962, Vol. III, p. 246).

In Figure 3.2 both the hypotenuse face of the prism and the point of observation are assumed to be perpendicular to the line of gravity—as if the hypotenuse face were resting on a table top while the observer is looking through one of the lateral faces. The structure of the light passing through the prism is geographically up–down reversed when the hypotenuse face is oriented perpendicular to the imaginary line of gravity and right–left reversed when the hypotenuse face is oriented parallel to the line of gravity. Helmholtz (1962, Vol. III, p. 60) describes this latter case as follows (see Figure 3.2):

> In looking through a prism of this sort [right-angle isosceles prism] in a direction parallel to the hypothenuse face . . . the ray of light *ab* is refracted at the side where it enters the prism so as to fall on the hypothenuse at *c;* whence it is reflected along *cd,* so as to emerge from the prism at *d.* If the points *b* and *d* are equally far from the hypothenuse face, the ray *ab* will emerge from the prism in the same direction *de* as it

---

surface [base] curves, thickness, and refractive power) as well as upon the prism's distance from the eye and its orientation before the eyes. Ogle's mathematical analysis is for the distortions produced by prisms with curved surfaces, whereas the displacing prisms used in adaptation experiments generally have plane surfaces. An analysis of the transformation of the direction of light rays passing through wedge prisms with a plane surface is given by Taylor (1966). Taylor is particularly clear in showing the optical origin of displacement and thus, of the differences between the apparent or perceived direction and the actual direction in which the viewed object is located (1966, p. 226).

had before it entered it. On the other hand, incident rays such as *ab′* and *ab″* which are not parallel to the hypothenuse face, and which after refraction are reflected from this face (at *c′* and *c″*), will subsequently emerge from the prism so that the incident and emergent rays, *ab′* and *d′e′* or *ab″* and *d″ e″* make equal angles with the hypothenuse face. Accordingly, under these circumstances a prism of this sort acts like a mirror; with this advantage, however, that the apparent direction of the central part of the reflex image remains the same as that of the object itself. When the observer looks through the prism in the direction *ab*, he sees objects on the other side of it "perverted" as to right and left, supposing the hypothenuse face is vertical, or perverted as to top and bottom, if this surface is horizontal.

WHAT IS REVERSED WITH REVERSING SPECTACLES?

This seemingly simple but thorny question has two kinds of answers. First, the observer's FV is reversed in relation to four constant points of reference: (*a*) the untransformed light outside of his or her FV, (*b*) gravity; (*c*) a fixed point of observation; and (*d*) the actual orientation of the observer's body. The second kind of answer is that the prism reverses the direction of the light that has passed through it relative to the light entering the prism: The phenomenal location and orientation of everything represented in the observer's FV is reversed in relation to its actual location and orientation. Each of the answers entails a new invariant[2] or constant for adapting, and the observer must come to terms with these new consistent facts.

The Field of View Is Reversed Relative to Four Points of Reference

First, the FV of the spectacle-wearer is reversed relative to the ambient array. The ambient optic array is now defined by Gibson as "a nested set of adjacent *solid angles*, not *rays*, each solid angle corresponding to one of the large faces or small facets of the environment [1974, p. 310; also cf. 1961, 1979, p. 308]." The ambient optic array constitutes

[2]Fieandt (1949, p. 344) introduced the concept of invariance (*Invarianz*)in his discussion of the influence of the (invariant) direction of the light in the perception of light and shadow when a surface with concavities and convexities is inverted. Gibson thinks of invariance as "the permanence in change or, in mathematical terms, the invariance under transformation [1966, p. 262, also, cf. 1967, 1979, pp. 310–311]." Permanent features of an array (informative variables of optical structure) that specify the permanent features of the layout are specified by what remains the same in the array during transformations over time (1966, p. 264). An invariant is a rule that specifies nonchange in change of an event during which structural or temporal dimensions of stimulation are transformed. Either recognizing or using the rule provides the perceiver with understanding or knowledge.

stimulus information about the structural characteristics of places, objects, events, people, and the self. Thus, regardless of what optic information is contained in the observer's FV, and whether he or she gained the information by eye, head, or body movements, the FV is optically reversed, whereas the light outside the FV at that moment in time is not.

Second, the FV of the spectacle-wearer is also reversed relative to gravity, a constant unaffected by the optical up–down reversal of the FV. Gravity remains for the observer a reference for the up–down direction (location and orientation) of places, objects, people, and events. Rooftops are not "falling," or "rising," or being "sucked into" the sky, regardless of how it might look to him or her. Yet, cognitive knowledge about abstractions like gravity does not seem to moderate the bewildering appearances experienced by an observer gazing through inverting or reversing spectacles (cf. Kohler, 1964; Stratton, 1896). Even though a falling ball looks like it is moving skyward to the spectacle-wearer, he or she can eventually visually confirm the gravitational fact that the ball moved groundward and came to rest there (see Figure 3.3).

Third, the FV of the spectacle-wearer is reversed relative to a fixed point of observation. The place from where an observer gazes at the environment and from where he or she regards himself–herself is the point of observation. Technically, a being with a binocular visual system occupies two points of observation. With reversing spectacles attached to the head, the observer's actual point of observation is behind the spectacles and remains constant relative to them; head and body

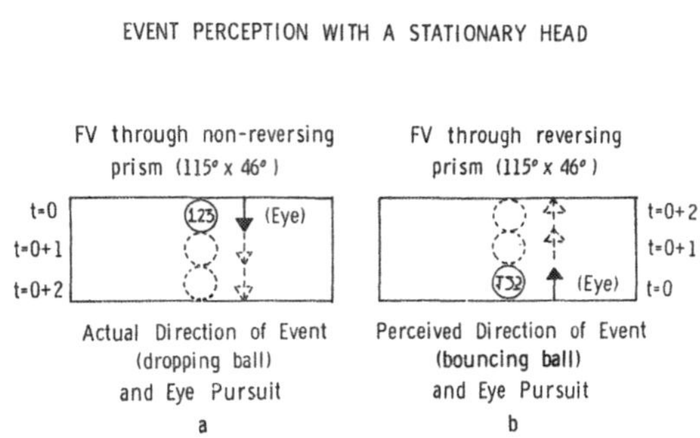

FIGURE 3.3. Event perception with and without reversing prisms attached to the observer's stationary head: (*a*) Actual and perceived direction of ball movement coincide; (*b*) perceived direction is opposite actual direction, thus a ball actually dropping appears to be "bouncing." The geographically upward pursuit eye movement required to follow this event is likely to elicit a skyward head movement by the spectacle-wearer, particularly if the event is rapid. (Note: These are immediate effects that may be altered by adaptation.)

movements, however, change the point of observation with reference to the environment.

Finally, the observer's FV is reversed relative to the orientation of his or her body. The observer's array sample is up–down reversed relative to his or her actual orientation, including the body parts, but especially relative to the real orientation of the head. Yet, insofar as the visible margins of the FV specify the orientation of the observer's head and insofar as the observer's body parts are, from time to time, optically represented in the reversed FV, his or her perception of the self should be affected.[3]

Postprism and Preprism Light

Structured light specifies the direction of the surfaces from which it is reflected. Since light within the prism-wearer's FV is reversed with respect to preprism light, it specifies the direction of *virtual objects in the FV* rather than the direction of *real objects in the environment.* Thus, reflected light appears to be coming from a direction in which the real surfaces are not located.

The Apparent Location of Objects Is Reversed

With spectacles, the phenomenal location of everything *within the observer's FV* is up–down reversed relative to its real location. The discrepancy between the direction of structured, reflected light before it enters the spectacles and after it has passed through them is lawful. This relationship has been diagrammed in Figure 3.4b and may be further described as follows. If a given object in the environment is geographically 15° below the point of observation, then the virtual object within the observer's FV will appear to be 15° above the point of observation, that is, at twice the angular deviation (30°) from its actual position in the environment. Thus, there is a bilateral symmetry of the real and virtual object that bisects the FV in the vertical plane.

The consequences of this new optical invariant on perception and visually guided action was vividly illustrated by the following observations: On Day 2, 18 hours after donning the up–down reversing spectacles during the Prism Study, I reported:

[3]Note that the principles of this analysis *are* transferable to other forms of optical transformation. You need only substitute "displaced" or "tilted" or "inverted" to check the claim. Since minification and magnification affect perceived size, the phenomenal size of seen body parts should be affected.

> *I'm approaching a tree branch, which turns out to be about 7 feet off the ground; yet, I am visually convinced that this branch will hit me in the face as I approach it. In order to avoid getting hit in the face by this branch, I reached down toward my knees to hold the branch aside. This happened once while I was walking and then again while riding a bike.*

On Day 11, after 142 hours with reversing spectacles, I observed:

> *Passing underneath an obstacle often provides visual information that it will hit me in the face, decapitate me, or hit me in the chest. Passing underneath a clothesline is particularly frightful. Though the line may barely touch the top of my helmet [which contains the reversing prisms] or can just be reached with an outstretched hand, visually I'm convinced it will cut right across my Adam's apple. Now, rather than reaching toward my knees to clear the obstacle out of the way, my reaction is to duck. The information that I will in fact clear the obstacle never comes; indeed, I anticipate impact and experience surprise when none is forthcoming. The same phenomenon is observed during bicycle- or car-riding where tree branches overhang the street. In the latter case (on Day 10) it appeared as if we were going to hit tree branches continually.*

Three hours later, I reported on what I called "clothesline decapitation":

> *I'm approaching a clothesline from 20 feet away, with my head cocked back. Given this head posture (and point of observation), the clothesline appears to be clearly higher off the ground than my head, that is, at this point my expectation is that I will clear it. As I approach, the line appears to begin to descend and finally it looks as if it would cut at the point of my Adam's apple if I were to proceed. In fact, the line is 1½ feet above the top of my helmet. I have retained my head in the cocked back position throughout this procedure. After a few trials with the* same *line, I no longer duck on approach.*

The Apparent Orientation of Objects Is Reversed

With spectacles, the phenomenal *orientation* of surfaces within the observer's FV is up–down reversed relative to their actual orientation. Thus, for example, the chin of a sculpture of a head (resting on a table), whose geographical center is in a straight line with the observer's point of observation, should appear phenomenally to be on the other side of where the real chin is located (i.e., on the same side of where its real head is located). The sculpture, and all else in the FV, should appear in reverse orientation to the real and remembered orientation of objects in the environment and to the observer's head, or vice versa.

Earth–Sky Light Intensities Are Reversed

The phenomenal direction of the difference in light intensity between sky and earth is reversed within the FV of the observer with up–down reversing spectacles. In an outdoor environment the intensity of light from the sky is always greater than from the earth (Gibson, 1966, p. 13). However, for the observer who looks through spectacles, the more intense light from the upper hemisphere is optically represented in the lower portion of the FV. Consequently, he or she must adapt to a new intensity invariant of the outdoor environment: the earth above and the sky below. When photographs are inverted, concavities (craters) turn into convexities (hills), and vice versa; the direction from which the more intense illumination arrives is thereby inverted. Moving about in a richly structured environment provides the observer with many more safeguards against perceptual trickery and error than does viewing the frozen, high-gloss world of photographs. Nevertheless, to adapt, the observer must successfully cope with the reversal of this earth-old constant: Hemispheric differences in illumination specify the surface of support below the feet and the sky above the head.

ADAPTING REQUIREMENTS FOR LOOKING AND ACTING WITH REVERSING SPECTACLES

To adapt, the spectacle-wearer must cope with a dilemma: The eyes have to respond to postprism light, whereas the rest of the observer must respond to the unchanged facts of the environment as represented in preprism light. For any given type of transformation, the extent and rate of adaptation are largely determined by the different kinds of eye movement (EM) control systems that direct action: the saccadic, compensatory, or the pursuit system. For example, in my experiment, catching an object, which requires coordinated eye, head, and arm pursuit, was never accomplished despite hundreds of trials spaced over 15 days. Riding a bike, on the other hand, was fairly successful on the first attempt (after 20 hours of having worn reversing spectacles); similarly, slow, visually guided reaching movements (for a doorknob) were competent on the second day (after 14 hours). (See Chapters 7–9 for further evidence.) Each adapting requirement may be regarded as constituting a *new kind of functional invariant,* a new set of "rules" for looking and acting, which describes how the visual system now *has to work* in conjunction with the motor system. An historical account precedes a brief analysis of these adapting requirements (see Dolezal, 1976, for a detailed discussion).

Looking from Behind Spectacles: History

Ewert was the first to note correctly that light, when passed through his inverting spectacles, produced what I have called unique adapting requirements for EMs as well as for combined eye-head and eye-head-body movements (1930, pp. 197-203, 1936, pp. 536-538). For example, he observed that "to fixate objects above the line of sight, the eye had to rotate downward, or to fixate points to the left of the line of sight, the eye had to rotate to the right, and vice versa [1936, p. 539]." Ewert also saw that head movements (HMs) had to be in the same direction as in normal vision if the observer's task was to bring a peripherally seen object into the center of the visual field (1930, p. 316, 1936, p. 539) and that consequently, "a conflict between the previously established eye and head reflexes results [1930, p. 316]." He further argued that "The reciprocal relationship which normally exists between eye and head reflexes, as a result of past conditioning, is now broken down [1930, p. 316]." Although Ewert was not quite explicit, it is safe to say that he was aware that not just fixations and saccadic and pursuit EMs were inverted relative to a viewed object but also that during lenticular inversion, compensatory EMs were also reversed relative to the direction of HMs. In 1930, he also said: "Normally, compensatory eye reflexes keep the eyes fixated on an object during head movement. Under disoriented conditions, however, due to the antagonism of the eye and head reflexes, the new compensatory eye movements could perhaps not keep pace with the head movement [p. 349]."[4] In 1937, Ewert was no more explicit as to the nature of this antagonism or how it is resolved. However, he again alluded to an antagonism "between normal head fixations and lenticularly induced eye movements, antagonism between eye movements of ocular and vestibular origin, and antagonism between body movements of kinaesthetic and vestibular origin and those of ocular origin [1937, p. 106]." With respect to combined eye-head-body movements, Ewert observed that "all bodily movements are now opposed to the new eye movements [1930, p. 317]."

Carr wrote, in apparent opposition to Ewert, that during lenticular inversion, "ocular habits remain the same, while antagonistic head movements are required for fixation [1935, p. 38]." However, the discrepancy can be cleared up. Ewert took the objective position of the distal object as his point of reference from which EMs and HMs are described,

[4]During a compensatory EM, the observer's eyes and head move in opposite directions; the eyes and their retinae thus remain stationary in relation to a fixated object during head and body movements.

whereas Carr chose light that has already passed through the inverting lenses as his reference. Both were careful and consistent in their description. Eyes respond to the directional characteristics of what I have called *postprism light,* not to the actual direction of objects. As Carr put it, the "eye reacts . . . to the direction in which the light enters the eye, or better, it reacts to the position of the retinal stimulus [1935, p. 36]."

Carr brought out two other important points. First, he observed that "Any object located in the optical axis of the lenticular system, i.e., in the center of the visual field, is correctly localized . . . [because] The object stimulates the same retinal point as in normal vision [1935, p. 35]." By implication, when both eyes and head are in the primary position (face front, gazing straight ahead), there are no functional differences with or without spectacles, at least not for the theoretical point at the very center of the FV. This theoretical "point" bisects the optical up from down and right from left. Second, Carr noted that during HMs, "All visual objects move in the direction of the head movements. . . . [and] that they move twice the distance and twice as fast [1935, p. 37]." (See my Table 3.1.)

Taylor derived five propositions that describe some important functional differences between wearing up–down reversing spectacles and freestyle viewing.

1. The field is perceived as inverted.
2. Perceived positions are stable under rotation of the eyes provided the head is stationary.
3. The field is stable under rotation of the head about the vertical axis.
4. Backward and forward tilting of the head has the effect that the field is perceived as sweeping past the eyes in the direction of the head movement but at double the speed.
5. Tilting the head toward a shoulder has the effect that the field is perceived as rotating about the axis of rotation of the head in the same direction as the head but twice as fast [1962, p. 176]."

Except for the fifth proposition, this account does not go beyond Ewert's and Carr's descriptions, although Papert has given Taylor's notation mathematical expression (Taylor, 1962, pp. 189–192). Papert also included the case of attaching inverting prisms onto the eyeball, in which case the field would be perceived as moving in the same direction as the EM and at twice the speed. HMs should now contribute to instability only to the extent that the eyes are carried with the head, according to Papert (Taylor. 1962, pp. 192–193).

Howard and Templeton offer the most complete diagrammatic and

TABLE 3.1

The Consequences of Optical Reversal and Inversion During Eye and–or Head Movements and Fixation: (1) Does the entire field of view, or stationary objects in it, appear to move?[a] (2) What relationship to the object must the line of gaze (fixation) maintain for fixation? (3) Is the eye pointed at the real object or the virtual object? (see Figure 3.4)

		Reversal (up–down)			Reversal (right–left)	Inversion
Prism, lens, mirror	With eye and–or head movement	(1) Apparent object motion	(2)[b] To fixate object	(3)[b] Eye pointed at	(1) Apparent object motion	(1) Apparent object motion
Attached to **head** of observer	Any eye movement	No	Line of gaze moves through equal and opposite angle	Virtual object	No	No
	Head movement					
	up–down	Yes	Line of gaze normal	Virtual object	No	Yes
	right–left	No	Line of gaze normal	Real object	Yes	Yes
	shoulder tilt	Yes	45° head movement = 90° visual field tilt	Virtual object	Yes	Yes
Attached to **eyes** of observer	Any eye or head movement	Yes	Line of gaze normal	Virtual object	Yes	Yes
Mounted **external** to observer	Any eye or head movement	No	Line of gaze moves through equal and opposite angle	Virtual object	No	No

[a]The geometrical relation–phenomenal observation rule appears to be: Object–world motion displaces twice as fast in the same direction as the eye or head movement (to whichever the device is attached).

[b](2) and (3) remain the same for right–left reversal and inversion, provided the apparent object motion is the same as for up–down reversal.

verbal description to date of the geometry of the relationship between movements of the eyes and head and the resulting "movements" of the retinal image when inverting and-or reversing spectacles are worn (1966, pp. 399–404). They distinguish among three cases: (*a*) When the spectacles are attached to the observer's eyes, (*b*) when they are attached to the head; or (*c*) when the device is mounted to a stationary object outside the observer. In addition to confirming the descriptions offered by the previously mentioned investigators, they discuss the relationship between the direction of EM or HM and movement of the retinal image for the three cases.

A careful reading of Ewert, Carr, Taylor, and particularly of Howard and Templeton (1966, p. 404) allows one to derive most of the contents of Table 3.1. It answers three questions (designated *a, b,* and *c*) about an observer who wears spectacles that up-down reverse, right-left reverse, or invert the available light as a function of whether the spectacles are attached to the observer's head or eyes or are mounted externally to the observer and as a function of the direction in which the observer moves his or her eyes and-or head. The terms *line of gaze* in Table 3.1 and *line of fixation* of Figure 3.4 (below) are interchangeable. Several of the elements of Table 3.1 are described in the next section.

Adapting Requirements of Reversing Spectacles

To function effectively, the observer must remain attuned to himself-herself and his or her environment in perception and action. When this "attunement" is disturbed, the observer seeks to reestablish it. We will consider four levels of looking and performing: (*a*) How the observer must hold and move his or her eyes in a stationary head to inspect an object or event of interest; (*b*) how the observer must hold and move his or her eyes during HM to inspect an object or event of interest; (*c*) how the observer must hold and move his or her eyes, head, and limbs for successful visually guided movements; and (*d*) how the relationship of the visible self within the environment is disturbed.

Holding and Moving the Eyes in a Stationary Head

To look at (foveate) an object lying on the ground, the observer wearing up-down reversing prisms attached to his or her head must point the eyes up (i.e., skyward) in the head. The observer's foveas respond only to the direction from which light emerges once it has passed through the prism and are therefore directed toward the virtual rather than the real object of the observer's attention (see Figure 3.4).

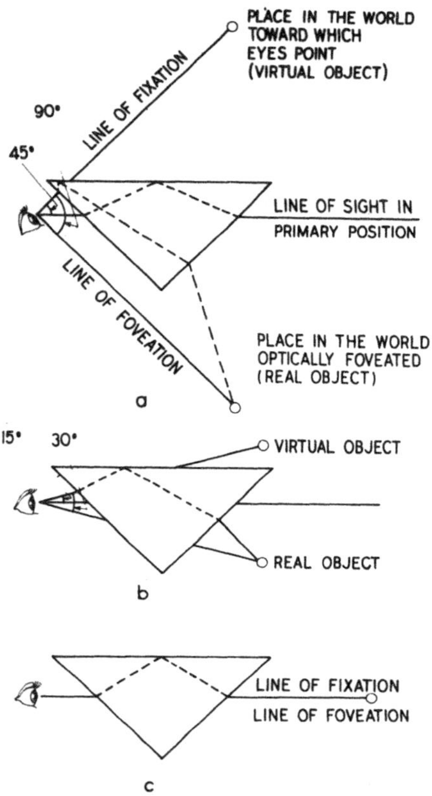

FIGURE 3.4. Unique adapting requirements for looking (fixating and foveating) with up–down reversing prisms.

Specifically, with prisms, the line of fixation and the line of foveation[5] are maximally separated or "out of phase" when the eyes assume an extreme up or down posture in the head (Figure 3.4a). Similarly, for successful *pursuit fixation,* the new rule for the observer with up–down reversing spectacles and a fixed head is to move the eyes in the direction *opposite* to the direction of the real motion of an object (see Figure 3.3).

[5]*The line of fixation* is the direction in which the observer must point the eyes within the head to foveally intercept light coming from a source external to the prism. The *line of foveation* is the direction in which light from a source external to the prism travels to the fovea when no prism is interposed between the source and the eyes. The line of foveation coincides with the direction of *preprism* light from, and specifies the direction of, the real object.

Holding and Moving the Head and Eyes

For successful eye-head pursuit fixation, the observer with reversing spectacles must move his or her eyes and head in opposite directions. Hence, the successful foveal pursuit of a falling object now requires an *upward* EM synchronized with a *downward* HM: indeed a unique requirement and an interesting case that violates the requirements of normal stabilization; errors in the direction of head pursuit and in pointing or catching any object in motion should result (cf. Chapter 8).

Understanding the optical, perceptual, and performatory consequences of up–down head movements for the observer with reversing spectacles attached to the head is vital.[6] As the observer raises the head, the leading (geographically upper) edge of the FV conceals places in the world visible the moment before, and the *trailing* (bottom) edge of the FV reveals places in the world concealed previously (Figure 3.5). Alternately, during down HMs, objects come into view at the top of the observer's FV and disappear from view at the bottom. As a consequence (it follows from the geometrical optics), the *rate* of revealing and concealing is *double* that of the normal situation: *The FV moves with the head but at twice the normal rate during up–down HMs.* Moving the head is a disturbing experience; the perceived motion of the surroundings is in the direction of the HM and twice as fast. In turn, these motions *in* and *of* the FV—these upheavals of the observer's visible phenomenal "world"—are perceived to be the cause of his or her own concurrently experienced bodily instability, vertigo, and nausea (see Chapters 7 and 12). The reversal of the compensatory EMs, discussed later, may well be an integral component of this bodily vertigo and especially of the nausea.

With spectacles, the *compensatory eye movements,* which maximize perceived stability of the environment during HMs, are reversed. Specifically, the normal, correlative relationship between neck-muscle, vestibular, and optical compensation—what I call *light-dependent compensation*—is reversed, that is, during an up–down HM, the eyes now have to move in the *same* direction as the head but twice as much. For example, when the observer fixates a place and then begins to move

[6]The discussion is easier to follow if the reader checks the phenomenology of these descriptions. Use the device suggested in the Introduction or cut a narrow slit into a piece of cardboard and hold it to the head and over the face so that it remains stationary with respect to the head during HMs. This rectangular FV will provide some appreciation for the relationship between the FV of the head and the environment. If the slit contained an up–down reversing prism, everything observed now would be up–down reversed. Some sense of this state may be achieved by putting the head between the legs, continuing to look through the slit, and moving the head up and down (by bending the knees) while in that orientation.

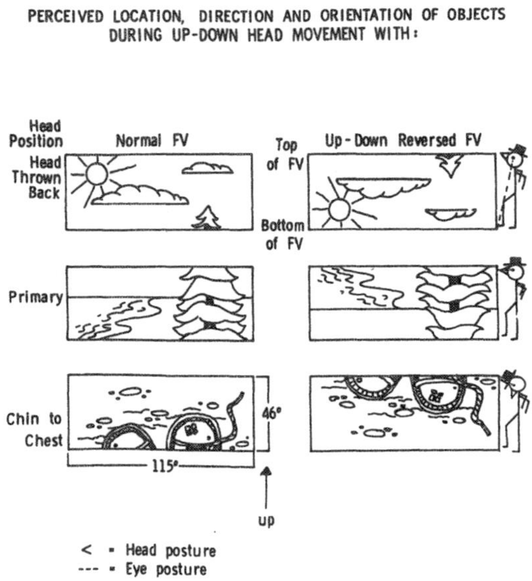

FIGURE 3.5. Perceptual consequences of normal up or down head movements (HMs) and with up–down reversing prisms attached to observer's head (rectangular 46° × 115° FV depicts the FV used in the Prism Study). During an upward HM with prisms, the leading edge of the top of observer's FV hides the scenery while the trailing edge of the bottom of the FV reveals it: just the reverse of the normal situation.

his or her head upward, the eyes *also* must move upward. This is so because light-dependent compensatory EMs are a response to the phenomenal *optical shifts* produced by the HM. The eyes attempt to pursue this observer-produced optical motion in order to remain foveally anchored to the shifting structure of the light reflected from the fixated place. To remain foveally anchored with spectacles, the observer's eyes have to (*a*) move ahead of the head; (*b*) move in the same direction as the head; and (*c*) move twice as fast as the head. The reversed relationship of compensatory EMs with respect to the head constitutes a new functional invariant, an *immediate optical requirement,* to maintain stabilization of the eyes relative to a foveated surface during up–down HMs (cf. Chapter 7).

During *tilting of the head toward either shoulder,* the slight counterrolling of the eyes (Helmholtz, 1962, Vol. III, p. 43) produced by light is assumed to modify or override vestibular–gravitational control of ocular countertorsion during lateral head tilt (cf. Chapter 7).

Right–left head movements contain varying components of an up–

down and onto-the-shoulder tilt motion. Hence, there should be some perceptual effect for the spectacle-wearer due to the difficulties described for vertical compensatory eye–head movements and due to the optical effects produced by slight counterrolling of the eyes with head tilt. (Note that with right–left reversing prisms [or inverting lenses] attached to the head, compensatory EMs would be reversed during *right–left* HMs. Moreover, right–left displacing prisms [base right or left] attached to the head should also modify compensatory EMs during right–left HMs.)

Adapting Requirements for Visually Guided Movements

The spectacle-wearer engages in unique eye–head and eye–arm movement *combinations* in order to effectively deal with the unique relationship between the optical facts and the environmental facts. For example, to point correctly, the observer must point at what he or she is *optically foveating* and not in the direction of his or her line of fixation (or where the eyes are pointed), as is usually done without spectacles. Thus, where the observer points his or her eyes and where he or she must point his or her arm at directionally incongruent or "out of phase."

In *eye–head–arm pursuit* of a moving object, the observer's eyes must move *up* in the head while the head and arms must move *downward* to foveate and catch a falling ball (cf. Figures 3.3b and 7.2). The observer is expected to reach toward the knees when the ball is overhead and overhead when the ball is at knee level. This is because the observer's arms are expected to be roughly in phase with the direction of the pursuit EM, and since the direction of this EM is out of phase with the actual location of the object at any moment in time, the direction of the observer's moving arm should be out of phase with the moving object. (For a photographic action shot of attempted ball-catching, see Figure 8.3).

Perceiving the Visible Self

With spectacles, the perception of the self is radically altered insofar as the observer has optical information about himself–herself, insofar as the borders of the FV constitute or specify information for head location and head orientation, and insofar as body parts are visible in the FV. The perception of self, particularly as regards the location and orientation of body parts, is assumed to be *reciprocally* related to the subject's perception of the environment and the location and orientation of the places, objects, people and events within that environment. Five predictions follow.

First, the landscape visible in the FV should appear phenomenally up–down reversed relative to (*a*) the visually remembered world; (*b*) the remembered orientation of the self in the total surrounding environment; (*c*) the visualized orientation of the self; and (*d*) the self-orientation experienced by means of nonoptic information (e.g., the haptically felt self, the acoustically heard self, and the nosmically experienced self).

Second, the relationship of the visible self with the environment should be disturbed. Although the content of the FV is up–down reversed with respect to both the surrounding environment and the actual orientation of the head, the observer has visual information that the head is up–down reversed and is expected to experience the confusion attendant to an up–down reversed head as part of the content of the reversed FV. For this reason, the orientation of objects, relative to self, should also be phenomenally ambiguous, confused, or judged to be "reversed" (cf. Chapter 9). (No prediction can be offered as to whether the observer will or can experience both an "upright" and "reversed" head simultaneously or in near simultaneity. Linguistic and conceptual confusions have to be ruled out before such a report can be accepted. When such confusions are cleared up, I doubt that any substance to such a claim will remain.)

Third, the observer's head should appear phenomenally up–down reversed to him or her. To adapt to a transformed world, the observer has to deal with a visually transformed body. Given that the only direct optical information for the orientation of body parts is contained in postprism light, the observer is expected to perceive the head visually as up–down reversed relative to its remembered visual image, relative to the remembered surrounding environment, and relative to the shoulders (if no visual information for shoulder orientation is available). The observer should judge the chin as phenomenally further away from the ground than the forehead or the top of the head. This is not too surprising when one considers that even the optical shifts of the observer's FV during up–down HMs *specify* an up–down reversed head with respect to the preprism environment. Moreover, the feet should be visually perceived as pointing toward the observer's midsection (at the level of the ground) and the hands, if placed on a table, actually pointing away from self, should appear, phenomenally, as pointing toward the observer (see Figure 9.1).

Fourth, recognition of objects, faces, and print should be disturbed with spectacles. I believe that the orientation of objects, patterns, and forms comes to determine the observer's phenomenal judgment of symmetry, "organization," and "good form." For example, recognizablility of static form (e.g., print), given that its uprightness in a definite frame of reference has been the standard, should be seriously impaired when uprightness in that sense is reversed.

Finally, event perception should be impaired. It is expected that the direction of ongoing events will be confused. If the observer experiences perceptual ambiguity as to the actual location and orientation of objects in the FV relative to those outside it and relative to the seen or remembered orientation of his or her own body parts and if the observer commits errors in the direction of HMs in tracking moving objects, then he or she should experience phenomenal confusion as to the true direction of ongoing events. For example, is that fly on the wall walking toward the ceiling or the ground? Remember, the fly optically enters the top of the FV and proceeds toward the bottom of the FV as it makes its way to the ceiling in the real world. Smoke from the cigarette in one's mouth should first appear at the top border of the FV and phenomenally "drift downward," toward the bottom edge of the FV.

In conclusion, it may be said that the observer adapts to a transformation's requirements. When gazing through reversing spectacles, he or she is confronted with novel, unique, phenomenal symmetry relations in everything, from static displays of print to dynamic events of smiles and walking movements. The observer must adapt to the discrepancy in appearance, between the perceived present and the visualized or remembered past, of textured object-surfaces, faces, smiles, print, and so on. I hypothesize that adaptation is to a new set of perceptual invariants, which influence the appearance and recognition of all that is seen through spectacles. Furthermore, while wearing spectacles, the observer makes perceptual discriminations of new distinctive features and learns performatory skills that are usable in his or her relation to *visualized* spatial array properties not in the FV. Consequently, I hypothesize that the observer's actions, such as reaching or orientation for locomotion, can be *vision based:* initiated and maintained by the observer's internal representations (memories, schemas), derived from the transformed visual information.

The subject also adapts to the discrepancy between the seen and the otherwise experienced, between the distorted FV and nonoptic information. Adaptation is to any observer-environmental fact specified by postprism light that is also perceptually available by means of acoustic, haptic-kinesthetic, gravo-ceptive, and nosmic information. For example, the observer might be confronted with a discrepancy between the seen and felt orientation of his or her own head, between the seen and heard location of someone's voice, between the seen and smelled location of a flower, and between the visually and haptically (gravitationally) perceived direction of the surface of support. Finally, adaptation must take place to the reduction in the extent of the FV. This factor is introduced by every spectacle ever used to transform an observer's FV, yet it has been greatly neglected in previous work. I will discuss it in the next chapter.

SUMMARY

In this chapter I detail to what the spectacle-wearer adapts during adaptation to optical transformation. Thus, I lay the groundwork for saying how and why adaptation occurs. There are new demands that an observer must satisfy in order to adapt: These *adapting requirements* for achieving consistent perception and skillful actions are derived from the unique and invariant relationship between light before it enters the prism (preprism light) and after it passes through (postprism light). A discrepancy is created by this optical relationship between where the direction of surfaces *appears* in the field of view (FV) and where those surfaces *are* in the environment.

Using up-down reversal as a paradigm case, I then describe what is reversed with reversing prisms. One answer is that the observer's FV is reversed with respect to four points of reference, which remain constant: (*a*) The untransformed light outside the observer's FV; (*b*) gravity; (*c*) the actual place from where the observer views himself-herself and the world; and (*d*) the actual orientation of the observer's body (and his or her memory of a nonreversed self and world). Another answer is that since the direction from which light is coming is optically reversed, the apparent location and orientation of everything visible in the FV is reversed: This is the optical invariant to which the observer adapts.

Three kinds of adapting requirements for successful looking and acting with reversing spectacles derive from the optical transformation imposed on the observer—perceptual, cognitive, and performatory. First, the optical invariant creates new *perceptual invariants* that are responsible for the strange appearances (seen through spectacles) to which the prism-wearer adapts. The observer has to adapt to the visually detectable discrepancy between the apparent and actual location and orientation of places, objects, people, events, and parts of the self. Naturally, the visible self is transformed no less than the observer's perception of the environment. The orientation of all visible body parts, especially the head, are perceptually up-down reversed relative to their actual and remembered orientation. The observer's task is to become acquainted, furthermore, with the distinctive features of smiles, walking movements, and print. These distinctive symmetry relations make identification, recognition, and consistent perception possible again. During adaptation, cognitive schematas based on the new sights are likely to become established before improvements in recognition of print, faces, etc. become measurable. Thus, the optical invariant necessitates new *cognitive adaptations.* Third, the optical constant also creates unique *performatory adapting requirements* for all combinations of eye, head, and limb movements used in looking and in visually guided action. Thus, the imposed transformation necessitates unique ways in which the observer must position his or her eyes relative to the head while looking through spectacles (cf. Figure 3.1) and novel ways in which he or she now has to coordinate eye movements and movements of other body parts to perform skillfully. Above all, the invariant rule that the spectacle-wearer now has to live by is that the eyes must respond to the directional characteristics of postprism light, whereas the rest of the observer must respond to the unchanged facts of the environment as represented in preprism light if he or she is to be competent.

A preliminary answer to our original question is beginning to take shape: The observer adapts to spectacle-wearing, an experience that has unique optical, perceptual, cognitive, and performatory consequences. He or she adapts to the differences between living with and without transforming spectacles. More specifically, if the observer adapts, it is because he or she is able to cope with the new optical invariant and with the resulting adapting requirements for looking, for perceptual recognition, and for visually guided action that confront him or her.

4

The Restricted Field of View: A Neglected Factor in Adaptation Research

Two quite different effects are produced by all spectacles used in adaptation research: transformation and restriction of the normal field of view (FV). Whenever an observer looks through a spectacle that optically displaces, tilts, inverts, reverses, minifies, or magnifies the contents of the FV, he or she is also exposed to a FV that is reduced in size and altered in shape. As a consequence, the subject's access to peripheral visual information is severely diminished. To date, no prism, mirror, or lens system has been constructed that even approximates the scope of the normal FV (Figure 4.1). Indeed, most experimenters have restricted the FV of their observers rather severely.[1]

[1]For example, Stratton's (1896, 1897b) monocular inverted field presumably subtended 45°. Brown doubts that Stratton computed the angular extent of his FV correctly. He says: "We have been unable by means of lenses to obtain a distinct monocular field as large as Stratton's, about 18° to 20° diameter being the largest we secured even with the assistance of the research department of a large optical company. The specification of Stratton's lenses is not given [Brown, 1928, p. 121]." Ewert also challenges the accuracy of that claim: "Stratton's . . . monocular field was reported to be 45° in size. We were unable to obtain as large an inverted field even with the aid of the research department of the Bausch & Lomb Optical Company, the Spencer Lens Company, and the Harvard University Physics Shop [Ewert, 1930, p. 201]." Also markedly restricted, the binocular, inverted fields of view obtained by Ewert (1930, p. 201), Peterson and Peterson (1938, p. 12), and

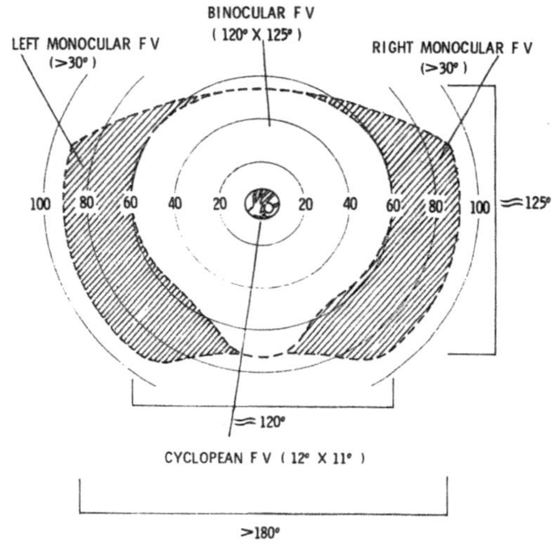

FIGURE 4.1. Normal, binocular and two monocular (shaded) fields of view with both eyes fixated (drawn to scale and projected onto the fronto-parallel plane). The restricted, 12° cyclopean FV that I experienced as the observer in the Tube Study is depicted in the center.

Adaptation to visual transformation cannot be clearly assessed unless one first isolates and measures the consequences of restricting the FV. To do so, the observer's FV must be limited in angular scope (and in shape) by the same amount before, during, and after exposure to the transformation. Of those experimenters discussed previously, only

---

Snyder and Pronko (1952, p. 49) were 34.5°, 34.5°, and 20°, respectively. The right-left reversed binocular FV used by both Grill in 1951, and by Kohler in 1953, measured 25° horizontally × 33° vertically. The up-down or right-left reversed FV used by Kottenhoff was 30° × 33° (Kottenhoff, 1961, p. 66). The tilted binocular FV employed by Brown in 1926 subtended a mere 10° of visual angle (1928, p. 122), and more recently, Redding (1973, 1975, Experiment I, and 1978) employed a monocular 10° FV. Similarly, all displacing prisms used in experiments since the time of Helmholtz have limited the size of the FV. For example, Cohen (1966) restricted a binocular field to 10° and to 15° × 10°. Redding (1973, 1975) created a 20° monocular field with Risley prisms. Even the largest laterally displaced FV ever reported, featuring a surprisingly large binocular FV of 90° × 60°, eliminated peripheral vision with side shields, according to the authors (Hay & Pick, 1966; Pick & Hay, 1964). Indeed, so unimportant seemed the restriction of the FV that many (displacement) experiments failed to even report the angular extent of the restricted and transformed FV (e.g., Helmholtz, 1867/1962; Kohler, 1964; Taylor, 1962; Wallace, Melamud, & Kaplan, 1973; and Wooster, 1923).

Ewert (1930) did so.[2] As will be shown later, major experiments abound that attributed their results to the optical transformation, even though they may have been due to the restricted FV (RFV).

ANALYSIS: LOOKING, ACTING, AND SELF-PERCEPTION WITH A RESTRICTED FIELD OF VIEW

Method of the Author's Tube Study

In order to document the effects of severely limiting the normal FV, I wore two paper tubes, which restricted my FV to 12° (Figure 4.2); like transforming spectacles, the tubes were attached to my head. A 12° FV corresponds to seeing no more than the head of a badminton racket at a 1-m (39-inch) distance; it fills the entire FV. Tubes were chosen for several reasons. First, the majority of the early investigators of long-term adaptation inserted their lenses into one or two metal tubes. Stratton used double convex lenses in one tube; Ewert used lenses in two tubes; Peterson borrowed Ewert's headgear; Snyder and Pronko had two unit-power inverting telescopes; and Brown, two right-angle prisms, one in front of the other. Second, the tubes are easy to construct and lightweight. Third, weight was an important consideration because I wanted to construct an apparatus that prevented sight of the hands and body to find out how the perceiver-performer would fare—simulating the condition of Held and Bauer's (1967) monkeys, which were deprived of the sight of their limbs with a collar around the neck. Thus, the tubes had to be long.

Observer: Then 29 years old, I served as observer and experimenter. My visual acuity was 20/40 for the left eye and 20/80 for the right eye. Binocular acuity was 20/40.

Materials: The FV was restricted by two tubes, which were fitted into a rubber diver's goggle (Figure 4.3). At a distance of 109 cm (43 in.) from the cornea, the visual field described an ellipse measuring 23 cm (9 in.) horizontally and 20.5 cm (8 in.) vertically (Figure 4.3). This area corresponds to a visual angle (Graham, 1965, p. 505) of approximately 12° × 11°, respectively. The weight of the tube system was 140 g (5 oz.).

Procedure: The general purpose of the study was to observe and

[2]Stratton did, apparently, measure his aftereffects in one experiment with the restricted FV (1897b, p. 469), and Snyder and Pronko (1952) took baseline but not aftereffect data with the restricted FV. Festinger, Burnham, Ono, & Bamber, 1967 (Experiments I–III) are among the few modern investigators who controlled for the limiting of the FV.

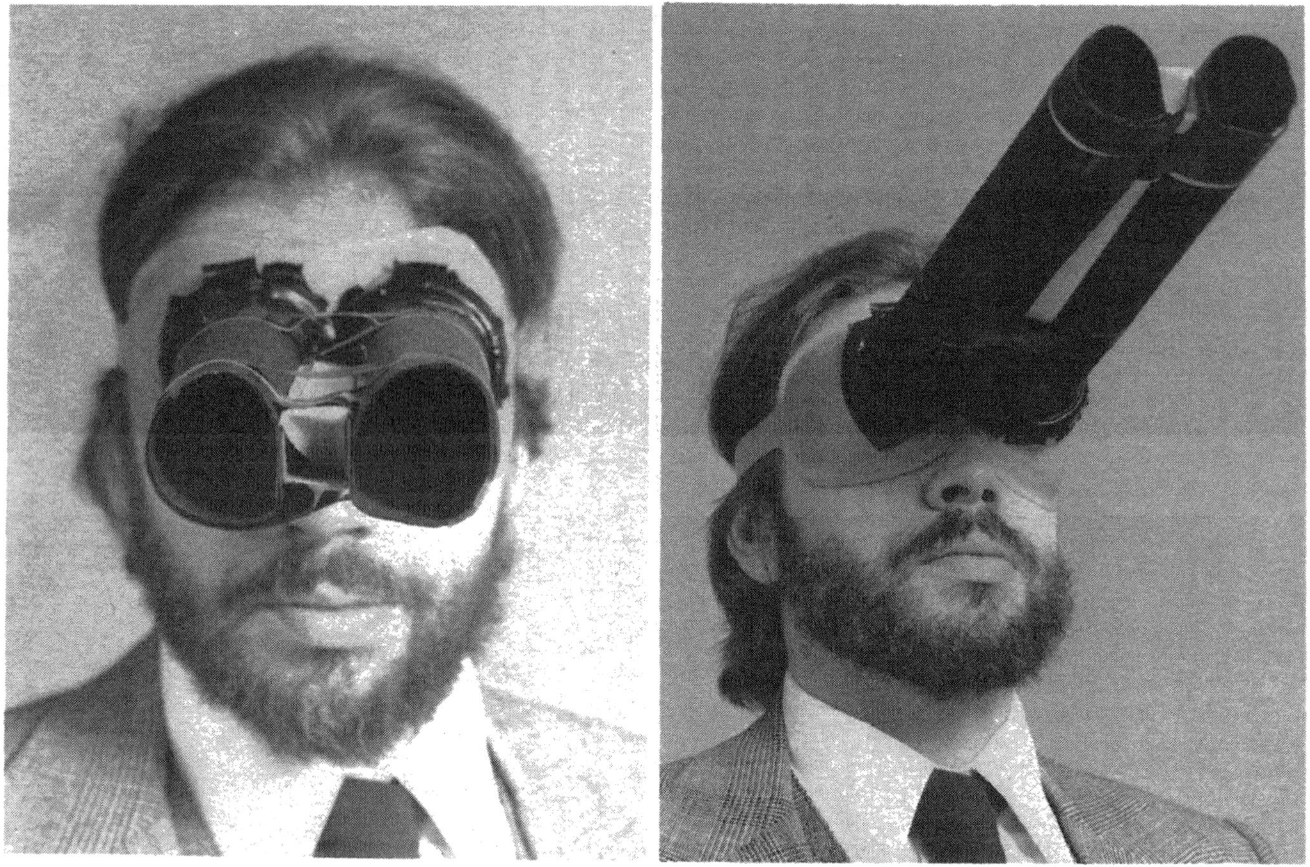

FIGURE 4.2. Tubes limiting the field of view used in the Tube Study. (Photos made 3/79.)

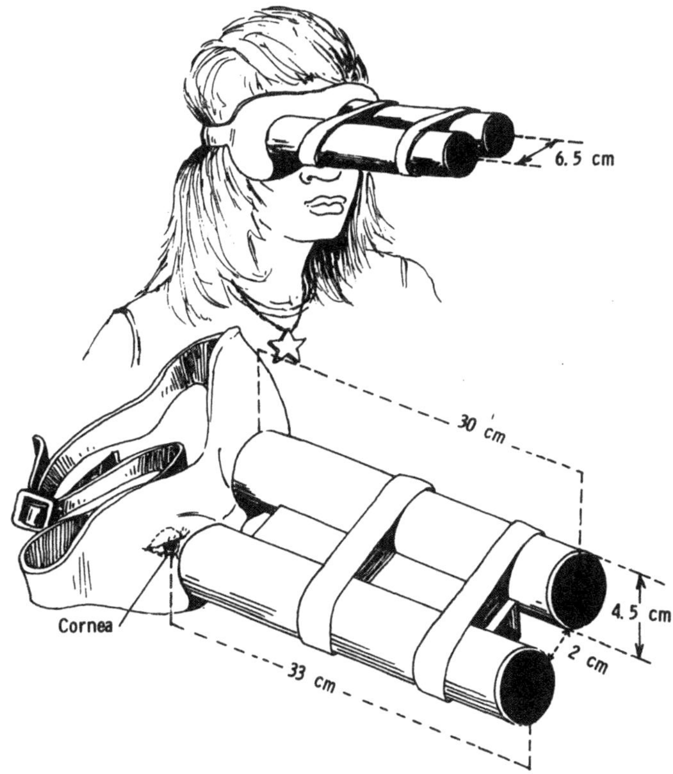

FIGURE 4.3. Description of tubes used to restrict the field of view.

describe the consequences of a restricted FV during everyday living. The duration of the study was 6 days (January 21–26, 1970). I wore the tube arrangement for 71 waking hours with a daily range of 11–14 hours. At all other times, I wore a light-occluding mask to prevent perceiving with anything but the RFV. Results are discussed in the final section.

Perceiving and Performing with a Normal and Restricted FV

The following analysis emphasizes eight functional differences for perceiving and acting between a normal FV and the 12° FV just described; these differences also hold for the FV restrictions inevitably created by any lens, mirror, or prism spectacle. First, unlike the normal FV, the RFV has obtrusively visible borders. When the observer fixates objects in the environment with restricting tubes, the visual field appears to be unitary, surrounded by one round border. Perceptually, he or she gazes "through" a cyclopean eye, apparently located in the center of the forehead (see Figure 4.1). However, when the observer accommodates for and fixates the end of the tubes or any object immediately beyond the end of the tubes, the perceived shape of the visual field is defined by two partially overlapping borders. If this perceptual situation were diagrammed, it would look like two intersecting circles. During head movements (HMs), the obtrusively visible borders of the FV sweep over places, objects, and people in the environment, revealing them at the leading border and concealing them at the trailing edge. This exposing and hiding of features of the environment is determined by where, how fast, and how far the observer moves his or her head. Moreover, since the often foveally visible edges of the tubes correspond to the borders of the observer's visual field, he or she is now more aware of the head-sweeping activity.

Second, when tubes are worn, successive fields of view of the head[3] have no visual information in common. *During* two successive HMs, the normal FV of the two eyes[4] and the FV of the head almost always contain some visual information contained in the preceding FV: each FV overlaps its preceding FV. I call this invariant fact *pan-overlap*. This statement holds true even for a RFV, although the absolute amount of shared optical information over time is smaller than with the normal FV. Then, at the *conclusion* of even an extreme eye movement (EM), HM-EM, or EM-HM, the large size of the normal FV virtually assures that some information will remain common to both the new and the previous FV. I call this *end-point overlap*. Indeed, by virtue of the large FV *Homo sapiens* enjoys, it is virtually impossible for the observer not to catch a glimpse of himself-herself and thus be continually informed

[3]The FV of the head (Gibson, 1966, p. 257) may be defined as the angular limits of detection of facts about self and facts about the environment as represented in the optic array at a given moment in time during which the observer's body is stationary while his or her head and eyes are free to move. The head's FV, then, is made up of any number of momentary head-eye or eye-head "samples". A sample is a finite portion of amount of optical structure obtained over a given span of time.

[4]The FV of the eyes (Gibson, 1966, p. 258) may be defined as the momentary sample of the available optic array obtained as a result of any eye movement while the observer's head and body are stationary. For the human perceiver, the FV of the eyes consists of the overlapping aggregate of the two fields of view of each eye, yielding the binocular FV. The FV of fixated eyes must be distinguished from the FV of mobile eyes; the latter commands a considerably greater area containing visible information (Haber & Hershenson, 1973, pp. 311-312; Helmholtz, 1962, Vol. I, pp. 93-94; Polyak, 1957, p. 633; Southall, 1964, pp. 747-750). Each FV contains two levels of information: (*a*) Retinally foveated optical structure and (*b*) peripheral, unfoveated structure.

about the location and orientation of body parts relative to the environment. With a severely RFV, on the other hand, a new constant predominates: At the conclusion of any two successive HMs that exceed the size of the RFV, none of the visual information available to the observer in the first FV will be available in the second FV. As yet, no systematic observations seem to exist on the angular extent of people's HMs in daily life. Everyday observations suggest that the most typical human HMs—with a normal FV—are between 15–50°; if the observer continues to exercise HMs of typical magnitudes with a RFV, the price he or she has to pay is nonoverlap of information, which, it turns out, sometimes causes misjudgments about head posture and visual disorientation in the immediate environment.

Does awareness of the continuity and unboundedness of the visual world[5] depend on end-point overlap of information in successive fields of view? I believe so. To orient himself–herself in the normal situation with a fixed body, the observer requires only 4 seconds to make 4 head samples that easily cover an area in the environment corresponding to 240°. To sample the same area with the 12° field used in the Tube Study would demand about 180 samples (fields of view of the head); even so, none of the samples would have had any optical information in common at the end of any HM (see Figure 4.1). The conclusion that the observer's capacity to gain simultaneous and successive contextual information is severely curtailed with a RFV does not overstate the case. In fact, if the observer executes HM–EM excursions that are larger than the RFV, he or she will experience no end-point overlap of optical information, and disorientation should result. The question arises, "What awareness of the surrounding environment can the observer have under such circumstances? Can we predict what his or her visual world will be like?" The Tube Study sheds some light on these questions.

Third, with a RFV, the observer must substitute HMs for large EMs (e.g., saccades and pursuit EMs) in order to see the environment;[6] a new way of looking is thus required. Consider the ecologically important fact

[5]The "visual world" (Gibson, 1950) may be defined as all aspects of the perceiver's body and the environment represented in light and detectable by a fully mobile observer. Our visual world is the result of perceiving an indefinitely large number of fields of view. The concept has as its counterpart the *visualized world*, the stored mental representations that the observer can rely upon for orientation and many other performances when direct optical information is unavailable.

[6]Evidence that confirms this post hoc expectation and actual finding of Tube Study was reported by Whiteside. He found that the number of HMs increased for flyers who wore goggles that restricted the FV. In subsequent tests, HMs occurred more frequently when the object of regard was eccentric by 20° or more (1957, p. 150) for observers wearing helmets with MK-8 flying goggles.

that, regardless of how large an EM the observer makes within the normal FV with a stationary head, some part of his or her observer-environment context of one FV of the eyes is necessarily present in the next FV. With the RFV, large saccades are now only useful in yielding information about the inside of the tubes or goggles.

The fourth difference between the normal and the restricted FV is that the observer's peripheral information for orientation and locomotion is reduced. Consequently, with a RFV, the observer must substitute HMs for normal peripheral vision in order to attempt to gain the information necessary for orientation and for visually guided action such as locomotion. It may well be that such activities require that some absolute amount (critical limit?) of optical information be available within any FV produced by a momentary eye-head posture. If that absolute amount of optical information does not contain sufficient *simultaneous* specification of the observer *relative* to his or her environment, then successful orientation, maintaining of bodily equilibrium, and locomotion may not be possible on the basis of optical information.

The fifth difference between looking and acting with a normal and a restricted FV is that with a RFV, the duration for which a moving object remains visible in the observer's FV is reduced. With 12° tubes and a stationary head, that time amounts to about one-fifteenth of what it would be with the normal FV. For rapidly moving objects, a RFV begins to function as a tachistoscope of sorts, impairing eye-head pursuit and event perception and often making recognition difficult or impossible. In the absence of the "lead time" provided the observer by an object entering the normal FV, the object may have gone out of the RFV before he or she can execute accurate pursuit movements; moreover, what is reduced with a RFV is the sheer *amount* of optical information, which often contains vital contextual observer-environmental information for the direction and velocity of the moving object relative to the observer. This is surely the case when the object—say, a ball—momentarily fills the RFV. Quite independent of the visual distortion introduced by any spectacle, the observer will have trouble telling the exact trajectory of the ball and hence where to move the eyes and head to visually pursue it, let alone catch it. If successful pursuit is to occur, HMs must supplement and "substitute" for EMs to a much greater extent than with the normal FV. Indeed, the size and shape of the RFV necessitate that the observer learn new techniques for accurate head-tracking.

As mentioned, the observer's opportunity for meaningful event perception is reduced. Many events vital to an observer go on in an area subtending more than the 12° of visual angle allowed by the tubes and more than in an area allowed by most transforming spectacles. Thus, with a RFV, we might expect that often only the beginning or the end of an event is noticed by the observer, leaving him or her confused about the *meaning* of this "partial" event. With a restricted FV, the spatial as well as temporal relationships that make up events are compromised; hence the possibilities for action, implied by events—their *affordances*[7]—are changed.

Sixth, with a RFV, the observer's visual information for his or her body parts is reduced or absent. When tubes are attached to the head, the observer's nose, head, shoulders, arms, and chest are no longer represented in any part of the array entering the observer's eyes; these parts no longer hide places and events in the world and therefore cannot provide the observer with visual information about head posture and about the relative positions of other body parts. Even when these parts became visible in the Tube Study, I saw a dissociated partial hand, unattached to a moving wrist, elbow, or shoulder joint. Transforming goggles typically do not preclude sight of the arms and chest. Yet, depending on the extent of the FV restriction imposed, the observer is deprived of some previously available optical information for the location and orientation of body parts. Visually guided actions will likely suffer disruption given this type of FV restriction; the observer must relearn to coordinate HMs with limb movements and intended limb movements with HMs. Less severe effects are expected for most modern distorting goggles. Yet, the point is made: The magnitude of such effects must be empirically determined and isolated before valid conclusions can be drawn about the magnitude of immediate effects or adaptations or aftereffects to *transformation*.

There is a seventh, largely unsuspected, difference between the normal and restricted FV. For the latter, the extent of optically driven compensatory EMs is reduced. With a RFV, a HM of only very limited extent can go on while the observer maintains fixation. That is, compensatory EMs now are restricted in angular extent by the angular scope of the FV restriction and "defeated" at some point of the HM-EM excursion.

The final difference between the natural situation and wearing tubes or distorting spectacles concerns pupil adjustment and accommodation: The overall intensity of the light entering the eyes will be less. Undoubtedly, greater than usual pupil dilation is the rule; also, more

[7]This idea may be represented by Aristotle's (cf. his *Parva Naturalia:* Great Books of the Western World, Vol. 8, 673–695, Encyclopaedia Britannica, Chicago, 1952) and by Hornbostel's concept of the unity of the senses (cf. Marks, 1978). The notion is also found in Koffka (1935). The position that so-called *nonvisual qualities* such as hardness, weight, edibility, ect. are contained in reflected light was made explicit by Gibson and is in sharp contrast to the probably more widespread and unfounded assumption represented by Gregory that "retinal images cannot directly monitor the strength of the chair or the palatability of the food. But the behavior is appropriate to the chair's strength or the food's quality though these, being non-optical, cannot be monitored by the eyes [1974, p. 260]."

abrupt pupil adjustments are called for when bright light suddenly enters the FV during HMs.

EVIDENCE: EMPIRICAL CONSEQUENCES OF RESTRICTING THE FIELD OF VIEW[8]

The analysis just completed suggests that exposure to restricting spectacles should yield important functional differences for (*a*) the looking activity of the visual system; (*b*) orientation; (*c*) perception of the seen self; (*d*) event perception; and (*e*) visually guided actions, including locomotion. The analysis strongly suggests that peripheral visual information is of great importance in these activities. It also predicts quite different consequences for attaching the restricting device to the eyes, to the head–eye system, or to the body (e.g., the shoulders) of the observer. Various visual "field" defects (e.g., those described by Polyak, 1957, or Teuber, Battersby, & Bender, 1960, and producing so-called *tunnel vision* or *scotomas* with central [field] sparing or central rests in bilateral homonymous hemianopia) represent examples of restrictions of the FV attached to the eyes, in the sense of being yoked to EMs. (A man-made device that might simulate tunnel vision would be a contact lens attached to each cornea to which was attached a narrow tube. The restricted field would sweep across the ambient array with every EM).

Results of the Tube Study[9]

The results may be summarized in terms of the immediate perceptual and performatory effects, adaptations, and aftereffects of restricting

[8]The findings and analysis of the Tube Study are also relevant to the constriction of the peripheral visual field experienced by observers under the following conditions: (*a*) As a function of acceleration, at positive g loads of 3–6.5 (e.g., Baker, 1965; Gillingham & McNaughton, 1977; White & Monty, 1965); (*b*) in response to hypoxia (e.g., Kobrick, 1975); (*c*) during hot and humid conditions (e.g., Bursill, 1958); and (*d*) due to hypnotic induction (e.g., Blum, 1975; Miller & Leibowitz, 1976). Visual–vestibular interaction in orientation of the self (e.g., Dichgans, 1977) is a special case; so are underwater distortions of object size and distance from self (e.g., Kinney, McKay, Luria, & Gratto 1970; Luria, 1969; Ross, 1975). Indeed, the FV restriction produced by diver's goggles may well account for part of the variance of these effects (see below; see also Welch, 1978, Chapter 12). Moreover, when peripheral visual information is reduced, orientation and locomotion of SCUBA divers and astronauts should be adversely affected.

[9]Confirmation for many of the short-term results was informally or unintentionally obtained. Approximately six colleagues and nonpsychologists insisted on trying the tube arrangement for 5–25 minutes, spontaneously reporting object minification, "shrinkage" of distance from self, and a cyclopean visual field when accommodating for places in the world only a few feet away. They experienced disorientation, loss of stability, and difficulty in walking. They also underreached for objects and overreached the ends of the tubes.

the FV. Some of the *immediate perceptual consequences* of restricting the normal FV were predictable, given the analysis just concluded:

1. I had difficulty keeping a moving object in the visual field, for example, in coordinated eye-head pursuit of a closing door.
2. I was surprised when objects or people entered the visual field while my head was stationary.
3. Event perception was impaired; for example, I was totally unable to follow the action in a movie until I moved back so that most of the screen was in my FV. Only then could I understand the depicted actions.
4. I became aware of small, rapid, involuntary HMs.

Several other effects were not as readily predictable:

5. Familiar objects appeared smaller and nearer to me than they had before I attached the tubes to my head; for example, I judged a quarter to be a nickel and a soup spoon to be a teaspoon.
6. I perceived that I was shorter than preexperimentally (e.g., I judged my eyes to be closer to the ground now; my *effective point of observation*[10] was several centimeters below what it had been.
7. At times, I experienced myself to be at the end of the tubes rather than 33 cm (13 in.) behind them (i.e., my functional eye seemed to be right behind the cyclopean FV); thus, my effective point of observation was several centimeters nearer to everything than it had been.
8. While gazing through tubes, I considered myself to be living in a *confined visual world,* rather like living in a dark cell with one, small, circular window.

[10]The effective point of observation is defined as that location (place in the world) from which an observer perceives himself-herself to be looking at himself-herself and at the environment. The effective point of observation is a phenomenal concept. Although the actual point of observation for a standing observer may in fact be 1.7 m (5 ft 7 in.) off the ground (i.e., the eyes are 1.7 m above the ground), the observer may, nevertheless, perceive himself-herself to be regarding the world and himself-herself from just .6 m (2 ft) above the ground, as indeed happened while I gazed through up-down reversing spectacles.

Incidentally, the social-psychological consequences of wearing tubes were dramatic. Family and friends became particularly disconcerted because they couldn't see my eyes. Indeed, their enforced inability to make eye contact, to be seen and watched by an observer but to not be able to see the eyes of the observer, agitated anyone who spent even major portions of 1 hour in my company. After extended periods of contact, particularly social activities typically involving much eye contact such as eating, several individuals expressed a desire to stop relating to me, suggested that I stop the study, or actually discontinued or avoided face-to-face encounters with me for some duration.

Some of the *immediate performatory consequences* were also predictable:

1. Many HMs were required for all activities, particularly for visual orientation and for carrying out all visually guided actions.
2. I experienced difficulties in maintaining equilibrium during locomotion; I was wobbly on my feet and bumped into objects, particularly doorframes.
3. I was mistaken about the posture of my head relative to my shoulders and body, and relative to the environment; for example, when my head was actually about 40° off to the side, I acted as if it were in the primary position and walked into a wall.

Several other effects were not as readily predictable:

4. I consistently *underreached* for objects and understepped intended places on the ground.
5. Yet, when I reached for the ends of the tubes attached to my head, I consistently *overreached.*

Some of the *perceptual and performatory adaptations* took place gradually over the 6 days of wearing restricting tubes and were predictable:

1. I continued to make very small HMs for one-half hour in carrying out all activities, even though this was no longer necessary once the tubes were removed.

Some other effects were less predictable than this.

2. For the first one-half hour after removing the tubes, familiar objects appeared huge; I was also greatly surprised at the great width of all corridors and the seemingly large size of rooms with which I was not thoroughly familiar preexperimentally.
3. Upon removing the tubes, I suddenly perceived myself to be taller than before (i.e., my head looked further from the ground than while wearing tubes).
4. For the first 20 minutes after removal of the tubes, I underreached (e.g., doorhandles) provided I closed my eyes just before the reach.

Discussion: The Importance of Peripheral Information

The discussion focuses on three effects of donning the tubes that I did not anticipate at the outset: I perceived that I now lived in a confined visual world; I underestimated object size and distance from self; I underreached objects and overreached the tubes. Adaptations and aftereffects are also briefly considered. The emphasis is on the information available to (normal) peripheral vision.

Living in a World Confined

In spite of the fact that theoretically all portions of the world could be inspected given enough sampling my dominant and most overwhelming perception was that I was living in an enclosed, limited, confined, or small visual world with the RFV. Even my great increase in head-scanning did not "make up" for the perceptual continuity available with a normal field. It is the lack of simultaneous, contextual observer–environmental information in any given FV, as well as in successive fields of view, that I postulate is responsible for the orderly appreciation of events, of causality, of object "constancy," and for the change from an unrestricted and coherent world to a visually confined world.

What happens to an observer's ability to orient himself–herself and to "construct" cognitive maps when peripheral vision is reduced? My ability to orient myself during the Tube Study was considerably better in a familiar room—the one of which I had a preexperimental cognitive map—than in an unfamiliar room. Furthermore, I had a great deal of difficulty in becoming aware of and "developing" a cognitive map of the unfamiliar room. These observations are underscored by the finding that, upon taking the tubes off (6 days later), I was not surprised by the layout of the familiar room but had difficulty believing that the unfamiliar room was actually the one in which I had spent several hours of active looking over the 6-day period; over and above the generalized judgment that this was a different room after removing the tubes, I judged it huge by comparison. I also had misjudged the orientation of many objects in the unfamiliar room relative to other objects and relative to its walls and windows. The perception and hence *conception* of the visual world is evidently dependent upon the size of the FV and the meaningfulness of the contextual information the observer can glean.

Size and Distance Underestimation

Why did familiar objects appear smaller and nearer to me than I remembered them to be? Six conditions may be jointly responsible. To discover whether, and to what extent, any of these factors account for the results would require several controlled experiments. First, it is possible that the tubes function as a reduction screen, "breaking down" size constancy, as was the case in Holway and Boring's famous experiment

(1941). Since the observer is deprived of context, he or she is forced to base size judgments on retinal image size—on the visual angle subtended by the viewed object. In short, perceived size is said to approximate the visual angle, which is Euclid's rule.

Second, I now had diminished information for the relative amount of environmental texture the viewed object intercepts and occludes (Gibson, 1966, p. 315). If progressively decreasing the scope of the FV decreases optical gradients of texture density and if a zero gradient specifies little, if any, depth, then the reduction of the size of the field may be a sufficient condition to produce object minification and distance underestimation.

Third, with a restricted FV, the observer may be provided with different or "new" information for the diminished size of objects, a window "framing" effect of the tubes (cf. Hagen, Jones, & Reed, 1978). Those objects beyond the "window" of the definite boundaries of the RFV are judged to be close to the window and small in size, thus "fitting into" the imposed frame. This frame acts even more powerfully than the porthole of a ship, which, as one approaches it, allows an expansion of one's FV; an expansion that is accompanied by an apparent increase in the size of everything behind the window.

Fourth, accommodation for a near object decreases the perceived size of any object further away (Koffka, 1935, p. 237). The effect is particularly vivid when one looks through tubes or a reduction screen. I suspect that underaccommodation accompanies the loss of texture-gradient information and the information provided by effectively superimposing picture-margins on relatively context-deprived objects. A contributory source of underaccommodation may be the cyclopean border of the FV. It cannot escape attention and may well act as a stimulus for a slight but constant change in accommodation. For example, as a passenger in a car on a rainy day, I perceived the windshield wiper as wiping across the cyclopean eye—very close to the end of the tubes—rather than across the windshield. I was surprised that the wiper did not dislodge the tubes. In reality, it was 30–36 cm (12–14 in.) beyond the end of the tubes.

Fifth, a change in the convergence of the eyes might well be associated with underaccommodation and might influence size–distance judgment in its own right. If the tubes act as a pseudoscope so that the eyes are induced to converge for distant objects as if they were closer, then the near fixation would cause objects beyond the plane of fixation to appear smaller and closer (Fischer & Kornmueller, 1930, p. 285; Wallach & Frey, 1972, p. 77). And further, the same diminution in apparent object size and distance from self would be expected if wearing tubes partially fulfills the conditions for micropsia, that is, even though an object is at distance X from the observer, he or she accommodates for distance X minus 1 and converges for distance X minus 2. The role played by these variables, and the RFV in its own right, in the size and distance distortions experienced under water bears further study. (Cf. Welch, 1978, Chapter 12.)

The last and sixth factor that may be correlated with underestimation of object size, and particularly with distance from self, is the observation that I judged the distance from my head-"eye" to the ground to be less than it had been prior to putting on the tubes. This perception may constitute visual information that I was now shorter than I had been. At least I believed I was looking from a place nearer to the ground. If perceived size and distance of familiar and unfamiliar objects is a joint function of the actual size and distance of objects relative to each other, as well as of the effective point of observation of the observer relative to the regarded objects, then the perceived shift in the observer's location should influence both size and distance judgments.

Underreaching Objects and Overreaching the Tubes

I consistently underreached for objects such as a doorhandle. Yet, when I reached for the ends of the tubes attached to my head, I consistently overreached. The visually directed underreaching is consistent with my report that places looked nearer to me than I judged or remembered them to be. If an object looks closer than it really is, then the observer should underreach it. Similarly, if the observer should perceive himself-herself to be closer to the object than he or she actually is, he or she should underreach. Convergence and accommodation for the distance of an object from the observer and fixation on the object may provide part of the necessary visual information for a correct reaching movement. Thus, assume that with tubes for whatever reason convergence-accommodation for an object 50 cm (20 in.) away is now at 45 cm (18 in.). If the intended distance of the observer's reaching movement is based on this convergence-accommodation information and if no correction is introduced between initiation and termination of the movement, than he or she should underreach.

Even though I underreached all else, I overreached the ends of the tubes whenever I tried to touch them. At times, I overreached the ends of the tubes by as much as 30 cm (12 in.), that is, by as much as the distance between my eyes and the ends of the tubes. This finding is consistent with my report that, at times, I saw myself as being very close to the end of the cyclopean tube. If the ends of the tubes are the observer's effective point of observation, then he or she should overreach them. When my eyes diverged and accommodated for a distance greater than the ends of the tubes, the unitary tube at times appeared longer than when I converged and accommodated to fixate the ends of the two tubes: The tubes then appeared very short, and I overreached least. To account for the overreaching of the tubes, it may also be necessary to assume that false convergence-accommodation information is supplemented by visual information, which tells the observer, effectively, that if the tube only looks about one-half to three-quarters of its actual length, then his or her point of observation is closer to the end of the tubes than it actually is. A detailed version of the above arguments may be found in Dolezal (1976, Chapter 5).

Adaptations to Restricting the Field of View

Both perceptual and performatory modifications to restricting the FV shared at least two characteristics. First, I was faced with a problem I had to solve. Second, I became aware of the inadequacy of my prevailing manner of coping with the new situation. The quest for a solution was generally initiated consciously. For example, I explored new strategies for HMs to aid walking: I surveyed the ground immediately in front of me with several, slow, sideway sweeps with frequent, short pauses; then I sampled the world at head level for obstructions. Walking was thus slowed considerably to allow for this extensive and continuous exploration. I adopted several strategies for different activities. It must not be supposed, however, that final success was simply the result of the systematic execution of particular HM sequences. I also had to pay careful attention to information from other perceptual systems. For example, to avoid walking into doorframes and walls, I began to attend to haptic information from the neck joint and muscles to keep track of head position. In conjunction, I worked at *memorizing* where I had moved my head (i.e., how far I had moved it from a given position). Overall, most adaptations were the result of a combination of consciously attending to the consequences of particular eye-head-body movements and making effective use of information without being aware of doing so.

Aftereffects of Restricting the Field of View

Two kinds of aftereffects may be distinguished. Both continued for brief periods in the face of the back-to-normal, observer–environmental conditions that did not require their occurrence. First, *perceptual* aftereffects consisted of totally novel experiences and might be best described as *contrast effects.* Thus, I experienced a sudden increase in my own height upon removal of the tubes. Also, familiar objects seemed greatly magnified relative to *any* remembered standard. Conscious control seemed to play no part in the progressive adjustments that eventually "returned" me to preexperimental perceptual judgments. Nevertheless, I was aware, for example, of repeated eye-scanning of the familiar objects that appeared huge, which seemed designed to enable me to confirm or disconfirm previous size judgments. After about 30 minutes, the now prevailing observer–environment condition again became the constant, for I could no longer make sense out of such questions as: "Does this telephone appear smaller or larger than at any time before?"

Second, *performatory* aftereffects consisted of actions that were carried out during the FV restriction and now persisted. These aftereffects might be best described as *carry-over effects*. Thus, I continued to execute small, head-scanning movements in spite of the fact that they were superfluous with a normal FV. Conscious control was very much a part of the progressive modification that returned my performatory competences to preexperimental levels. For example, I noted that I was employing HM techniques that were now dispensable and consciously inhibited their occurrence, substituting EMs for HMs. Another carry-over effect was that I continued to underreach doorhandles for the first 20 minutes after removing the tubes, but only if I closed my eyes just before reaching, thus preventing corrections during reaching.

CONCLUSION: TRANSFORMING AND RESTRICTING THE FIELD OF VIEW HAVE SIMILAR CONSEQUENCES

Restricting the normal FV to 12° by the use of tubes attached to the head had profound consequences on visual perception and on visually guided actions. Many perceptual misjudgments and performatory difficulties were experienced, apparently because the observer's opportunity for obtaining optic information was severely limited (*a*) by the diminution of peripheral information and (*b*) by the lack of overlap of information in successive fields of view of the head. The evidence indicates that both are important for the kind of coping we tend to take for granted in everyday living: (*a*) Orientation in the immediate environment; (*b*) equilibrium and balance maintenance in locomotion; (*c*) complex, visually guided action; and (*d*) veridical perception of events, the self, and the layout of the visual world.

Some of the results of long-term, spectacle-wearing experiments are strikingly similar to those of the present study, which merely restricted the normal FV with paper tubes. Yet, many of their results have been generally attributed to the optical inversion, tilt, and reversal (Brown,

1928; Kohler's protocol quoted in Kottenhoff 1961, Stratton, 1896, 1897b). I offer three examples.

Diminished Peripheral Information

I believe that orientation and event perception are impaired by diminished peripheral information. Stratton's report of 1897 will serve as the first example:

> Objects were, however, taken more or less isolatedly; so that inappropriateness of place with reference to other objects even in the same visual field was often, in the general upheaval of the experience, passed by unnoticed. I sat for some time watching a blazing open fire, without seeing that one of the logs had rolled far out on the hearth and was filling the room with smoke. Not until I caught the odor of the smoke, and cast about for the cause, did I notice what had occurred [1897b, p. 345].

I submit that Stratton's failure to notice was not as much related to the inversion of his visual field as to a lack of available context in peripheral information—an "isolation" of objects from one another and from their surrounding environment.

I believe restricting the FV interferes with adaptation to transformation for another reason. It creates competition between the central and peripheral portions of the retina. Throughout Stratton's account, it becomes increasingly clear that his attention was directed to remembering and "picturing" parts of the environment and body parts not immediately in the visual field and that those visual images misled him to act (e.g., reach) on their bases. In fact, Stratton continually comments on the imagery (remembered visual perception) outside his immediate FV.[11] He says:

> Similarly, the actual visual field was, for the most part, taken by itself and not supplemented, as in normal vision, by a system of objects gathered and held from the preceding visual experience. Sporadic cases occurred, in which some object out of sight was represented as it had just been seen; but in general all things not actually in view returned to their older arrangement and were represented, if at all, as in normal sight. Usually this was the case also in picturing an unseen movement of some part of my body [1897b, p. 345].

[11]Although Walls (1951, p. 84) thought that Stratton was an eidetic imager and somehow unique in his ability to "visualize" past scenes, Kohler also reports obtrusion of visual imagery and preexperimental visual memories of objects and places in the environment not represented in the immediate visual field. For examples, see the protocol of his 1953 right–left reversing prism study; his FV was restricted to 33° × 25° (Kottenhoff, 1961, p. 69). My own experience substantiates the occasional obtrusion into consciousness of visual memories.

And again:

> But the detailed filling of this outline was far less complete than is usual in my case in normal sight. A large number of important things in the room simply did not arise in my mind until their relation to the field of seen things had been brought home afresh by perception. During the first days of the experiment ideas of objects frequently arose in opposition to the new sight-perception; now they either did not arise at all, or came in the newer form [1897b, p. 464].

These observations lead me to speculate that restricting the FV interferes with adaptation because the peripheral area of the retina (and the portions of the visual system subserving it), which is no longer stimulated by light due to the FV restriction, competes with the more central, still-stimulated area of the retina (and the portions of the visual system serving it). The peripheral, unstimulated portions compete with foveal portions of the visual system for attention and "recruit" stimulation by evoking visual images and visual memories, thus slowing the course of adaptation. The restriction of the FV might, in fact, be partly responsible for the persistence of the visual imagery of places and body parts outside the FV.

A second, and by no means mutually exclusive likelihood is that the relatively context-deprived central FV evokes stored vision-based memories in an effort to "supplement" the context-less array. However, my phenomenal experience does not support this idea. If anything, the RFV aided focused attention on the limited information within its well-defined borders.

No Overlap of Information in Successive Fields of View

I believe that the lack of optical information overlap in successive fields of view is responsible for the observer's disorientation in his or her immediate surround and in incompetent visually guided locomotion. Brown's (1928) report will serve as the second example:

> It was harder still to perceive and react to groupings of furniture whose spatial relations were not previously known. In the rooms in which the subject spent most of his time, where the arrangements of furniture were nearly constant, learning to "see" them correctly was almost, but not entirely accomplished. In visiting the laboratory, the tables, chairs, and apparatus had been rearranged after the subject had put on the goggles and an accurate idea of the new arrangement was never correctly formed. Cautious groping around the room was here necessary and only a slight improvement in this adjustment had occurred by the end of the week. Contact with unknown groupings of objects on the floor always caused some initial bewilderment [p. 135].

Note that the size of Brown's tubular FV (10°) was very similar to mine (12°). His observations comparing orientation in a familiar and unfamiliar room correspond rather well with my own. Whatever someone with a normal FV typically does within his or her immediate, visible surrounding—becoming aware of it, learning to "see" it correctly, "developing" a cognitive map, or achieving an accurate idea of the layout—neither Brown nor I managed to do veridically or competently. Brown attributes his findings to the 75° clockwise optical tilt of the FV produced by his spectacles.

Again, I submit that in the absence of the appropriate control for the restriction of the FV, the results quoted may not be unequivocally attributed to optical tilt. Rather, the great difficulty in procuring end-point overlap of optical information common to successive head-samples (fields of view) may be directly responsible for the orientation difficulties experienced by both perceivers and may simply insure a very different (perception of the) visual world.

The third example further substantiates that the lack of information overlap for successive percepts rather than the optical transformation per se are responsible for the observer's disorientation. Kohler described orientation in his visual world in these choice phrases:

> [In contrast to the old optical view of the world, the spectacle-world is] in fact like a cobweb, in which each time only a single thread comes to awareness which one follows to a particular point in order to arrive at another point by means of a different thread. A scheme or survey of the entire web seems to me impossible [Kottenhoff, 1961, p. 69].[12]

Kohler's metaphorical use of the word "thread" and his observation that he could not gain a general view of the fabric of the cobweb could not have been more appropriate had he intended to describe the frustration of trying to determine the layout of his environment, faced as he was with confinement to his restricted FV and the lack of shared end-point overlap in his optical information.

While walking about in the city of Innsbruck with right-left reversing spectacles, Kohler reports:

> Finding one's way about is not only impeded because the perceived image does not correspond to the old conceptual scheme of representation (Vorstellungsplan) but

[12](Im Unterschied zum alten optischen Weltbild ist die Brillenwelt) in der Tat so wie ein Spinngewebe, wobei jedesmal nur ein einziger Faden bewusst wird, den man bis zu einem bestimmten Punkt geht, um dann auf einem anderen Faden an einen anderen Punkt zu gelangen. Ein Plan oder eine Uebersicht des ganzen Gewebes scheint mir unmoeglich. (My translation.)

> also because I headed in the wrong direction at curves and intersections without noticing it at first [Kottenhoff, 1961, p. 70].[13]

Again, I submit that Kohler's disorientation, seemingly "fragmented" layout perception, and failure to notice errors in the direction of oriented locomotion cannot be unequivocally attributed to right-left reversal of his FV. His inability to gain an overview of a substantial portion of his visual world appears to contribute to his disorientation and to his "not noticing at first" having turned into a wrong street. The imposed restriction of the FV may well suffice to account for such observations. Perhaps both the optical characteristics of the spectacles and a restricted FV produce, independently, the many consequences described above. However, in the absence of the appropriate control, any mutually exclusive claim must be tempered.

In summary, the evidence presented shows that the consequences of restricting the normal FV to 12° can produce effects astonishingly similar to those reported, for example, by Stratton, Brown, and Kohler, who attributed these effects to inversion, tilt, and right-left reversal of the FV, respectively. In the absence of the appropriate control for the restriction of the FV that is necessarily imposed by transforming spectacles, other interpretations seem plausible: (*a*) The observed phenomena are not produced by the optical transformation but only by the restriction of the FV; (*b*) both factors act independently to produce the observed effects; or, (*c*) both factors interact.[14]

[13]Das Zurechtfinden is nicht nur deshalb erschwert, weil das gesehene Bild mit dem alten Vorstellungsplan nicht uebereinstimmt, sodern auch deshalb, weil ich an Kurven und Kreuzungen die falsche Richtung einschlage, ohne es zunaechst zu bemerken. (My translation.)

[14]*Methodological Note.* Holding the size and shape of the FV constant during the pretest, exposure, and posttest is not necessarily a sufficient safeguard against confounding the effects due to the restriction and transformation of the FV. If the experimenter takes baseline measures with control spectacles that only restrict the FV (or sets displacing prisms at zero diopters) before exposure to the optical transformation, he or she does not eliminate the effects that may be due to the FV restriction; the experimenter may merely confound the baseline data. He or she must make sure that the dependent variable(s) measured during the pretest reach an asymptote. The logic of this procedure is clear: If the experimenter measures a baseline that consists of an immediate effect of the restriction and then introduces the observer to the transformation, changes in the observer's behavior may still occur that are due to the restriction while the observer's FV has also been transformed. If so, the transformation will have been introduced prematurely. The idea is that validly measuring adaptation to an optical transformation necessarily entails measuring adaptation to the limiting of the FV created by the transforming spectacles. The most informative sequence of testing for adaptation is laborious: Measure the observer's behavior with (*a*) normal FV, (*b*) restricted FV, (*c*) restricted *and* transformed FV, (*d*) restricted FV, and (optionally) (*e*) normal FV.

SUMMARY

In this chapter, I treat a widely neglected but important factor in adaptation research: the restriction of the field of view (FV) created by any light-transforming device and the consequent reduction in peripheral visual information. Taking as a paradigmatic example a 1-week study in which I limited my normal, 180° × 150° field of vision to 12° with two paper tubes that were attached to my head, I described my perceptual experiences and actions in an everyday environment. The most striking overall finding of this Tube Study was that I observed effects startlingly similar to those reported by other investigators but they attributed these effects to optical inversion, tilt, and right-left reversal of the FV. Thus, with the restricted FV, I was generally disoriented, experienced dizziness during rapid head movements, and had difficulty maintaining bodily equilibrium during walking. I also bumped into obstacles such as doorframes, was unsure about the location of my head, had difficulty keeping a moving object in my FV, was unclear about the layout of unfamiliar places, and was unable to form a representative cognitive map of them. Finally, I did not always understand the meaning of ongoing events such as scenes depicted on film.

In this chapter I also analyze the differences between looking, acting, and perceiving the self with a restricted and a normal FV. Two main differences emerge from which all others follow. First, restricting the FV reduces the observer's useful, peripheral visual information commonly used in visually guided behavior. Second, restricting his or her FV reduces or eliminates information that is commonly shared by any two successive fields of view as the observer moves his or her head and body. This lack of visual information overlap interferes with the perceptual continuity that normally provides the optical context necessary for meaningful and accurate perception of the unbounded world and for successful visually guided actions, including orientation and locomotion. A vivid illustration of this consequence of limiting the normal FV was provided by the fact that as the tube-wearer I perceived myself as living in a *confined visual world.* Another influential difference between living with a normal and a restricted FV is that the duration for which a moving object remains visible in the observer's FV is reduced. Coordinated eye-head pursuit as well as event perception were thus impaired. Further, I was surprised when people or objects entered my visual field while my head was stationary.

Not only is the importance of peripheral vision for functioning effectively in one's natural ecology broadly documented, but restricting the FV is shown to have important consequences in its own right. For example, familiar objects appeared smaller and nearer to me when I was wearing the tubes than I remembered them to have been. Also, I consistently underreached for objects and understepped intended places, as if my *effective point of observation* had shifted toward the end of the tubes. This possible explanation was substantiated by the finding that I consistently overreached whenever I intended to touch the end of the phenomenal cyclopean tube. Adaptations to and aftereffects of these effects are discussed.

Many past experiments, especially long-term studies, that attributed their results to the optical transformation imposed on their observers should be reevaluated. This conclusion is encouraged by the need for methodological rigor and by the weight of evidence. The methodological point is clear: In every spectacle experiment, the experimenter must limit the size (and shape) of the FV by the same amount before, during, and after exposure to the transformation. Only then is he or she permitted to conclude that the results are due to the effects produced by the transformation, unconfounded by the effects due to the restriction of the FV as such. The evidence from the Tube Study also suggests that restricting and transforming the FV have similar consequences because peripheral visual information commonly used in a wide array of visually guided actions is diminished in both.

5

Living Transformed: Method of the Prism Study

In this and the next five chapters I describe a study of long-term adaptation to up–down reversing of the field of view (FV) in which I was both experimenter and observer. The study had three aims:

1. To provide an accurate description of the facts: how I as the observer perceived and acted in my world transformed
2. To extend the data base for a theoretical analysis of how information first confuses and misleads the observer and eventually enables him or her to adapt successfully to the optical transformation
3. To provide a prototypic example of this sort of experimentation in such a way that (*a*) its method is transferable to the study of other forms of optical transformation; (*b*) its results may generate hypotheses for future investigations; and (*c*) its theoretical analysis may be applicable to a wide array of transformation phenomena

In this and the next chapter I deal with aim 3(a); in Chapters 7–10, with the others.

METHOD OF THE AUTHOR'S PRISM STUDY

Observer

Then 29 years old, I served as observer and experimenter. My visual acuity was 20/40 for the left eye and 20/80 for the right eye. Binocular acuity was 20/40.

Procedure

The principal method of data collection was the observation and description of my perceptual experiences and behaviors over the 5 weeks of the experiment. The critical stage alone—during which I wore up-down reversing spectacles—produced over 9 hours of cassette tapes and yielded a typed protocol of 165 double-spaced pages.[1] The observations were then arranged in naturally occurring descriptive categories and presented in table form. Much of the data contained in the original protocol appear in Chapters 7-10. Photographs were also taken (Figures 5.1-5.4 and Figures in Chapters 7-9 and Appendix B).[2]

The experiment was conducted from July 3 to August 6, 1971, in Greece. The place is a tiny village (St. John's of Kissos) that faces the Aegean Sea, with Mount Pelion behind it (Figure 5.1). The village is located roughly 350 km (220 mi.) northeast of Athens, 250 km (155 mi.) south of Thessalonica and 40km (25 mi.) east of Volos. Its commercial part (shops, restaurants) is spread along approximately 920m (1000 yd.) of ocean front and has one paved strip of road running parallel to, and about 92 m (100 yd.) away from, the water front. Most of the residents live in houses dug into the mountain which rises steeply 140-185m (150-200 yd.) from the ocean. A combination of cement stairs and narrow paths lead up to these houses. I lived in one of them during the study. My seen environment while wearing up-down reversing spectacles, unlike the quaint one just described, can be viewed in Figure 5.2 (photographically up-down reversed to simulate my phenomenal experience).

[1]Dolezal, H. Long-term perceptual and performatory adaptation to wearing up-down reversing prisms in the real world. Unpublished monograph, Cornell University, 1971. Tapes and protocol available from the author.

[2]Unless specifically indicated, all photos in this book are "action" shots, taken during the experiment (i.e., I did not pose for them in order to simulate the recorded results: They are data). Photos that were taken later or that were simulated are followed by the date of their shooting.

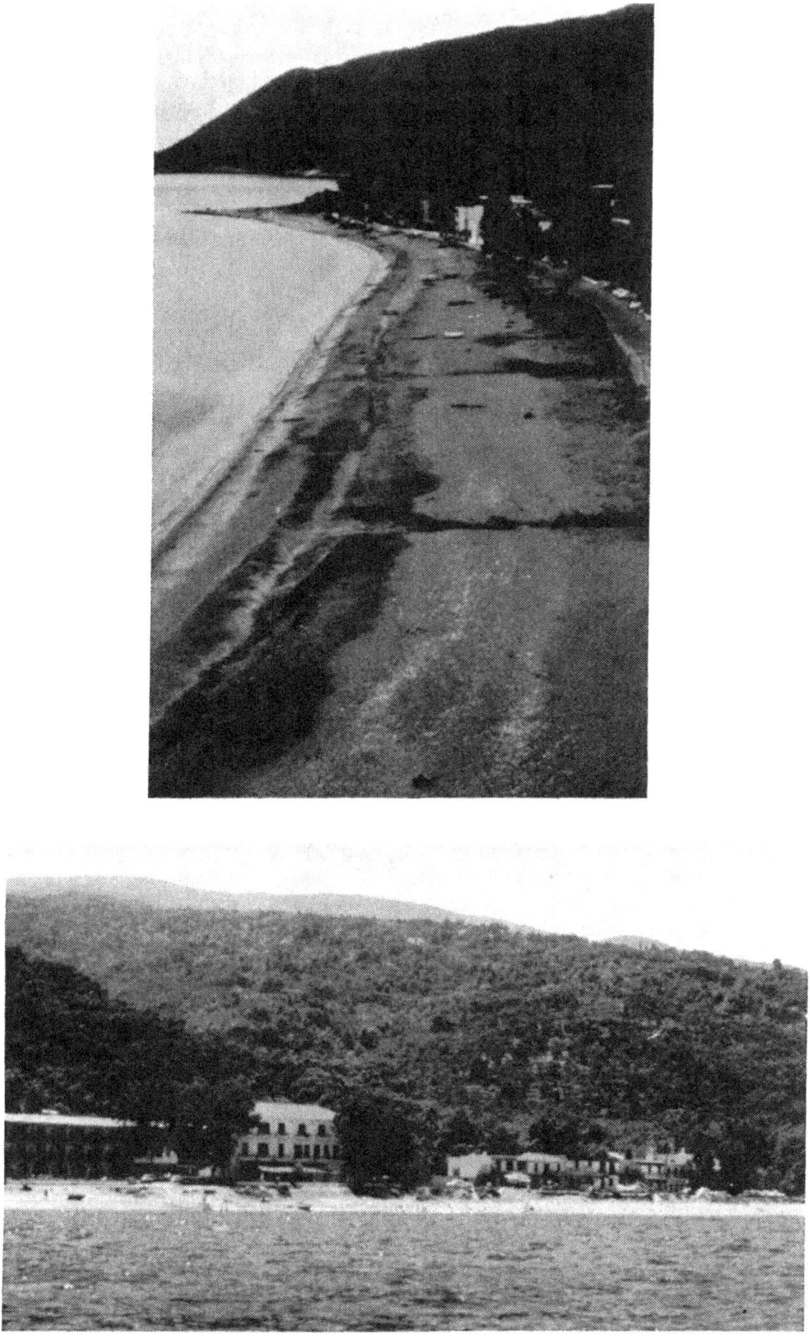

FIGURE 5.1. Site of the 5-week Prism Study: St. John's of Kissos in Greece.

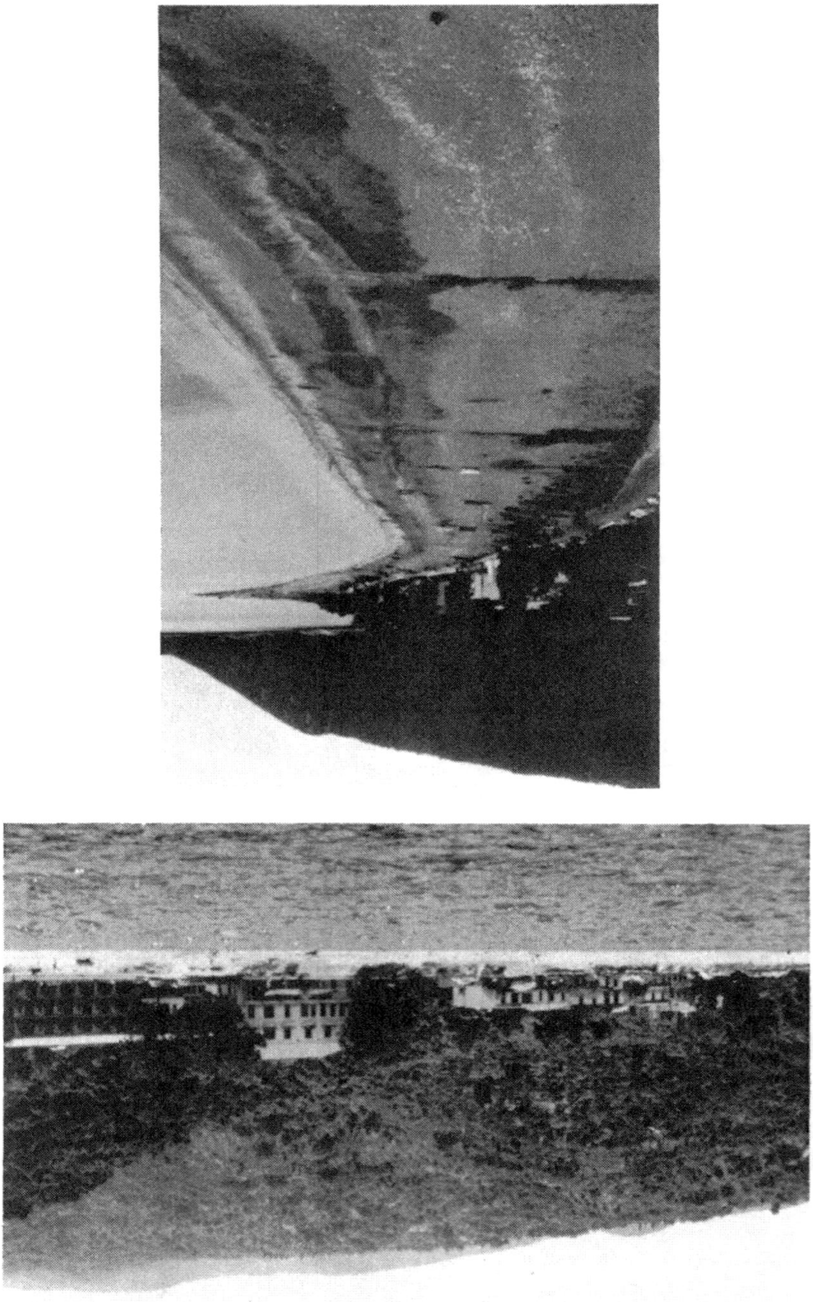

FIGURE 5.2.

Design

The time-course of the Prism Study is shown in Table B5.1 of Appendix B. As can be seen, the study took about 5 weeks (488 waking hours) and consisted of six stages, the main one lasting 211 waking hours or 15.2 days. The design is presented in Table 5.1.

Stage 1: Adaptation to Increased Weight and Size of the Helmeted Head

Table 5.1 shows clearly that this control stage was necessary to distinguish which effects were in fact due to the increased weight and size of the head and how to avoid attributing these effects to either the restriction of the FV or to the optical up–down reversal later imposed by the prisms. Once I had evidence that adaptation had taken place—had reached an asymptote—I initiated the next stage. I wore a modified football helmet with a counterweight mounted in front. The counterweight was identical in weight and very similar in mass distribution to the prism units that were to be inserted during Stages 2–4 (see Figures 5.3 and B5.2 of Appendix B). Relevant baseline observations were taken.

Stage 2: Adaptation to Restricting the Field of View

The counterweight was replaced by a nonreversing prism to avoid attributing effects that were in fact due to the FV restriction to the optical up–down reversal (see Chapter 6). The FV yielded by the reversing spectacles of Stage 3 was identical to that provided by the nonreversing prism and is the largest FV ever used in a reversal or inversion study. The only difference between the nonreversing prism unit of Stage 2 and the reversing prism unit to be used in Stage 3 was that in the nonreversing prism, the silvered surface had been removed so that light entered my eyes as it would through a Porro prism (see Figure B5.3 in Appendix B). Looking through the Stage 2 spectacles was perceptually like looking through a thick piece of glass. During the entire period in which restriction of the FV was a relevant variable (Stages 2–4), I wore a light-occluding mask after removing the helmet in the evening and before replacing it in the morning to prevent perceiving with anything but the

---

FIGURE 5.2. Where the Prism Study was conducted, phenomenologically speaking (photographically up–down reversed to simulate the observer's experience). Note that it not only takes longer for the viewer to determine the point of observation for the scene depicted when it is reversed but that the observer is also uncertain as to where he or she is viewing the scene from—a fact of observation that makes orientation quite difficult. To enhance a simulated viewing the reader should look at these scenes through a sheet of paper rolled into a tube that does not permit sight of the borders of the photograph.

TABLE 5.1
General Plan of the Prism Study

Stage of study	Duration of stage[a]	Wore helmet/ no helmet	Type of prism system used (if any)	Size of field of view[b]	Weight of helmet system[c]	General purpose of this stage: (to observe)
1	4 days (50 hours)	Helmet	Skiing goggles plus prism-counterweight	Almost normal	3.8 kg (8 pounds, 6 ounces)	Adaptation to **weight** and **size** increase of observer's functional head
2	5 days (73 hours)	Helmet	Nonreversing prisms	Small (46° × 115°, vertical × horizontal plane[d]	3.8 kg	Adaptation to **restricting** observer's **field of view**
3	15 days (211 hours)	Helmet	Up–down reversing prisms	Small (46° × 115°)	3.8 kg	Adaptation to **up–down reversing** observer's field of view
4	5 days (60 hours)	Helmet	Nonreversing prisms	Small (46° × 115°)	3.8 kg	Aftereffects of **up–down reversal**
5	2 days (30 hours)	Helmet	Skiing goggles plus prism-counterweight	Almost normal	3.8 kg	Aftereffects of **restricting** observer's **field of view**
6	4 days (64 hours)	No helmet	None	Normal	Not applicable	Aftereffects of **weight** and **size** increase of head

[a]Total number of waking hours during each stage (total for all stages: 488).

[b]Size of field of view of Sector A: (upper prism); 18°; Sector B: (lower prism): 28°; total size of field of view for both prisms: 46°.

[c]Weight of helmet without prisms or counterweight: 2.4 kg (5 lbs. 6 oz.); weight of either nonreversing or reversing prism: 1.4 kg (3 lbs.); weight of prism-counterweight substituted for prism unit during Stages 1 and 5: 1.4 kg (3 lbs.).

[d]Began wearing occluding mask at night (and a walking stick and tape recorder during the day).

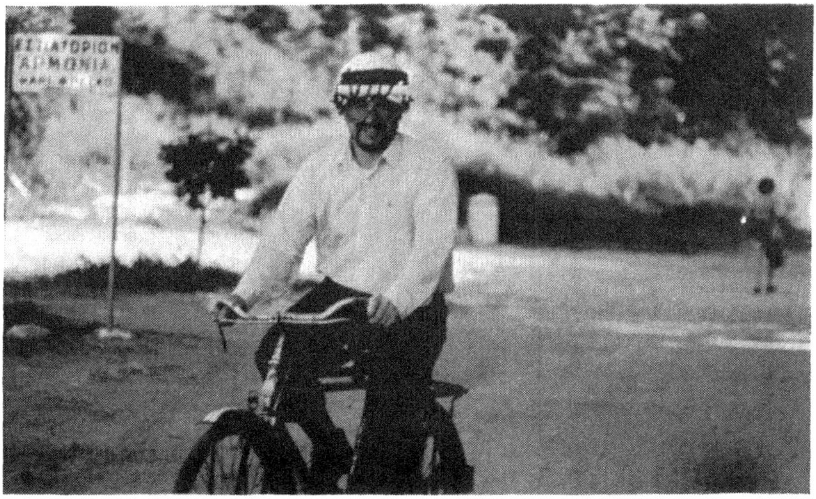

FIGURE 5.3. Adaptation to the increase in weight and size of the observer's *functional head,* produced by the helmet. Photo shows the front counterweight (white metal bar above the observer's eyes) of Stage 1, for which nonreversing prisms were to be exchanged during Stage 2 and reversing prisms, during Stage 3.

restricted FV. On Day 2 of Stage 2, I also began carrying a walking stick (which I suspected I might need during Stage 3) and a portable tape recorder (Sony TC 120) slung over my shoulder. I did so to familiarize myself with these additional changes. The recorder was used to record all verbal descriptions of observations during Stage 3. (I had anticipated that I would not be able to write them.) Relevant baseline observations were again collected.

Stage 3: Adaptation to Up–Down Reversing the Field of View[3]

During this, the main stage of the experiment, only transformed light entered my eyes (see Figures 5.4 and B5.1a in Appendix B): The nonreversing prisms worn during Stage 2 were now replaced by up–down reversing prisms. As the experimenter, I wanted to describe a maximum number of different immediate perceptual and performatory

[3]Places in the world visible in the vertical plane, relative to Stages 2 and 4, given a constant head posture, did not correspond exactly. Specifically, if one could arrange a simultaneous viewing through both the nonreversing and reversing prisms, the two fields of view would overlap 26°, with the reversing spectacles showing 20° more of the *geographically upper* portion of the world.

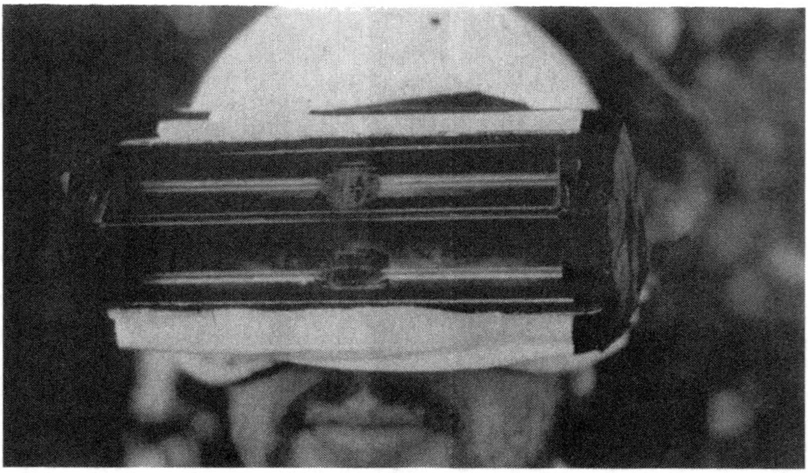

FIGURE 5.4. Adaptation to optical up–down reversal. I, the observer with up–down reversing prisms of Stage 3 of the Prism Study. Note appearance of the eyes. That's how others' eyes looked to me when seen through the prisms.

consequences of, and adaptations to, wearing reversing spectacles attached to the head (see Chapters 7–9). I was able to meet these requirements by simply following my daily routine as normally as was possible, which insured a maximum of heterogeneity and diversity of activities. Thus, including everyday necessities and banalities—which turned out to be anything but that—I repeated some 50 planned observations daily. These may be divided into three classes. First I will discuss *perceptual judgments and actions.* I described the experienced results of assuming different head positions and of engaging in different head movements. Results included judgments of the relative magnitude of perceived world (FV) motion and self-movement; judgments of the slant of the ground and the size and distance-from-self of objects; my knowledge of the location and orientation of objects and body parts, especially of my own head; and adaptations of typical eye–head and body movements. (Described in Chapter 7.) Second, I also described and regularly engaged in the following *visually guided actions:* (*a*) Orientation; (*b*) locomotion; (*c*) sitting down in a chair; (*d*) bicycle-riding; (*e*) swimming; (*f*) pointing; (*g*) reaching; (*h*) grasping; (*i*) lifting; (*j*) pushing; (*k*) pulling; and (*l*) twisting objects in all planes; (*m*) ball throwing, catching, kicking, and heading; (*n*) getting dressed; (*o*) eating; (*p*) pouring; (*q*) drinking; and (*r*) operating the tape recorder. Visually guided activities that were not repeated daily included: (*a*) Water-skiing; (*b*) riding a mule; (*c*) driving a car; (*d*) playing tennis; (*e*) hiking up the mountain; (f) rowing a boat; (*g*) diving; (*h*) testing for transfer or practice to the unused hand in eating; (*i*) localization by sound, smell, and temperature; (*j*) playing chess; (*k*) writing; and (*l*) trying to shake hands. Indeed, the first three were one-time opportunities. (Described in Chapter 8.) Third, I also described the following observations and activities, paying especial attention to *visual perception of the self,* relative to the visible environment (mostly while my head and body were stationary): (*a*) Recognition of facial features and expressions of familiar persons and strangers; (*b*) watching movies; (*c*) reading typewritten material in four different orientations; (*d*) telling time; (*e*) pictorial and nonpictorial tests of the orientation and location of body parts, especially the head (Chapter 9); (*f*) visual imagery with closed eyes; and (*g*) noting the effects of sleeping on performance after prism exposure (described in Chapter 12).

Stage 4: Aftereffects of Up–Down Reversing the Field of View

I inserted the nonreversing prisms after removing the reversing prisms to ensure that all aftereffects would be correctly attributed to adaptation to the up–down reversal rather than to a sudden increase in the size of the FV. Moreover, I kept the helmet on my head to ensure that aftereffects attributable to the increased weight and size of the functional head would not be erroneously attributed to the aftereffects of up–down reversal (see Chapter 10).

Stage 5: Aftereffects of Restricting the Field of View

I removed the nonreversing prism unit of Stage 4 and put the front counterweight and skiing goggles in its place. Hence, the size of the FV was again nearly normal after having been restricted for 25 days or 344 waking hours. The helmet again remained on my head to ensure that all aftereffects would be correctly attributed to the restriction of the FV rather than to the sudden decrease in weight and size of the functional head (see Chapter 10).

Stage 6: Aftereffects of Weight and Size of the Helmeted Head

I simply removed the helmet to which I had adapted for 30 days or 424 waking hours (see Chapter 10).

Backup Systems

There were a few instances during Stages 2–4 when it was highly impractical or dangerous to keep the helmet on the head: (*a*) When taking a shower; (*b*) while the helmet was drying after a swimming and diving session; and (*c*) once while water-skiing. Hence, a backup had been constructed for these relatively rare and brief occasions. When switching from the helmet system to the backup system, I closed my eyes as an obvious control measure. For Stages 2 and 4, this alternate system consisted of a diving mask, the glass portion of which had been taped with black masking tape in such a way that when I looked through the mask: (*a*) The size of the FV was identical to that of the nonreversing spectacles used in Stages 2 and 4 and (*b*) for any given head posture, the same places in the world were visible as with the nonreversing spectacles of Stage 2 and 4. The weight of this backup was only .45 kg (1 lb.), and it was used for not more than a cumulative total of 2 hours during any stage and for no more than about 15 minutes at any one time. For Stage 3, the backup consisted of one right-angle (up–down reversing) prism, set in a plastic harness adjustable to any head size. The size of the FV was only 37° × 115°; the weight, only 1.4 kg (3 lb.). This backup was used about 5 hours during Stage 3 and not for more than 20 minutes on any one occasion.

Apparatus: Prism

All prisms in this study were silvered, right-angle "tank prisms" measuring 69 × 49 × 167 mm (2.72 × 1.93 × 6.57 in.), hypotenuse face × lateral face × length, respectively. They were obtained from Edmund Scientific Company, Barrington, New Jersey 08007, stock number 806. In addition to yielding a large FV in the horizontal plane, the main advantage of using one long prism rather than two smaller, separate prisms (one for each eye) is that one large prism block avoids the special problems of binocular disparity: viewing with each eye discrete light-samples that fail to overlap or match optically.[4] Two of these prisms were joined hypotenuse face to hypotenuse face to maximize the size of the FV yielded in the vertical plane.

Two sets of two prisms each were joined. One set served as the up–down reversing prism unit used during Stage 3 and the other as the nonreversing prism unit used during Stages 2 and 4. Once the hypotenuse faces of the two prisms were joined, a block of glass resulted

[4]This has been a problem with experiments (described in Chapter 4) using a binocular arrangement of lenses or prisms (Porro, Risley, Amici Roof prisms, etc.) that reverse or invert the FV because a single block of glass such as the one used in the present study has not been used. Displacing prisms not cut from a single piece of glass or plastic for the two eyes, or not arranged and held in place carefully, also produce binocular disparity and irregular distortions with head movements.

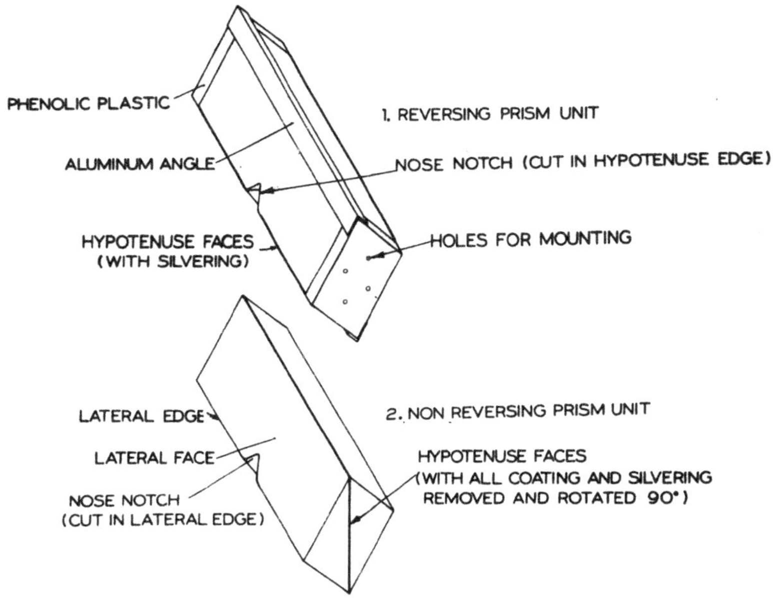

FIGURE 5.5. Reversing and nonreversing prism units. The former was used in Stage 3, the latter in Stages 2 and 4.

with the dimension of 49 × 49 × 167 mm (1.93 × 1.93 × 6.57 in.). Figure 5.5 presents all this graphically. A more detailed description of the apparatus used in the Prism Study is featured in Appendix B. It should make experimental replication possible.

SUMMARY

This chapter features the method of the Prism Study, a 5-week experiment during which I wore up–down reversing prisms affixed to a football helmet and lived as normally as possible in an outdoor environment. The study consisted of six stages. Stage 1 determined the effects of and adaptations to the increase in weight and size of my functional head, produced by the wearing of the football helmet into which the prisms were to be inserted. Stage 2 ascertained the effects of and adaptations to restricting my field of view (FV), another factor in need of independent assessment before the experimenter exposes the observer to the crucial test.

During the third and critical stage, my FV was up–down reversed for the first time. I described the effects and adaptations of three classes of activities as accurately, clearly, and with as much linguistic consistency as possible: (*a*) Perceptual judgments and actions, especially during head movements; (*b*) visually guided actions; and (*c*) visual perception of the self. I collected data by speaking my observations into a portable tape recorder that I carried. Some of the changes in my perceptual experience and my progress in performances were also measured and photographed. Later, the tapes were transcribed and constitute the protocol, major excerpts of which are reported throughout the book.

Stages 4–6 measured, in order, the aftereffects of up–down reversing the FV, restricting the FV, and adding weight and size to the observer's head with the helmet. The up–down reversal was, of course, discontinued at the end of Stage 3. The weight of the entire helmet system, 3.8 kg (8 lb. 6 oz.), was held constant during Stages 1–5. Also, the size of the FV, 46° vertical × 115° horizontal, the largest reversed or inverted field ever used, was held constant during Stages 2–4. The apparatus, especially the prisms, is described here and in Appendix B with added detail. My aim is to provide a prototypic example of this type of long-term experiment so that its method will be transferable to the study of other forms of optical transformation.

6

The Prism Study: Control of Influential Variables

Before he or she assesses the effects of the optical transformation, the experimenter must control two sets of experimental variables: the weight and size of the spectacle and the restriction of the field of view (FV). Accordingly, this chapter describes the effects of and adaptations to increasing the weight and size of the observer's *functional head* by the donning of a helmet that later contained the prisms and restricting (but not reversing) the observer's FV. The observer's eye(s) or head (whichever is used) must support the weight of an attached transforming lens, mirror, or prism while the observer is stationary and during movement. An observer's perception is changed insofar as the frame, tube, or goggles containing the optical element protrudes from his or her head, extends the room needed to move the head freely, and becomes visible in the FV. The observer is thus provided with novel optical information for head posture and head movements (HMs)—much like Cyrano de Bergerac's nose. To attach a prism to an observer's eye(s), the experimenter must affix it to a contact lens (Taylor, 1962); "slipping" of the cup relative to the eye and extension of the device from the eye, which may interfere with blinking, also become factors in the adaptation process that are in need of experimental control. The typical welder's goggles now customarily used to carry displacing or tilting prisms probably do not weigh enough or stick out far enough to influence the observer substantially. Hence, experimental control of these secondary variables is not nearly as important as control for limiting the observer's FV. Nevertheless, it should be noted that some previous studies have altered the perceived weight and size of the functional head or eyeball and have ignored the potential influences of these variables.[1]

My own study is an obvious extreme due to the necessity of inserting the large and heavy pair of prisms into a football helmet to keep them securely attached to my head. Ideally, the optical elements the observer wears should not move relative to the head (or eyes) and should be placed so as to minimize discomfort during long-term exposure. Since each prism pair weighed 1.4 kg (2 lbs.), a sturdy, counterweighted frame of some sort was required. Thus, what was expected was not only a dramatic increase in the weight placed on top of the observer's head but also a considerable expansion of the size (width and length) of the maneuverable head. Consequently, changes in the power output of the neck musculature needed to move the observer's head could be safely anticipated; the observer's facility in moving in confined spaces, such as through narrow and low doorways, might also be expected to change.

[1]For example, studies of attaching (displacing) prisms to one or both eyes were carried out in 1959 by Taylor (1962; his experiment III), Smith (1966), Festinger *et al.* (1967; their experiment IV) and by Slotnick (1967, 1969). Changes in functional head weight and–or size were affected, for example, by Stratton (1896, 1897b, 1899), Brown (1928), Ewert (1930, 1936), Peterson and Peterson (1938), Snyder and Pronko (1952), Snyder and Snyder (1957), and by Kohler (1964). Stratton (1896, 1897b) inserted his convex inverting lenses into a tube that extended (an unreported distance) beyond the head. In 1899, Stratton wore a mirror arrangement that was supported by a frame that extended upward from the shoulders and left his head free to move. One mirror was positioned 25.4 cm (10 in.) above Stratton's head; it extended 50.8 cm (20 in.) beginning at the back of his head; it therefore extended about 30 cm (12 in.) beyond his face. A second 61 cm (24 in.) mirror extended diagonally downward and outward from the above-the-head mirror, thus hiding Stratton's face from an onlooker. Therefore, Stratton's functional head–upper body was "extended" vertically by 25 cm (10 in) and by a little more than that horizontally. Brown's (1928) tilting prisms were inserted into two brass tubes extending 6.5 cm (2.5 in.) beyond his face. Ewert's (1930, 1936) lenses were inserted into two tubes that extended about 15 cm (6 in.) beyond his head; the entire apparatus added about 184 g (6.5 oz.) to the weight of the head of each of Ewert's observers. Peterson and Peterson (1938) borrowed Ewert's lenses. Snyder and Pronko's (1952) and Snyder and Snyder's (1957) binocular headgear contained four lenses each, stuck out from the head, and clearly increased the weight of Snyder's functional head. Finally, one of the up–down reversing systems used in the Innsbruck studies (Kohler, 1964; Kottenhoff, 1961) consisted of an up–down reversing mirror designed by Kundratitz; it is essentially a visor attached to a head gear and it protruded from the observer's head just above the eyebrows.

ADAPTING TO WEIGHT AND SIZE OF THE FUNCTIONAL HEAD

Method

During Stage 1 of the Prism Study, which lasted 4 days, I wore a modified football helmet fitted with a front counterweight equal in weight to the prism unit that was to be inserted during the next stage. The weight of the entire system was 3.8 kg (8 lbs., 6 oz.). Instead of prisms, I wore clear skiing goggles yielding a FV almost normal in size. Normally, my ear to ear distance is 16.5 cm (6.5 in.). With the helmet, this distance was increased to 20.3 cm (8 in.), or 25.4 cm (10 in.) including the screws that protruded from both sides. My front-to-back head distance, which is normally 20.3 cm (8 in.), was increased to 33 cm (13 in.) with the helmet (from the front weight to the rear counterweight).

Results

Head Weight: Effects and Adaptations

The actual weight that the muscles of the neck, shoulders, chest, and body had to bear during the study was increased by 3.8 kg (8 lb., 6 oz.). The main effects of, and adaptations to, bearing this weight on the head were:

1. I was aware of a new momentum that caused me to "overshoot" the intended extent of my right–left HMs. I recorded this effect for the last time after 8 waking hours and noted that the effect ceased by the fourth day of this stage; what seemed to be a ballistic HM going beyond its intended limit became accurate again. The increased moment of inertia of the head seemed to have been taken into account by the system that controls neck-muscle activation. This was true for HMs initiated by me as well as for HMs elicited by events in my peripheral FV.
2. Extreme excursions and retaining the head in an extreme posture were strenuous, tiring, and hence consciously minimized; yet, after only 7 hours, the fact that I had a 3.8 kg helmet on my head began to go unnoticed during periods of head immobility. After about 46 hours assuming even extreme head postures was fairly comfortable.

3. Initially, all activities necessitating HMs (e.g., eating, pushups, ball-playing, swimming, walking, and bike-riding) were more taxing and debilitating than preexperimentally. After about 36 waking hours, I was frequently unaware of the helmet weight during virtually all activities, and most activities went on with an ease and competence that made them roughly indistinguishable from preexperimental levels.
4. When I was in water, and therefore subject to decreased gravity, I reported:

Relative to sitting and walking, during swimming helmet seems surprisingly light as concerns perceived pressure on head and perceived work neck muscles must do to support this weight. Yet, swimming is noticeably more strenuous and slow than preexperimentally.

5. Walking, swimming, and other gross bodily movements lacked balance and coordination at first. For example, I reported: "I have to be quite careful about walking on narrow mountain paths: I must stop frequently and look down; this HM must be executed slowly." After about 36 hours most activities went on with an ease and competence roughly equal to preexperimental performance.
6. The weight of the helmet produced noticable downward pressure on top of my head. Consequently, I repeatedly lifted the helmet briefly throughout the experiment to gain relief. Between the sixth and forty-seventh hour of this stage, I reported:

Pain on top of head builds to a "pain-crescendo" every 15–30 minutes. At the end of such a time-segment, the pressure becomes unbearable, and I need to lift the helmet—just a few centimeters without removing it. Lifting the helmet in this fashion for 5–15 seconds is exceedingly restful and helps me "get through" the next 15–30 minutes. During periods of lifting or removing of the helmet, there is an initial perception of "lightness" of my head, an exaggerated ease of head, arm, and body mobility; [while swimming, especially, there is] a perception of enhanced strength of my feet and particularly of my hands.

Head Weight: Aftereffects

Shortly after removing the helmet for the day and before placing it on my head each morning, my head seemed lighter and felt less massive during HMs than while I was wearing the helmet. I did not notice any overshooting or undershooting of the head without the helmet.

Head Size: Effects and Adaptations

The actual size of my functional head was increased by 54% in width and 63% in length. The main effects of, and adaptations to, the increase in the size of the head were: (*a*) I immediately perceived my *functional head* as being wider and longer than it was preexperimentally; this remained invariant as long as I had the helmet on my head. (*b*) I consciously avoided walking between persons or upright obstacles when there was not sufficient room for approximately two persons to pass; this behavior persisted even when the helmet was removed. Some sort of adaptation was further indicated by the observation that when my head itched, I repeatedly and unhesitatingly scratched the top of the *helmet* (the summer heat and perspiration it exacted made itching frequent).

Head Size: Aftereffects

I began to measure the aftereffects of adaptation to the increase in the size of the functional head long before I had expected to do so: a striking case of serendipity. On the first day, I removed the helmet after wearing it for 10.5 hours. Then, with eyes open, I grasped my head between my hands to rub my itching scalp. To my amazement, my head felt quite small to my hands—hardly larger than a large grapefruit. Based on this observation, I immediately began a series of hand-based and other head-size judgments that were repeated twice daily *during* Stage 1: before putting the helmet on in the morning and after removing it in the evening. On occasion, these judgments were also made before or after a shower, when the helmet was removed. Hence, they are designated aftereffect judgments. During each series of head-size judgments, three methods of determing the size of the head were used individually, or any two of them were combined and applied concurrently. Also, any resulting combination of judgments was spaced minutes apart ("individual judgments") or tried in quick succession ("successive pairs of judgments"). All possible combinations (14 in all) were tested during each series and are shown in Table 6.1, along with the results. The order of testing was randomized within as well as across all judgment sessions. These aftereffects will be described in detail because of their relevance to the phenomenon of "visual capture" (Tastevin, 1937): the dominance of visual over haptic information when, for example, the size of an object is judged by touch to be smaller than it actually is because the observer views it simultaneously through minifying lenses. Moreover, these data speak to the broader issue of the stability

TABLE 6.1
Aftereffects of Wearing the Helmet: Visually and Haptically Judged Size of the Head

Condition number	Eyes open with observer looking into a mirror/eyes closed	Hands grasping head/not grasping head	Did this condition immediately follow previous condition?	Type of judgment of head size[a,b,c]	Descriptive statement of results
Individual judgments					
1	Eyes open	Grasping	No	Visual + haptic	At first, head feels smaller than it looks; then, suddenly, looks and feels normal.
2	Eyes open	Not grasping	No	Visual only	Head looks normal in size (as pre-experimentally).
3	Eyes closed	Grasping	No	Haptic only	Head feels smaller than pre-experimentally; particularly true of front portion (head feels pear-shaped).
4	Eyes closed	Not grasping	No	Haptic judgment without hands	Head size is indeterminate.
Successive pairs of judgment					
1	Eyes open	Grasping	No	Visual + haptic	Head looks and feels normal.
2	Eyes open	Not grasping	Yes	Visual only	Head looks normal.
2	Eyes open	Not grasping	No	Visual only	Head looks normal.
1	Eyes open	Grasping	Yes	Visual + haptic	Head looks and feels normal.
1	Eyes open	Grasping	No	Visual + haptic	Head looks and feels normal.
3	Eyes closed	Grasping	Yes	Haptic only	Head is felt to **shrink;** onset: 2–5 sec.; duration: 3–15 sec.

3	Eyes closed	Grasping	No	Haptic only	Head feels small.
1	Eyes open	Grasping	Yes	Visual + haptic	Head is felt to **grow** into hands; onset: 2–5 sec.; duration: 2–8 sec.
1	Eyes open	Grasping	No	Visual + haptic	Head looks and feels normal
4	Eyes closed	Not grasping	Yes	Haptic judgment without hands	Head at first feels normal; then, indeterminate.
4	Eyes closed	Not grasping	No	Haptic judgment without hands	Head size is indeterminate.
1	Eyes open	Grasping	Yes	Visual + haptic	Head looks and feels normal.
2	Eyes open	Not grasping	No	Visual only	Head looks normal.
3	Eyes closed	Grasping	Yes	Haptic only	At first, feels normal; then, smaller than normal.
3	Eyes closed	Grasping	No	Haptic only	Head feels small.
2	Eyes open	Not grasping	Yes	Visual only	Head looks normal.
3	Eyes closed	Grasping	No	Haptic only	Head feels small.
4	Eyes closed	Not grasping	Yes	Haptic judgment without hands	At first, head feels small; then, indeterminate.
4	Eyes closed	Not grasping	No	Haptic judgment without hands	Head size is indeterminate.
3	Eyes closed	Grasping	Yes	Haptic only	Head feels smaller than normal (i.e., smaller than pre-experimentally).

[a]Visual judgments. I tried to determine, and remember for comparison, the "seen" size of my head by looking at it in a mirror.

[b]Haptic judgments. I determined the "felt" size of my head by lightly grasping it between the slightly cupped palms of the hands, placed so as to follow the contour of the head, wrists facing each ear and fingers meeting on top of the head. Operationally, the judged distance between the palms of the two hands is the basis for haptic head size. I closed my eyes during these judgments.

[c]Haptic judgments without hands. I determined the "felt" size of my head by voluntarily moving ("wiggling") the scalp and ears. My hands did not touch my head.

and veracity of visual and haptic-kinesthetic information about seen and felt body parts (cf. Chapter 11).

Discussion

Weight and Size of the Head: Perceptual and Performatory Adaptation

The results show that, on one hand, adaptation to the increase in total weight of the helmeted head was characterized by progressively less awareness of that increase when I was stationary and eventually even during gross motor action. I also eventually performed as if I were not loaded down with the helmet gear. Adaptation to the increased size of the functional head, on the other hand, was characterized by persistent awareness of increase in functional head size, which clearly aided competent action. Thus, I avoided collisions and was persistently careful when walking close to people and obstacles. Objectively, the increase in both weight and size of the functional head remained a constant. Pheonomenally, however, the increase in weight ceased to be attended to whereas the increase in size became a perceptual constant. Both changes were dealt with competently in action.

Head Size: Aftereffects

The aftereffect results indicate that the present method brings out the malleability of our perceptual apparatus when that method is used to judge conflicting information about the size of our own body parts or about the apparent extent of separation between stationary limbs, even in the absence of optical transforming devices. Six main aftereffects are discussed.

First, why did I feel that my head was smaller than my preexperimental (remembered), haptically judged head when I grasped it with eyes closed? The reason may be simple. Throughout the day, I had to lift the helmet slightly and hold it for a few seconds between my cupped hands to ease the pain and pressure. On the first day, I lifted the helmet every 15–30 minutes or between 20–30 times. On these occasions, my hands were in fact 20.3 cm (8 in.) apart. Once the helmet was removed and I grasped my head, my hands were only 16.5 cm (6.5 in.) apart—a 19% decrease in the distance between the hands. On this basis, we may expect that all with-hands judgments are, at least in part, a function of the perceived difference between the width of the helmeted head and the head without helmet. This perceived difference may be called a *successive contrast effect.* The haptic information that I had for noticing that my hands were less than 20.3 cm (8 in.) apart when judging head-width may have come primarily from my shoulder and elbow joints.[2] Adaptation requires that the observer perceive the helmet as part of his or her head. Hence the new functional head feels bigger. When a portion of this larger "head" (helmet) is removed, the real head feels smaller.

Second, why was I unable to say whether my head felt smaller, larger, or the same as my preexperimental head when judging head size by passive haptic means only (i.e., by the "feel" of the head without touching it)? By itself this observation is puzzling. However, the finding that I judged my head to be quite small when using my hands to estimate head size, whereas I did not judge my head to be smaller than preexperimentally when I did not use my hands, suggests that "head size" judgments are really judgments of the phenomenal decrease in the distance between the arms-hands, with shoulder joint information for successive arm position (Goldscheider, 1898) as their likely basis. Hence, passive haptic judgments ("wiggling" of the skin covering the skull) yielded indeterminate judgments of head size. What remains unaccounted for is the unequivocal phenomenal "localizing" or "transfer" of what is presumably the judged distance between the hands to the clear experience of a smaller head size. Why the head feels smaller is still puzzling.

Third, why did I judge my head size veridically when looking in the mirror? We can account for this result by assuming that visual judgments—unlike haptic judgments—are not based on the discrepancy between the judged width of the helmeted head and the head without helmet. This assumption may be supported by the fact that I did not compare directly my mirror judgments of the head without helmet to my mirror judgments of the helmeted head. It seems that independent knowledge is derived from the haptic and visual system about the size of our body parts and that this knowledge is not "mixed" and does not

[2]This aftereffect result bears some similarity to the so-called *figural aftereffects in kinesthesis* findings of Koehler and Dinnerstein (1947). They found that following active thumb-finger exploration of a fixed separation, the apparent separation with a smaller test object is decreased, that with a larger one increased (also, cf. Walker & Shea, 1974). In spite of essential similarities, the present observations are concerned with the static separation of the distance between the two hands (or with the apparent felt size of a body part), whereas Koehler and Kinnerstein were dealing with the perception of the parallelity and width of the edges of an object between the moving fingers of one or both hands. The present period of exposure (*statiation* in their terminology) was 20–30 times for 5–15 seconds each over a 10.5 hour period, often with hours elapsing between exposure and test, whereas Koehler and Dinnerstein's satiation duration for most experiments was one 30-second period (1947, p. 203) prior to comparison with the test object.

"transfer across" perceptual modalities: A direct comparison is required before a perceived discrepancy is resolved in such a confrontation.

Fourth, why did I describe my head as being normal in size when I looked at my head in the mirror and felt it with my hands at the same time? This result is puzzling since when I saw my head in the mirror without touching it, I said it was normal in size; yet, when head-width judgments were made with the hands only, I said my head felt quite small. These two results suggest that I should have experienced a discrepancy during *simultaneous* visual and with-hands judgments. Why did I fail to report such a discrepancy? The finding suggests that when the observer has simultaneous access to both optic and haptic information, he or she primarily attends to, and bases perceptual judgments on, the visual rather than the haptic information, a case of *visual capture.* The observer may be trying to accomplish two quite different tasks: visually judging the size of the head and haptically judging the extent of the separation between the hands.

Fifth, why did I feel that my head shrank (or the distance between my hands decreased) as soon as I stopped looking at my head in the mirror? Why this vivid *apparent haptic motion?* Perhaps visual judgments of head size are veridical, whereas with-hands judgments of head width are successive contrast judgments. My observation that the head was felt to shrink once I closed my eyes—once visual information for head size was removed—suggests that the dominance of visual information may, in part, be a dominance of attending to visual information: shifting attention from haptic to visual information. (To be sure, this is a guess at what sort of "dominance" visual information exhibits over haptic information rather than a statement about why visual information should be dominant.) Once the visual information was unavailable, I was free again to attend to the haptic information for head-width, as if "released" from the demand of the preponderant visual information. Both this and the following phenomenon may be called *dynamic visual capture.*

Finally, why did I perceive my head "grow into" my hands (or my hands to be "pushed apart") as soon as I opened my eyes? The same explanation as in the phenomenal shrinking case is appropriate, only in reverse. When only hand-haptic information was available, I judged my head to be quite small. All mirror judgments of head-width were totally unaffected by hand-haptic information. Thus, once I opened my eyes and visual information for head-width was made available to me, the hand-haptic information began to "yield" to the comparatively large visual standard. I felt my head "grow into" my hands. The haptic perception seemed to undergo a progressive change, essentially conforming to the available visual information.

The most unexpected results were the vivid apparent haptic motions, including apparent shrinking and expanding of the head during a quick succession of visual and haptic judgments of head width. That such vivid discrepancies between visual and haptic perceptions of the size of a body part can be produced without the use of optical magnification or minification has both methodological and theoretical appeal. The apparent haptic shift observations appear to constitute confirmation for the phenomenon of *visual capture,* the dominance of visual over haptic information (Hay, Pick, & Ikeda, 1965; Tastevin, 1937). Ultimately, adaptation of head size during Stage 1 consisted of acquiring two distinct sets of head size: a seen head size that was veridical whether the helmet was on or off and a relatively smaller felt head when the helmet was off.

ADAPTING TO RESTRICTING THE FIELD OF VIEW

Method

The data and analysis of the Tube Study made clear the importance of the restricted FV as a variable in its own right and in need of control. Consequently, I measured this adaptation during the 5 days of Stage 2 of the Prism Study. I inserted the nonreversing prisms into the football helmet, which yielded a 46° × 115° FV. The angular extent of the FV was identical to that imposed by the reversing prism unit that would be inserted at the beginning of Stage 3.

Results: Effects and Adaptations

The main effects of, and adaptations to, restricting my FV were:

1. I frequently bumped into door frames and table edges and tripped over obstacles underfoot. These effects ceased after about 32 hours.
2. My gross coordination and balance were poor; both improved progressively.
3. I was startled or surprised when someone entered my FV by passing on either side of me and even when my own arm entered my FV. After about 40 hours such events lost part of their startle value.
4. I became acutely aware of engaging in a great deal of extreme head lowering and raising, now necessary for visual orientation

and for the efficient visual guidance of walking, eating, sitting down, dressing, writing, and bicycle-riding. Although this active head exploration persisted, I ceased to be aware of it. Moreover, maintaining the extreme chin-to-chest position came to feel quite "natural" and comfortable after some 40 hours of living with the restricted FV.

5. Generally, my pace of living slowed down relative to Stage 1, that is, I simply did not get as much done as I had done preexperimentally. For example, I read less and ate more slowly; activities such as dressing and showering became a huge chore.
6. When the information was not readily accessible visually, I now relied greatly on the haptic system to gain information about the world and my actions in it. For example, I reported:

In sitting down I "felt" for the edge of the sitting surface of the chair with the back of my thighs before I trust myself to sit. In finding objects which have fallen close to my body, or to locate spilled food, haptic search is preferred to extreme chin-to-chest position HMs and to body twisting necessitated for visual localizing.

7. With the restricted field, I became aware of continual up–down tremors of my head (of an approximate frequency of 4–7 per second) while I attempted to keep it stationary. This finding was made possible by both the restriction of the field and the windowlike shape and distinctness of the borders (occluding edges) of this novel FV. These head tremors were generally not obtrusive. They are probably not noticed in the natural viewing situation because the borders of the FV are too indistinct, being noticed, at best, peripherally.

Discussion and Conclusions

To date, investigators have not raised the question as to whether the initial perceptual confusions and errors in action suffered by spectacle-wearers should be attributed to the optical transformation or to the restriction of the FV. The results show that restricting the FV appears to produce some of the same effects and adaptations as transforming it. For example, I bumped into door frames and table edges; tripped over obstacles underfoot; experienced instability and loss of balance, particularly while walking; and was startled when I saw my arm enter my FV. These effects are particularly interesting in view of the fact that previous investigators (Brown, 1928; Held & Bossom, 1961; Held & Rekosh, 1963; Kohler & Kottenhoff, 1961; Peterson & Peterson, 1938; Stratton, 1896, 1897b) have described very similar effects, as if they were a consequence of the distortion of the FV. (These experimenters did not use a control stage for the restriction of the FV produced by their lens, prism, or mirror spectacles.) As it turns out, imposing the up–down reversal on the observer's already restricted FV *again* produces disorientation, dizziness, poor equilibrium, and a great variety of disturbing sights and incompetent action. In general, then, it seems that both restricting and transforming the observer's FV produce a good many similar effects; in addition, transforming his or her FV has consequences in perception and action that cannot be caused by simply restricting the FV (described in Chapters 7–9).

Several principles derived from the Tube Study found support in the results from the Prism Study. First is that restricting the FV reduces the observer's useful peripheral information, normally used for visual guidance. Thus, I had to substitute HMs for normal peripheral vision. The size of the FV and the requirements of successful action determine the direction, extent, frequency, and timing of HMs in orientation, walking, eating, swimming, sitting down, etc. With respect to sitting down, for example, I landed on the ground instead of on the chair unless I engaged in many extreme HMs to visually guide my movements—stepping closer, turning, and lowering myself onto the chair. Thus, when peripheral vision is denied the observer, he or she must learn new rules for coordinating HMs with intended limb movements. Importantly, the observer cannot visually anticipate many sights about to become a foveal reality. Hence, not only is the sheer amount of visual guidance decreased, but a delay is often in effect between initiating an action and visually perceiving it. This time-lag may be called a *visual guidance delay* or *visual anticipation delay*.

One strategy I used to minimize this delay was to turn or lower my head so as to have the hand in the FV prior to a reaching movement and to affect coordinated head–eye pursuit of the reaching hand. Such adjustments precluded being visually surprised by my own limb movement and enabled me to introduce corrections during a reach. In walking, too, I had to lower my head frequently until my chin touched my chest to sample the portion of the world directly in front of my feet; I then had to raise my head in order to pay visual attention to landmarks of the terrain that would guide my efforts at orientation. Only by continuous up–down head exploration could I both successfully negotiate the places and obstacles not in the immediate FV and manage to follow the chosen path. Yet, even upon having detected an obstacle underfoot, I still frequently stumbled unless my actions were carried out with direct visual guidance (i.e., using information about the relative position of the obstacle and the observer).

Several adaptations appeared to be a joint function of the weight of the helmet system and the novel way in which I had to move and hold my head to carry out many actions, including the perceived progressive freedom, ease, and comfort of all HMs and the experience that maintaining the extreme chin-to-chest head posture, at first strenuous and painful, eventually came to feel quite natural and comfortable. I suggest that there is a rule that unites these examples of adaptation. Awareness of a new prevailing condition persists if, and as long as, it can be an aid to competent action. However, if awareness interferes with competent action, it ceases and is effectively "nullified" by a process of internal and external adjustments. Adaptation of perception and action proceed because a new set of observer–environment functional invariants become available to be responded to: The observer discovers, establishes, and follows new and effective rules for action.

The second principle is that restricting the FV reduces or eliminates information commonly shared by any two successive fields of view as the observer moves his or her head. Special problems for *event perception* are posed thereby. For example, on Day 2 of Stage 2, after 25 hours of living with a restricted field, I reported: "someone had the audacity to put his fork into the salad bowl of my companion at the dinner table. When I raised my head to look up, I discovered, to my surprise, that it was my companion who was holding the fork." In this, as in many other situations, I failed to understand the *meaning* of this partial event. What I was lacking was the broader event-context that provides all the necessary information about the significance of the events. Hypothetically, there are nested units of such observer–object context, observer–place-in-the-world contexts, and observer–event contexts. Simultaneous information about the spatiotemporal interplay of these contexts may be requisite to understanding an event. That is, perceptual meaning may be implicit in relatively simple invariants (e.g., information for a looming object) as well as in very complex "situational" invariants, which may be called *event perception structures.* In order to diminish the number of misunderstood or initially incomprehensible events that might evoke surprise, I increased the frequency of exploratory HMs. An extension of this account à la Neisser (1976, 1978), Hochberg (1968), and Hochberg and Brooks (1978, Chapter V.4) is clearly fruitful.

The following conclusions seem warranted:

1. Getting concurrent optical information during an action or event in the world is thwarted in proportion to the decrease of the observer's FV.
2. General visual orientation in the observer's immediate environment is directly dependent on a minimum amount of concurrently visible observer–environment information.

3. Understanding the meaning of a visually perceived event is similarly dependent on the observer's simultaneous accessibility to the layout-context within which the event occurs. This includes perceiving the onset as well as termination of an event or an action.

SUMMARY

Using Stages 1 and 2 of the Prism Study as a paradigm, I consider the effects of and adaptations to (*a*) the increase in weight and size of the observer's *functional head,* created by the football helmet that would later contain the reversing prisms, and (*b*) the restriction of the field of view (FV). Both sets of variables must be controlled and measured independently to enable the experimenter to validly evaluate the results of the critical Stage 3, which followed these baseline measurements: optical up-down reversal.

The actual weight of the head was increased by 3.8 kg (8 lbs, 6 oz.), and its effects were assessed over a period of 4 days: My head shot beyond the object I intended to look at in my right or left peripheral FV; walking, swimming, and other gross bodily movements at first lacked balance and coordination and debilitated me considerably. Both effects ceased so that after 36 hours of adaptation, most activities proceeded with an ease similar to preexperimental performance. Perceptually, I rarely noticed the added weight, yet I remained aware of my increased head size and avoided collision: it became a perceptual constant.

Similarly, the actual size of my head was increased by 54% in width and 63% in length. I visually perceived my functional head as being wider and longer than it had been in the past. I consciously avoided walking between any obstacles unless there was enough room for about two people to pass. Adaptation to the helmet was further indicated by the fact that whenever my head itched, I scratched the top of the helmet repeatedly and without hesitation.

The important issue of the dominance of visual over haptic information (the so-called *visual capture phenomenon)* was explored quite serendipitously and without the use of transforming lenses, which magnify or minify viewed objects. As early as the end of the first day of wearing the helmet, I experienced several startling aftereffects upon comparing the felt and seen size of my head while removing the helmet before bedtime. For example, when I grasped my head between my hands, it felt tiny compared to its remembered, haptically judged size. Further, when I grasped my head first and then looked in the mirror, I felt my head "grow" into my hands until it was visually and haptically judged to be normal, or I felt my hands being pushed apart. Analogously, when I judged my head size by first looking into the mirror (while holding my head) and then closed my eyes, either the distance between my hands was felt to decrease or my head was haptically perceived to shrink until it was judged to be quite small. These instances of vivid *apparent haptic motion* are examples of what may be called *dynamic visual capture.*

From this evidence, I was also able to draw conclusions about the stability and veracity of visual information and the malleability of haptic-kinesthetic information for knowledge of the bodily self. Independent knowledge is derived by the haptic and visual systems about the size of our body parts. This knowledge is apparently not "mixed," "averaged," or used interchangeably: A direct confrontation is required before a discrepancy is perceived and resolved. A static haptic perception becomes "fluid" within seconds, stabilizes again, and conforms to the available visual specification of head size. A *dominance-of-attention* in favor of optic information appears to aid this process of conversion. The newfound haptic standard is seemingly "held captive" by concurrent optic information, a hunch supported by the fact that this new standard is reversible and that the haptic system's former standard is readily recovered.

The consequences of restricting my normal FV to a 46° vertical × 115° horizontal FV were then assessed over the next 5 days. Several such effects had been ascribed to optical inversion, reversal, or tilt by previous investigators. For example, I frequently blundered into doorframes and table edges; my balance and motor coordination were poor; I had difficulty orienting and performing visually guided actions like walking, eating, and sitting down; and I was startled when something, even my own arm, entered my FV. This latter observation, as well as the head-size data, suggests that the mapping of even our own body parts in our awareness needs constant visual input. Moreover, the vital importance of the pervasive yet unobtrusive control of peripheral vision was underscored by these data. These effects ceased or stabilized after 30–40 hours of living with the limited FV, and I learned to function competently again before the critical stage of the Prism Study was initiated. For example, I improved my ability to visually anticipate many sights about to become foveally available. I also relearned to coordinate my head and limb movements. Yet, my pace of living remained slowed. These findings represent a beginning for understanding the interplay of central and peripheral vision in many visual–cognitive search tasks.

7

Conquering Instability in a World Transformed

During Stage 3 of the Prism Study, I replaced the nonreversing prisms in the helmet with the reversing prisms. When I, as the spectacle-wearer, moved my head, I saw my environment in motion even though it was not. Concurrently, I misjudged the actual rate, direction, and extent of my head movements (HMs). What information the observer uses and how he or she uses it to adapt to these and related phenomena of *visual instability* is my main concern.

RESULTS OF THE PRISM STUDY

1. During head and body movements, I initially experienced a swaying of the entire visual scene, accompanied by perceived bodily unsteadiness, disorientation, a sense of vertigo, and nausea. After 6 hours of spectacle-wearing, I took a 4-hour nap, after which I no longer experienced nausea. However, the seen swaying of the entire field of view (FV) (briefly, "world motion") remained as marked for 7 days, though it gradually bothered me less. I also perceived progressively less self instability. Finally, I came to experience a phenomenally stable environment and a stable self during normal HMs. After 10 days of adaptation, I again experienced severe nausea, vertigo, and motion sickness

[more properly, "being moved sickness"] while a passenger in a car [passive] condition; minutes later, I drove that car and experienced no discomfort [active condition].

2. On the third day, I noticed that the world motion was accompanied by a joggling or jerkiness that made recognition of focal details (e.g., facial recognition) very difficult. This effect persisted for the entire period remaining in Stage 3 and was most disconcerting when both the object viewed and I were moving

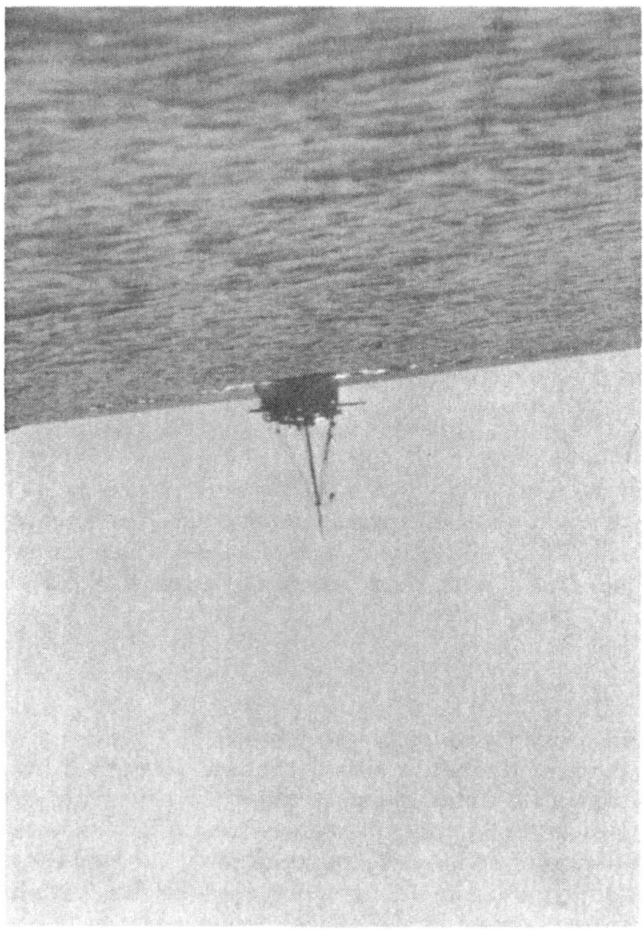

a

FIGURE 7.1. The visual consequence of tilting the head toward the shoulder with up–down reversing prisms (photographically up–down reversed to simulate the spectacle-wearer's experience): (*a*) Head tilted by about 4°, field of view (FV) seen as tilted 8°; (*b*) head tilted 13°, FV tilted 26°. Note the difficulty of determining the observer's point of observation and how that contributes to the already powerful infor-

and least obtrusive when I was stationary and the regarded person or object moved. This *joggle effect* disappeared whenever I arrested all movements, of course.

3. Exact conscious knowledge of where my head was postured relative to the primary position was often not available. When the FV did not contain salient features of the environment, such as the horizon, I also experienced disorientation. This effect persisted for at least 14 days. Figure 7.1 shows the perceptual result of

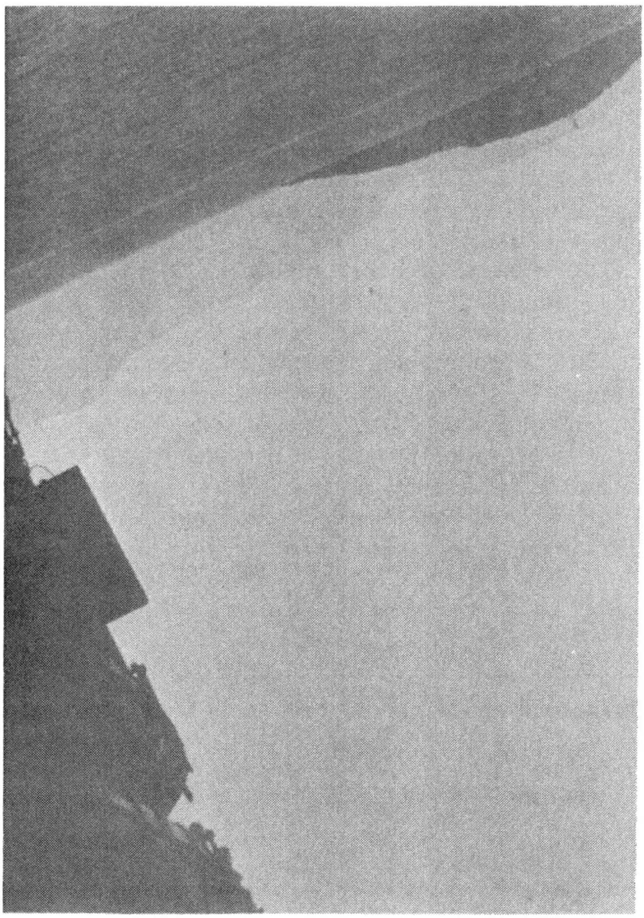

b

mation for disorientation during head tilting. In actuality, I took the photograph as I "stepped" from a larger ship with lifeboats (depicted on reader's lower left) into a dinghy: a most precarious maneuver, indeed. View through FV restricting tube for full impact.

tilting the head toward one shoulder by about 4° (Figure 7.1a) and by about 13° (Figure 7.1b): The *apparent* tilt is double the actual head tilt.

4. Visual overestimation of distance from self and underestimation of the size of objects varied with head posture. The clear discrepancy between visually and haptically judged height of objects was resolved by the sixth day. Some of these as well as other results from the protocol are presented in Tables A7.1–A7.6 of Appendix A.

Immediate Effects: The Visual Seesaw

Undoubtedly the most pervasive and striking consequence of HMs with reversing spectacles is the *seesaw effect:* world motion and concurrent self instability. During extremely slow up–down HMs (one pair every 6–10 seconds), I reported that places and objects in the world were sweeping past my eyes in the *same direction* as my HMs but at a much greater speed than observed normally. During head-turning, I reported a great deal of unsteadiness and apparent tilting of places and objects relative to myself, suggesting that I was unable to turn my head on a vertical axis without tilting or raising and lowering it a bit as well. During up–down HMs comparable or faster in speed and extent than those executed normally, the seesaw effect became overwhelming. Nausea and disorientation resulted. At first, I was totally unable to describe or point to the direction of this global upheaval or to sort out the rate, direction, and magnitude of my own HMs relative to the global upheaval I perceived or was caught up in behaviorally. I was unable to distinguish my perceived world instability from my perceived self instability.

Observer's Direct Report

Immediately upon placing the helmet containing the up–down reversing prisms on my head, I reported (1/0–1/6)[1]:

Any HM, but particularly rapid and repeated HMs, result in immediate and complete disorientation, sweating, tachycardia, trembling of the limbs, a sense of

[1]This time code gives the following information, taken from the taped transcript: Day of Stage 3 of the Prism Study when a given phenomenon was first reported; number of waking hours—to the nearest one-half hour—since donning up–down reversing prisms; day of Stage 3 when the observation was last recorded; and number of waking hours since donning spectacles. Thus, (1/0–1/6) means that the observation was first reported on Day 1, within the first one-half hour, and was last recorded on Day 1, 6 waking hours later.

vertigo, and a strong inclination to vomit. During up-down HMs, the whole visual world appeard to be swinging or swaying rapidly [past my eyes]. [At the same time] I perceive myself to be wobbly on my feet and in danger of falling to the ground. Whenever I make any quick HM which contain a tilt or up-down component (this includes right-left HMs which contain a tilt component), I almost fall down, almost get sick to my stomach, and become quite giddy or "lightheaded." The experience is comparable to being seasick; neither the world nor the observer appear to be, or can be made to remain, stationary during (up-down) HMs. The ground comes up to meet me, and I see and feel myself being pushed toward or approaching the ground in a totally novel way. In short, my visual and behavioral world is destabilized. It should be noted that it would take me minutes to ascertain and describe in what direction, relative to my own HMs, the world appears to be moving. I seem to respond to the optical information directly and immediately without stopping to think or say or point to what is up or down relative to what. And in spite of the fact that there is a sense in which I both know and perceive that I am not experiencing an earthquake in which houses collapse and earth and sky are in upheavel, I respond as if that were the case. As yet, I have no perceptual-performatory appreciation of the fact that I am causing this world-self upheaval. My knowledge is helpful only insofar as I can decide to stop moving my head or to close my eyes. (When I close my eyes [1/1-1/6] my head ceases to "swim," and the nausea gradually subsides.) That is, at this point I do not distinguish, visually or otherwise, between the rate, direction, and magnitude of my own HMs and the global upheaval I perceive and am caught up in behaviorally.

A bit later (1/1-1/6) I stated:

My head feels quite "light"— as it does normally after overexertion or drinking— and at various times, particularly after any quick and-or large-excursion head movement, I have the definite feeling I'm going to vomit.

I noticed similar effects when tilting my head (1/0-1/7.5):

Tilting my head onto either shoulder produces much the same self-world instability as produced by up-down HMs described above under the same time code. In addition, during a 90° head tilt, the up-down reversing prisms now function as right-left reversing prisms.[2] Moreover, during a 90° head tilt, the perceptual and performatory consequences of wearing up-down reversing prisms are the same as wearing right-left reversing prisms without tilting the head.

Regarding changes in body position, I recorded the following (1/2.5-1/7.5):

[2]Note that tilting the head with, versus without, reversing prisms constitutes a useful analytic tool in investigating the relative contribution of optical, vestibular, and neck-joint-neck-muscle influences in the production of compensatory, torsional, and nystagmoid eye movements.

Standing up from a sitting position causes great world and self instability. The global *upheaval of the visual world is perceived to be directly connected with the more "focal upheaval" in my stomach, the "rubberiness" of my legs, and my steadiness on the ground. In sitting down, the floor is perceived to come up to meet me, and I perceive myself to be falling toward, or* [as] *being pushed toward, the nonstationary ground. Generally, ordinary HMs during sitting down, standing up, or walking spell two simultaneous affordances: the affordance of the world* and *oneself being unstable. An unstable self in an unstable world is treacherous to behold, and a treacherous way of being and living. I experience extreme global flux not only in the world but also within myself.*

Gradual Modifications: Solving the Head Movement Connection

Conquering visual instability and its paralyzing disorientation is a process with a vivid experiential history and consists of two adaptations: (*a*) Overcoming nausea and (*b*) quieting the seesaw effect. The first sign of adaptation was that nausea disappeared after sleeping. I no longer experienced any nausea, tachycardia, or sweating during normal and slower than normal up-down HMs. The experience was that of a radical change, not of an attenuation, as if the previous apparent connection between the visual seesaw and these bodily discomforts had simply been eliminated. However, the judged magnitude of the world and self instability remained as great, (i.e., as noticeable) as it had been immediately after putting on prisms.

The second sign of adaptation was that I noticed that my HMs caused the phenomenal swaying of the visual world. However, it took me 7 days, or 87-odd waking hours of wearing prisms, to notice a clear decrease in the rate of world motion. Moreover, I no longer perceived world motion to be the cause of my experienced bodily instability: HMs came to be judged as self-produced rather than induced by untoward environment forces. Head movement rate also became a progressively better indicator of the speed of the experienced swaying of the FV.

Observer's Direct Report

Following a 4-hour nap (after wearing the up-down reversing prisms for 6 hours) I observed (1/6–1/7.5):

I no longer experience any *nausea, stomach discomfort, tachycardia, or sweating during normal HMs. All other aspects of world-self instability remain unaltered. This means that even though this self-world instability is just as great in perceived magnitude—just as noticeable as ever—it bothers me less than before. This may be partly because I have learned to keep my head as steady as possible during walking and other activities necessitating HMs. In fact, executing 10 kneebends or pushups rapidly again destabilizes my visual and behavioral world dangerously, returning me to presleep nausea, etc.*

My impression of walking also changed in the direction of self stability after sleep (1/7.5–1/11):

The perception, as I'm walking along, is almost an exact copy of watching this action on film after recording it with a hand-held camera. Except perhaps, that the rapidity of perceived flow gradients is comparable to seeing a small plane landing at roughly 100 mph. What I perceive is stunningly similar to taking a camera and putting it on the hood of a car (as in the film Bullitt*), or attaching a camera to the tip of a ski (as in the film* Downhill Racer*) and then watching this film on a panoramic screen.*

Much later I reported a similar experience during head-tilting (4/45–7/87):

Tilting my head onto either shoulder, particularly as I'm walking along, vividly reproduces visually what one observes when one rapidly banks in a small airplane.

(1/13–5/71):

No evidence of self-world instability while my eyes are closed *during up-down HMs, either while standing or walking a few steps. However, on Day 5, while walking [inside the house] in complete darkness and rapidly moving my head up and down or alternately tilting it into either shoulder, I became quite unsteady on my feet.*

Upon waking on Days 2–7 of Stage 3, I reported modifications consonant with those after the first sleep period (2/13.5–7/87):

Today (Days 2–7) global up-down HM-coupled world motion is as noticeable as yesterday, but it bothers me less. That is, global world instability is as great in judged magnitude for a given HM, but these HMs no longer seem to afford perception of self-movement or self being moved in a dangerously inappropriate way. In short, observer-induced movement seems to have decreased markedly; there is no sign of nausea, but vertigo is still noticeable with normal HMs. I'm much less prone to sway or lose balance during or following HMs now. All ill effects decrease progressively for a given HM rate and magnitude.

Somewhat later (2/20–4/51):

After any kind of strenuous activity (brisk walking, pushups, bike-riding, ball-playing, or prolonged swimming), I am much more likely to become disoriented, shaky, and generally unable to function effectively.

Similarly, later yet (4/48–13/168):

> Rapid *up–down HMs produced marked and disconcerting global self–world instability.*

Similarly, I reported (4/48–7/87):

> *Rapid onto-the-shoulder head tilts produce marked and disconcerting global world instability. This is true whether I'm stationary, walking, swimming the crawl, or riding a bike.*

Even later, nausea could still be evoked (5/66.5–5/66.5):

> *HM and object motion synchronized: I went to a park and decided to see what would happen if I moved my head in phase with a swing (i.e., up and down as the swing with a child on it went toward and away from me as I stood just out of range of the swing's full excursion). I observed for 5 minutes, moving my head in rhythm with the swing at the rate of 1 up–down HM pair per second. To begin with, I pretty much lost all sense of knowledge of HM. When I turned away, I experienced the same sort of stomach upset and dizziness that I had experienced on Day 2 of Stage 3. There was no confusion about the fact that there was movement in the world but decidedly a decrease of knowledge of my own HM as I was watching the swing.*

On the third day, I began to notice a new phenomenon, which remained a factor throughout Stage 3 (3/30–15/200):

> *Global up–down HM-coupled world motion now has "superposed" on it the tremulous motion of* focal *detail. This (Day 3) is the first time I have become aware of this phenomenon. This joggling about of places and events which I foveate becomes particularly obtrusive when I'm moving—be it walking, bicycle-riding, water-skiing, mule-riding, or being driven in a car. This jerkiness is quite similar to gazing at the scene while joggling one's eyeball. The effects of this joggling of the scene are manyfold, but most importantly,* focal *rather than* global *information about objects and events is destroyed or obscured. This means that the perception of micro-structure is impaired, while the perception of global layout and sequence-of-event information remains relatively intact. Concretely, [while I move] this is the reason for impaired feature recognition, particularly at a distance of more than a few feet; for mistaking one person for another—only gross or global features can be utilized as identifying information; for deciding whether, or if, a person more than a few feet away is smiling and so on [and depends on the nature of my body movements.] This apparent joggling about of places and objects is quite comparable to watching a film sequence which (1) has been taken with a shaky hand-held camera or (2) when film is slipping as it is run through the projector—the projected image appears to "flutter" or "tremble" or quiver or scintillate or vibrate at a high rate of oscillation.*

A noticeable milestone seems to have been reached on the seventh day (7/87–15/200):

> *I'm again able to detect self-produced ego movement (particularly up–down HM) and to distinguish it from perceived global world motion. More and more, I'm becoming visually aware of my own HMs; the perceived global world motion is less disturbing and less noticeable than my own HMs. Whereas previously [during Stage 2] the perceived world motion appeared to be the direct product of my HMs, now a HM of a given extent and rate of speed no longer produces a global world motion of the same magnitude as before. Judged global world motion has finally decreased slightly (Day 7) and continues to do so.*

With respect to tilting the head, I reported (8/100–13/168):

> *Onto-the-shoulder head tilting produces global upheaval which is just as vivid as ever but less disconcerting as concerns self instability.*

Final Accomplishment: Visual Stability

I adapted to the untoward effects of bodily movement in that I came to experience a stable self and a stable phenomenal world during normal HMs. Thus, the end-product of the adaptation process was that after about 200 hours of living with reversing prisms, I again experienced the FV as "sweeping over" the total environment for a wide range of rates of HM. This "sweeping" was clearly experienced as gaining new vistas in a stationary environment by means of self-initiated HMs. Only when I moved my head more rapidly than typical in everyday life did the component of phenomenal world instability become dominant over the awareness that my HMs were self-generated.

Observer's Direct Report

The following observations serve to illustrate the specific nature of HM-coupled or HM-contingent adaptation (9/115–15/200):

> *During relatively slow and moderate up–down HMs, I'm visually only aware of my own HMs. No global world motion is discernible. Now, during progressively faster up–down HMs, the optical information is apparently made up of two components: perceived world motion and self-produced HMs. Today (Days 9–15) the judged proportion of perceived world motion to self-produced HM during up–down HMs is roughly 1:5 to 2:5 for world motion to 3:5 to 4:5 for observer HM. It is quite clear that these well-defined margins of my FV are sweeping across the scene rather than the scene being "in motion"; the former component is much more obtrusive. The faster I move my head up and down, the greater becomes the component of "the*

world is in motion" until, when I move my head very rapidly—which I need not do for any ordinary purposes—the global world motion component becomes dominant.

Tilting the head yielded the following report (9/115–15/200):

> *During* very slow *onto-the-shoulder head-tilts the judged proportion of world motion to observer HM is about 3:5 to 2:5; that is, during this kind of head-tilt, the information specifies a 3:5 component for "the world is in motion" to 2:5 for "I'm moving my head." Progressively faster rates of head-tilts produce a nonlinearly increasing (greater and greater) component of "the world is tilting"; the component of "I'm moving my head" (the margins of my FV are sweeping across the scene") increased slightly over the days.*

My final report on the phenomena engendered by HMs (15/203–15/203):

> *Global world motion no longer produced by slow up-down HMs but definitely produced by standing and raising and lowering self on toes: Here, perceived global world motion and focal joggling about of the world begin to mix. Note that one unavoidable component of normal locomotion is the same as raising oneself on one's toes and sinking down again, only in walking, this component is not begun and concluded in the same place. During walking, only focal joggling of foveated details is noticed now.*

DISCUSSION: THE INFORMATION FOR VISUAL STABILITY

Control of bodily balance, locomotion, and adequate orientation in his or her visible environment (cf., Gibson, 1958, 1966, 1970, 1972, 1979; Howard, 1974, 1978; Howard & Templeton, 1966; Lee, 1978; Richards, 1975; Ryan & Ryan, 1940; Sandstroem, 1951; Schilder, 1935) and, indeed, the very survival of a creature rest on two important and closely related perceptual achievements: (*a*) Distinguishing self-generated movements and events from motions and events originated in the environment and (*b*) experiencing a relatively stable visual world during eye and–or head and body movements. The latter is known as *visual position constancy* (VPC[3] (Rock, 1966, 1975; Shebilske, 1977; Welch, 1978[4]). As we

[3]The phenomenon of experiencing a stable visual world during *eye* movements (and an invariance of the apparent direction of seen objects despite changes in fixation while the head is stationary) is generally labeled *visual direction constancy* (VDC) and will be discussed in Chapter 8. Experienced world stability during head and body movements, known as *visual position* (of objects) *constancy* (VPC), is the subject of this chapter. The distinction between VDC and VPC was emphasized by Shebilske (1977).

[4]Welch (1978, p. 159) described Stratton's loss of visual position constancy as a "form of visual rearrangement," but it is not. Stratton's "swinging of the scene," described later, was an inevitable consequence of moving his head while wearing inverting lenses. It was a unique adapting *requirement*, as I have shown in Chapter 3 and will show further on.

have seen, achievement (*a*) represents the observer's successful adaptation to the seesaw effect and achieving VPC is synonymous with restoring visual stability. Therefore, the spectacle-wearer who regains VPC conquers instability in his or her world transformed.

Normally, the visual, haptic-kinesthetic, and vestibular systems cooperate (Gibson, 1966; Hornbostel, 1925; Marks, 1978) to provide the observer with the information needed for adaptation. Therefore, following a brief historical survey of experiments on the perceptual relearning of position constancy, three kinds of covarying information—optical, kinesthetic, and vestibular—will be considered in analyzing how the observer achieves visual stability during movements.

Historical Precedent: Stratton and the Constancy of Visual Position

Stratton was the first to describe prismatically induced visual instability, calling the seen displacement of the FV the "swinging of the scene." On the first day of his 8-day study, he looked through a set of monocular inverting lenses subtending, very probably, no more than 25° and wrote:

> When I moved my head or body so that my sight swept over the scene, the movement was not felt to be solely in the observer, as in normal vision, but was referred both to the observer and to objects beyond. The visual picture seemed to move through the field of view faster than the accompanying movement of my body although in the same direction. I did not feel as if I were visually ranging over a set of motionless objects, but the whole field swept and swung before my eyes [1897b, pp. 343–344].

About 7.5 hours later, Stratton reported:

> Whether as a result of the embarrassment under which nearly all visually guided movements were performed, or as a consequence of the swinging of the scene described above, there were signs of nervous disturbance, of which perhaps the most marked was a feeling of depression in the upper abdominal region, akin to mild nausea. This disappeared, however, toward evening; so that by half-past seven it was no longer perceptible [1897b, p. 346].

On the third day, Stratton observed:

> Head-movements were still accompanied by a slight swinging of the scene, although in a markedly less degree than on the first day. The movement was referred more to the observer, so that it seemed to be more a moving survey of stationary objects [1897b, p. 349].

Several investigators subsequently observed similar effects, confirming Stratton's observations. They include Brown (1928, p. 134), Ewert (1930, p. 351), Kohler (1951, p. 17; 1964, p. 31), Kottenhoff (1957, p. 153), and Peterson and Peterson (1938, p. 25). Only Snyder denied experiencing a "swing effect" or nausea (Snyder & Pronko, 1952, p. 125) but did report the expected aftereffects, including dizziness and nausea (1952, pp. 142–143). None of these investigators have been able to say much beyond asserting that the perceived "swinging" stops after 3–6 days of wearing the lens, mirror, or prism device and that an aftereffect occurs upon removing the spectacles, specifically, that "swinging" is now noticed *against* or opposite to the direction of head rotation.

The Constancy of Visual Position

More recent investigators have attempted to take the phenomenon into the laboratory for more detailed analysis. The most prominent of these is Wallach. He and his co-workers have labeled the problem the *constancy of visual direction* (i.e., "the fact that the displacement between the visual field and the head is evaluated in such a way that the stationary environment is perceived as stationary during head movement [Wallach & Kravitz, 1965a, p. 217]."[5] Thus, Wallach and Floor (1970), Wallach and Frey (1969, 1972), Wallach, Frey, and Romney (1969), and Wallach and Kravitz (1965a,b, 1968) have shown, via a series of ingenious studies, that the relationship between the direction and magnitude of HM-coupled "field motion" is experimentally modifiable.[6] Wallach and Kravitz (1968) reason that "Only if the relative displacement of the environment closely approximates that which is normally produced by head movements is the environment perceived as stationary [p. 299]." From their results they conclude that "the amount of head turning is normally taken into account in the perception of motion or rest of the environment [1968, p. 299]." However, these conclusions, as stated must be viewed with caution because a small, luminous spot, moving on a screen in a ratio relationship with the rate and direction of the observer's HMs in an otherwise dark room, does not constitute displacement of the normal-sized, and highly textured FV of the head, let alone an environment. This caution, already forecast by Duncker (1929), is underscored by recent evidence that shows that perceived self-motion versus the

[5]Wallach and his co-workers apply the label *constancy of visual direction* to the same phenomenon that most writers have called *visual position constancy* (see Footnote 3).

[6]The cited work of Wallach and his co-workers is collected in Wallach (1976) and further reviewed in Welch (1978). Interesting extensions of Wallach's early work, successfully pushing the limits of human flexibility in adapting to radically altered HM-contingent optical motion, have been reported by Hay (1968, 1971) and Hay and Goldsmith (1973).

seen motion of textured, illuminated, and moving visual scenes is importantly a function of the size of the FV stimulated and whether the foveal or peripheral—the more motion-sensitive FV—was stimulated (Dichgans, Held, Young, & Brandt, 1972; Dolezal & Held, 1975; Fischer & Kornmueller, 1930; Held, Dichgans, & Bauer, 1975). More recently, Wallach and Canal (1976) used a small fixation point superimposed on a stationary or moving patterned field as large as 48.5 × 39.3°. The complex optical information provided in the Prism Study requires an analysis of the several adaptation relationships among head–eye compensation and eye–head pursuit movements.

Distinguishing Self-Produced Movements and Environmental Motions

Some characteristics of optical information in the array always covary predictably with the static position of the observer's eyes, head, and other body parts as well as with their dynamic translations during movement (Gibson, 1966; Ebenholtz, 1977). As the observer's head moves, objects and events undergo a continuous relational flow of pattern transformations over time (Gibson, 1966; Johansson, 1977), which specify the direction, rate, and extent of his or her movement. Indeed, the perspective transformations produced by self-generated movements are optically different from the perspective transformations produced by events in the environment (Gibson, 1966, 1979). Consequently, the observer has direct optical information to distinguish movements of the self from optical motions and events originating in the environment.

Immediate Effects and Adaptation: Using Optical Invariants to Restore Visual Stability

The optical characteristics of the reversing prism dictate the new relationship that now exists between the objective rate, direction, and extent of the observer's head–eye movements and the optical image motions (displacements) they produce. In particular, as the observer moves his or her head, the FV moves at twice the rate of the HM and in the same direction as the head because the light that has passed through the prism moves through twice the angle of head rotation. Figure 7.2 illustrates two examples of this new reality. For example, if the fovea of the reversing-prism-wearer is to remain on target during a 15° lowering of the head, the fovea has to move through twice the angle and in the direction of the HM (or 30°) to do so (Figure 7.2a.2.). The regarded object

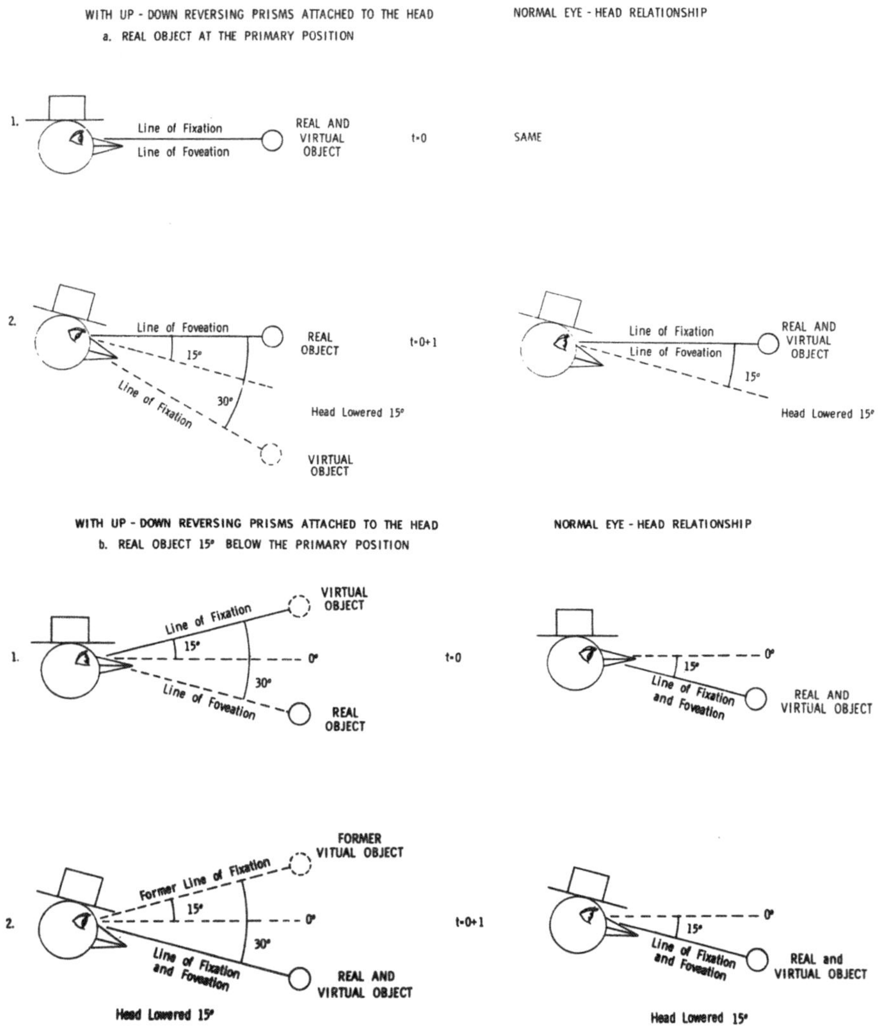

FIGURE 7.2. Direction and extent of (foveal) eye rotation necessary to maintain fixation during a 15° head inclination with and without up–down reversing prisms attached to the head (see Figure 3.4).

appears to move 30° in the direction of the HM. Figures 3.3 and 7.1b may afford additional explanatory realism.[7]

Thus, three parameters of seen world motion are altered for the spectacle-wearer: its apparent rate, direction, and extent. Concurrently, the apparent motions of the FV erroneously specify the rate, direction, and extent of the observer's own head (and body) movements. During the Prism Study, my adaptation consisted of eventually experiencing a stable world. That included gaining a clear awareness that the rate, direction, and extent of my HMs were directly responsible for, and proportional to, the rate, direction, and extent of the motions of my FV rather than that world motion produced my instability.

Optical Rate Information During and After Head Movement

During head and body movements, the spectacle-wearer is faced with *misleading* optical information about the true rate of motion of the FV and about the true rate of movement of the head. Thus, a new optical invariant obtains between the rate of HM and the rate of shearing of optical elements along the borders of the FV—the rate of revealing and concealing of features of the environment. Even though the optical constant during movement is misleading as to the true state of affairs, it specifies a *consistent relationship* between rate of HM and seen FV motion and, as such, becomes part of the information for adaptation. The observer accepts perceptually this new standard for "resetting" the visual system. In the process, he or she learns a new rule: HMs are responsible for the world motion and world motions are *seen* to be the result of how rapidly (and in which direction and how far) the observer moved his or her head. Visually perceiving that the FV of the head is sweeping over the environment, rather than that the world is sweeping past the eyes, is tantamount to perceptual adaptation in this situation. The observer identifies the origin of the visual seesaw and thereby "splits" it, as it were.

The observer could cope with the distressing consequences of HMs in at least two ways. First, world motion might continue to be quite as noticeable as ever but possibly would come to be understood by the

[7]I speculate that the larger the inverted or reversed FV, the more severe the visual seesaw should seem because peripheral receptors of the retina are particularly sensitive to motion information. Anyone who has ever been exposed to a rollercoaster "ride" displayed on a panoramic screen knowns how much more of an ego-motion effect is brought about than by watching the same display on a TV screen (or when viewed through tubes that restrict the FV).

visual system not as an upheaval originating in the environment but as one commenced and terminated by the way the head is moved. The observations of the Prism Study are consonant with this interpretation. Apparent world motion remained rather similar in judged magnitude for 7 days but gradually I perceived it as the result of my HMs. The optical information I formerly registered as world motion came to be registered for what it really specified, movement of the head.

The second way for the observer to adapt is to cease to notice any world motion during HMs and to perceive, again, stability of rooted objects and places in the visible environment. This solution represents an extension of the first solution—a final accomplishment that was, in fact, only approximated in the Prism Study. Perceived self stability was similarly only approximated, becoming quite adequate for comfortable and competent action under all circumstances except during purposely exaggerated HMs. There are several reasons why perfect object-directional constancy was not observed and should not be expected. First, even in everyday life, HMs of unusual rapidity yield perceptible shifts of the visible environment. Second, the process of adaptation must reckon with the fact that the *frequency* of most ordinary HMs ranges between 0.5–5 Hz (Raphan & Cohen, 1978, p. 537). A correspondingly wide range of accelerations and decelerations directs the head. Third, the *direction* of HMs used in an observer's natural ecology is variable, as is the uniformity of the direction of any individual HM. Fourth, the *extent* of normal HMs also varies widely. Finally, all these parameters are greatly modulated by bodily movements, particularly by locomotion and by the specialized skills required in different sports. Yet the observer adapts, suggesting a general flexibility of the visual system that allows for the learning of higher order rules or correspondences that apply to a wide range of HM rates rather than the learning of single piecemeal correlations or conditioned associations of particular HMs with particular rates of field motion. Put another way, the visual system appears to favor flexible covariation of input and feedback to tight coupling. This suggests that our visual scheme of HM–world stability of rate (and direction, as we will see) is only one of many possible ones the human brain can accept as common. This *perceptual accomplishment* is powerfully reminiscent of the learning of a linguistic rule that has broad applicability, yet implies exceptions that violate its use.

An important *performatory task* was to move my head at a rate that prevented vomiting and-or compromising my equilibrium. I had, and consciously exercised, some control over the rate at which I at first moved my head.

Optical Direction Information: New and Old Invariants

As with rate information, the observer is faced with two kinds of misleading and covarying direction information *during* HMs. First, the FV appears to move along with the head. Second, the head appears to move in the same direction as the seen FV motion and thus opposite to its actual direction. This constitutes a new perceptual invariant in that during up–down HMs, the occlusion–disocclusion relationship is reversed; that is, as the observer raises his or her head, the leading or geographically upper edge of the FV *conceals* places in the environment visible the moment before and the trailing or bottom edge of the FV reveals places in the environment concealed previously, and vice versa. Furthermore, as the observer raises his or her head, this optical information misleads the observer to visually anticipate seeing the geographically lower portions of places and objects within and just outside the FV; likewise the observer expects to see their upper portions when he or she lowers the head. This optical information also misleads the observer to *see* that he or she is raising the head when he or she is, in fact, lowering it, and vice versa.

Adaptation cannot proceed if the observer continues to rely exclusively upon this new invariant. What information does the observer use to adapt then? He or she uses an *old* perceptual invariant that still specifies the true direction of HM and FV motion: Whenever the head is lowered, the ground and the observer's feet eventually become visible; whenever it is raised, the sky eventually becomes visible. Thus, the observer gains end-point information about the true direction in which he or she *has moved the head.* He or she perforce compares the visual information available during and after a HM and notices that the information available during a HM is *contradicted* by the veridical information that becomes available at the termination of the HM. I hypothesize that the observer uses this old constant to stop moving the head in the wrong direction (discussed later). Perceptually, the contradictory information during the HM comes to be judged in line with the veridical invariant: The apparent direction of hiding and revealing of places in the environment comes to *mean* that the observer *is moving* the head in the appropriate direction. Similarly, if, at the *completion* of every downward HM the ground becomes visible even though the perception *during* the HM was that the observer moved the head upward (and that the FV displaced upward), then the simplest way to resolve that conflict between the two kinds of optical information is to begin to perceive or judge the direction of that field motion and HM as *downward.* Thus, the direction of the optical transformation experienced during a downward HM should come to *mean* that a downward HM is in progress and should lead, eventually, to the visual expectation that the ground will come into the FV, even before it does. Thus, one form of adaptation observed in the Prism Study consisted of a *visual meaning change.*

To adapt, I postulate, the observer eventually makes consistent use of the optical information available *after* the completion of a movement rather than the information available *during* a movement. Why? First, and foremost, the observer makes preferential use of old invariant information because, rather than specifying a confusing and contradictory state of affairs, the facts as they are in his or her ecology are verdically represented by that information. No observer believes that he or she is looking at the sky when the FV is filled with gravel and the tips of shoes, no matter in what direction he or she perceived the head to be moving and no matter how powerful the expectation was of seeing sky. Second, end-point information is more reliable because it is typically available for much longer periods of time and permits opportunities for simultaneous comparison judgments not available during a movement. Indeed, one major obstacle to judging the direction of the visual seesaw is that the rate of optical flow *during* a normal up–down HM is so rapid and obtrusive that it does not register; at least it is not consciously comprehended. All the observer knows at first is that something is radically wrong. Third, the opportunity for comparing the afferent consequences of efferent output are far greater at the completion of a movement rather than during that movement: The visual system can leisurely collect confirmation or disconfirmation for several parameters of motor commands (viz., the rate, direction, extent, and velocity of the movement of any body part), giving the observer a kind of optical "knowledge of results." Fourth, the optical information available during a HM is contradicted by vestibular, neck-joint, and muscle information; once the head is stationary, however, no such contradictory information obtrudes itself, and the observer can fully attend to and act upon the optical information. For these reasons, it would seem that the observer has a better chance to attend to optical postaction information, to discover what it specifies, and therefore to use it as a guide to future action. End-point information can also serve as a guide to identify and "relabel" the misleading perceptual meaning of the optical transformations witnessed *during* action, as I have shown. Adaptation finally succeeds because the new sights are reconciled not just with old visual knowledge but with information from other perceptual systems, which remain untouched by the optical transformation.

The observer's important performatory task is to make no errors in the direction of intended HMs (see Chapter 8). During the study, I seemed to be at the mercy of optical information, which at first misled me. Once I had learned to judge perceptually and then anticipate the relationship between the true direction of the optical flow and my HM, these errors ceased.

Extent and Rate Information Mediated by Duration of Movements?

I believe that the length of time it takes before any familiar landmark or any stationary body part enters the observer's FV as he or she moves the head from one point of observation to another is a familiar, memory-coded time constant. For example, normally the observer knows how long it takes before the feet or the horizon line become visible, given any known head posture and familiar rate of HM. He or she may well use these constants to gauge the extent and perhaps even the rate of a given HM because such "time-to-arrival" constants are not *directly* affected by the prism's optical transformation. Whether this old duration-distance equation can still be used by the observer is questionable because, with reversing prisms, getting unequivocal information about the extent of HMs is complicated by a misleading new invariant: More of the environment is seen to sweep past the eyes than normally, and concurrently, the head is seen to cover more area and–or appears to go further than normally during any slice of time. The extent of either the HM or world motion is difficult to determine because it is confounded by direction and rate information. What favors the role of the old duration invariant in adaptation is that the rate, extent, and duration of any given HM covary with one another and with the visual angle "covered" by the HM in the FV, from one point of observation to the next.

Whether the duration of a HM comes to be misjudged because the observer misjudges the rate (and extent and direction) of both the HM and world motion is unclear. Potentially, at least, the observer has available veridical information about the rate of a HM once terminated because he or she can compare rate information *during* the HM and duration information *after* completion of the movement (i.e., how long it took for the head-eye system to arrive at its new position). The observer continues to get information for the time required to traverse, say, the distance between the horizon and his or her feet while moving the head at an intended rate.

In summary, the information for a stable self and a stable phenomenal world during the observer's HMs is optical. In adapting to the dynamic effects of optical transformation, the visual system learns that new invariants have predictable consequences and that old rules either still hold or have new and predictable accompaniments. Thus, HMs of a given rate, direction, extent, and duration produce corresponding motions of the FV and soon, correspondingly familiar HMs. To adapt, the observer surmounts discrepancies between what he or she perceives while moving and *after* that action has been completed.

Observer Unaware of Kinesthetic Information for Head Movement

Vestibular, but especially visual, information specifies relations between the observer and the environment; haptic-kinesthetic information—primarily derived from the joints, muscles, viscera, and skin—also helps to specify the location and orientation of body parts relative to one another. For the observer wearing any kind of transforming spectacle, a new covariation exists between the rate, extent, and direction of an eye movement, and hence retinal image motion, during a given HM—the retinal sweep—and vestibular and neck-muscle input. During HM and adaptation, the observer eventually learns that a retinal *sweep,* accompanied by covarying vestibular and neck input, *means* a HM instead of a retinal nonsweep with vestibule and neck input. Overall, it is the consistency of these new covariations during the observer's HMs that helps make adaptation possible.

To the extent that optic information inaccurately specifies HMs of the prism-wearer, kinesthetic information contradicts the visual information. As the evidence of the Prism Study indicates, however, in the face of the obtrusive visual information, I had difficulty even attending to the information from the neck joint and the neck muscles for the rate and direction of HM. Only a very deliberate effort was able to provide conscious and usable kinesthetic information about *where* I had moved my head. Kinesthetic information about the rate or direction of HM *during* a HM was never consciously picked up. My observations appear to bear out the hypothesis that kinesthetic perception and adjustments of haptic perception are, at best, an incidental accompaniment of the resolution (within the visual system) of misleading, contradictory, and discrepant visual information. That is, when the observer has concurrent access to both optic and kinesthetic information, he or she bases perceptual judgments and actions primarily upon the predominant visual, rather than the haptic-kinesthetic, information. None of my evidence denies, however, that information from the haptic system is demonstrably important, especially when the observer's reliance on visual information is curtailed (e.g., when the eyes are closed).

Proprioception and Proprioceiving: Misleading Concepts

The old and honored distinction between *perception* and *proprioception* makes assumptions about the nature of perception that are misleading. The solution I propose is to abandon the concepts of *proprioception* and *proprioceiving* in favor of a unified and more accurate descriptive system of *perception* and *perceiving*. Since all processes of gaining information about oneself and the environment are postulated to be perceptual, I deny that we have any need for the concepts of *proprioception, kinesthesis, sensing,* or *introspecting* as *replacements* for descriptions of perceptual processes. Specifically, the many functions formerly attributed to processes of proprioception should be attributed to the visual, haptic-kinesthetic, auditory, and other *perceptual* systems and to the processes of perceiving, in general.

It was Sherrington (1906) who introduced the terms *proprioception, interoception,* and *exteroception* and implied a strict separation of the world into inner and outer, into two distinct sources of stimulation with corresponding sensations. This separation, in turn, was meant to imply two distinct modes of sensing. The difficulty with this proposal is that the two presumed distinct processes of perceiving and proprioceiving, one directed at the world and the other at oneself, do not correspond to the facts of anatomy, function, or everyday experience. First, it is contrary to anatomical fact that any "sense" or perceptual system is so constructed that it cannot provide the observer with information about himself-herself *as well as* about the environment. There are no interoceptors as opposed to exteroceptors in that sense. Organisms obtain information about themselves and the world via every perceptual system. Every form of energy to which perceptual systems of a given observer are attuned typically specifies, simultaneously, facts about the self relative to the environment as well as facts about the environment relative to the self. This is so whether the observer produces that energy (e.g., by calling out) or whether the source of the energy is external to him or her. Therefore, every perceptual system serves not only awareness of the environment but also awareness of the self. Second, the actions of hypothetical interoceptors and exteroceptors cannot be functionally divided into the self-detecting and the world-detecting. The common condition in the ecology of organisms is a functional simultaneity of world-detection or perception, and body-detection or perception, demanded by the availability of mutually supportive perceptual information. Third, it is contrary to everyday experience that an observer does something fundamentally different when picking up information about himself-herself rather than about the environment. *Effective* information, whether its source is the observer or the environment, is always duoreferential in the sense that is *relational*. What I deny is that in primarily attending to self, one is sensing or introspecting or prorioceiving or making use of kinesthesis, whereas in primarily attending to one's environment, one is perceiving. In both cases, the observer is perceiving.

Even in recent books and articles on adaptation, the term *proprioception* (literally "self-perception") is rarely defined clearly or used consistently. Sometimes *proprioception* is made to refer to various sensations and feelings about body and limb positions (e.g., Day & Wade, 1968, p. 292, Rock, 1966). *Proprioception* is also equated with *kinesthesis* as either the sensations arising from the joints, tendons, and muscles or, regarded in behavioral terms, as the discrimination of the position and movement of actively or passively moved body parts (e.g., Day & Wade, 1968, p. 292, Howard & Templeton, 1966, p. 71). At still other times, *proprioception* has been defined as "sensing the location of a body part, always relative to the felt location of the rest of the body [Harris, 1963a, p. 12; similarly, Welch, 1969, p. 305]" or is regarded as efference-derived cues about relative position of body parts, including conscious or unconscious appreciation of eye position (Harris, 1965). *Proprioception* has also been replaced by the general term *body position sense* to imply that both afferent input and efferent outflow may be responsible for felt knowledge of the position and movements of body parts (Welch, 1978, p. 24). I consider all the above uses as forms of *perception* and as functions of the haptic system. I believe that the language of perception suffices to describe all these facts adequately.

Immediate Effects Revisited: Reversed Compensatory Eye Movements (CEMs) and Nausea

Two important effects that followed the donning of the reversing spectacles in the Prism Study remain to be discussed. I will go into some detail because the findings are new and the issues are complex and basic to many practical problems (e.g., motion sickness, orientation during weightlessness) beyond adaptation to spectacles. During HMs, I experienced nausea and my compensatory eye movements were now opposite in direction to normal CEMs. I was obtrusively conscious of the nausea; the reversed CEMs escaped my direct conscious appreciation during the Prism Study but I directly observed the phenomenon in 1971 and measured it in 1973 in two subsequent studies in which other observers wore reversing prisms.

I experienced nausea during up–down and tilt HMs for the first 6 hours of wearing reversing spectacles. One might well reason that the optical information responsible for the disturbing, vertigo-producing FV motions also induced my nausea. However, after a 4-hour sleep period, which followed the first 6 hours of wearing prisms, I no longer experienced nausea during normal HMs. Yet, I judged the magnitude of the motions of my FV to be just as great as before the period of sleep. Therefore, optical motion information can be only partly responsible for the observed nausea. An explanation for the nausea I experienced can be sought, however, in the conflict created between the prism-produced motion information, which directs the observer's eyes to move in the same direction as his or her head while the vestibular signals attempt to "drive" the eyes in the opposite direction. To trace this argument, we first must take a look at the nature of normal CEMs. Second, I will report on my observations and on the work of other researchers, notably Gonshor and Melvill Jones (1971, 1973, 1976a,b), who measured the aftereffects of this reversal of normal CEMs.[8] Third, I will suggest how optic and vestibular information create nausea.

Three Mechanisms Control Normal CEMs

The ability to maintain one's eye posture relative to an item of interest in the environment during head and body movements insures that the observer remains visually oriented and enables him or her to control the balance of the body. When the observer turns the eyes and then the head to attend to an object in the peripheral FV, the eyes remain "on target" following the original saccadic EM. If the head carried the eyes with it, the direction of gaze would greatly overshoot the target (Piercy, Poeck, & Held, 1976, p. 267): Thus, the observer's eyes move in the direction opposite to the HM, remaining stationary with respect to the object. Such head–eye coordinations are known as *compensatory eye movements*. The main perceived effect of CEMs is the apparent immobility of the fixated object relative to its environment and relative to the subject's point of observation and gaze line.

History

Raymond Dodge was the first to photographically measure CEMs (1903, 1921). He distinguished between two types: First, coordinate CEMs for active HM with no fixed latency between the onset of the HM and EM. These are controlled by central nervous system mechanisms

[8]As early as 1966, Franklin (1966) presented some evidence consistent with the suggestion that atypical CEMs play a role in apparent motion perception during HM and that CEMs may be modifiable.

(1921). Second, the reflexive or reactive CEMs for passive head rotation in the dark with a latency of about 50 msec and controlled by vestibular innervation from the inner ear (1923a, p. 24). According to both Dodge (1923b, p. 169) and Woodworth (1938, p. 587), the function of both types of CEMs is maintaining fixation during head and body movements.

Three Guarantees for CEMs

Ordinarily, three mechanisms work together and guarantee CEMs, that is, "When the head moves, the vestibular system responds and acts in concert with neck and visual receptors to produce the induced eye movements [Cohen, 1974, p. 482]." First, in what I will call *light-dependent stabilization,* CEMs are controlled by the visual system; they are dependent on the presence of structured light though independent of active head-turning. Second, in *vestibular compensation,* CEMs are controlled vestibularly and are independent of the presence of any light or of the observer's active participation in head- or body-turning (Dodge, 1921; Wendt, 1936, p. 323). Third, in *neck-muscle compensation,* CEMs are affected by afferent innervation from the neck joint and muscles and are independent of the presence of light but dependent on the observer's active head-turning (Wendt, 1951).

Neck Muscle–Eye Compensation. The relative contribution of neck-joint and muscle input to the eye muscles is difficult to assess. Evidently, neck-joint and muscle innervation (via the first and second cranial nerves) overlaps and may modulate the function of light-dependent and vestibular CEMs (Wendt, 1951). Note that the position of the head relative to the observer's body rather than the movement of the head with respect to environment are signaled. To find out about the level of independent contribution of the neck afferents in people, one would have to test a person suffering from bilateral loss of vestibular function during active and passive head-turning while in the dark or in the presence of unstructured light. All in all, the neck-muscle contribution to oculomotor control is believed to be small (e.g., Carpenter, 1977; Dichgans, 1975; Jung, 1973). Miles and Fuller (1974) and Smiles, Hite, Hyams, & Junker (1975) have shown that, in monkeys at least, assistance provided by the neck muscles is relatively small.

Vestibular–Ocular Compensation. The normal CEM–HM relationship persists even when there are no visible objects to fixate (Dodge, 1921). As summarized by Fleming, Vossius, Bowman, & Johnson (1969), "the eyes continue to move out of phase with the head in complete darkness and when the eyes are closed [p. 846]." It is clear that the quickest source of information for EM compensation for head rotation is the vestibular apparatus. Three distinct processes act in series to activate the eye muscles: During normal head turns the onset and velocity of the HM is signaled to the semicircular canals. Eighth-nerve fibers carry these frequency-coded impulses to the oculomotor nerves via the brainstem and the cerebellum (Cohen, 1974, p. 523). Finally, the transduction of these frequencies into eye deviations takes place (Carpenter, 1977). However, in order to isolate the vestibular component of CEMs, the experimenter must make sure that the observer does not move the head relative to the body lest neck-joint and neck-muscle input contribute to the CEM.[9]

Light-Dependent Stabilization.[10] Some investigators have held the view that CEMs are reflexive in nature (e.g., Alpern, 1969; Howard & Templeton, 1966, Ch. 3). The present approach and evidence to be presented argues that whenever a textured environment is specified in the available light, the appropriate CEMs need not be compulsory reflexes. Rather, ocular stabilization requires only structured light and appears to be controlled by processes utilizing the optical rather than the vestibular information. Thus, a person with bilateral loss of vestibular function still displays CEMs during active head-turning (Howard & Templeton, 1966, pp. 135–136). Moreover, in the visual system of the rhesus monkey, at least, CEMs reappear after several weeks following both bilateral ves-

[9]The finding (Bizzi *et al.*, 1971) that a CEM (in the monkey) does not occur if the head is fixed or braked just after the onset of a HM does not necessarily support the conclusion that vestibular stimulation is necessary for CEMs to occur or that optical control is insufficient. The sudden absence of *optical* information for relative motion between the head and eyes and between the head and the environment may suffice to inhibit the CEM.

[10]Light-dependent stabilization should not be confused with optically induced *eye-head* nystagmus (*optokinetic nystagmus*), or with vestibularly induced ocular nystagmus (*vestibular nystagmus*). *Light-dependent CEMs* refer to ocular stabilization relative to a place in the world during active or passive head or body movement, characterized by sinusoidal, angular acceleration that is immediately followed by angular deceleration (Guedry, 1965a, p. 68). The fixated object usually remains stationary. *Optokinetic nystagmus,* on the other hand, generally refers to the elicited ocular following of a simulated *moving* environment or event while the observer's head and body are, at least initially, stationary. Depending on the velocity of the optical event (e.g., a rotating merry-go-round, a passing train, or a waterfall) the eyes will "lock onto" and "follow" the optical flow and pursue the event (slow phase) until the eye can no longer move in its orbit; it will then flick back (quick phase), resetting its position with respect to the viewed event, and take up its pursuit once again. The angular acceleration is typically followed by a long period of constant angular velocity. *Vestibular nystagmus* involves the same ocular events—slow and quick phases—but is distinct in that it typically refers to the response of the eyes being turned at constant velocities or accelerations. The rotation is frequently in the dark with the observer's head stationary relative to the body. I believe that optokinetic nystagmus displays important differences from vestibular nystagmus, particularly with respect to their quick phases. The quick phase of nystagmus may be seen as equivalent in function to the rapid whipping around of the head during visual spotting by dancers (see Chapter 12).

tibulectomy and dorsal root rhizotomy, thus obviating both vestibular and neck-joint and neck-muscle control of EMs (Bizzi, Kalil, & Tagliasco, 1971; Bizzi, Kalil, Morasso, & Tagliasco, 1972).

In summary, to remain oriented, the observer nullifies the effects of his or her normal HMs by matching the velocity of the eyes to that of the head and thus maintains the position of the retinas constant with respect to the environment (Carpenter, 1977, p. 25). This system of "holding movements" (Carpenter, 1977, p. 8) is also commonly, though I believe misleadingly, called the *vestibulo-ocular reflex* (VOR). The designation is misleading if by *reflex* we mean an activity whose characteristics are not, or cannot be, modified by environmental influence. I will argue that far from being reflexive, CEMs are closely dependent upon *optical* information that exerts a modifying and even overriding influence on the phylogenetically older vestibular control system. What has been called the *VOR* is far from being a reflex, I believe. More likely, the VOR is the vestibular and visual systems working in concert. The basis of that cooperation probably is vestibular and visual *information*. Its function is to ensure that the perceiver can maintain his or her gaze successfully "anchored" to a place of interest in the environment. The observer thereby remains visually and vestibularly oriented to the environment. *Visual orientation* maintains a meaningful relationship of the observer's body to the visible surround for action. *Vestibular orientation* assures control of balance of the body, the latter constituting (at very least) a highly desirable and often necessary condition for continued visual orientation. The vestibular system alone is frequently insufficient to sustain adequate directional orientation and equilibrium of the body: The essential contribution of visual information for maintaining or regaining self-orientation has been discussed by Dichgans (1977), Duncker (1929), Gibson (1950), and Lee (1978).

Reversed CEMs: Optic Dominance over Vestibular Control

Reversed CEMs are an immediate optical *requirement* if the observer with reversing spectacles is to maintain successful ocular stabilization to features of the environment. Indeed, eye rotations that normally compensate for head rotations by moving in the opposite direction prove ineffective in maintaining foveation once the observer views the object through reversing prisms. Additionally, the normal VOR would now cause the observer to lose the object from the FV. With reversing prisms attached to the head, the observer's eyes now respond to postprism light and consequently, the eyes now have to move in the *same* direction as the observer's head. Proper compensation for HMs thus occurs. For example, with reversing prisms, the observer saccades geographically downward to *foveate* an object 15° *above* the line of sight in the primary position. He or she then begins to raise the head to bring the object into the center of the FV. To continue foveating the object, his or her line of fixation has to move through an equal and opposite angle to that of the head. As the observer begins to raise the head, the virtual object at which the eyes are pointing appears to move geographically upward. Hence, to remain foveally "anchored" to an object, the eyes must (*a*) move in the same direction as the head; (*b*) move ahead of the head; and (*c*) move twice as fast as the head. What we have normally is a compensatory slow phase and an anticompensatory quick phase. However, with reversing prisms attached to the head, the slow phase becomes anticompensatory, whereas the quick phase becomes compensatory.

Consequently, a conflict exists between a HM and EM to the extent that the direction of a HM vestibularly governs the direction of its coupled EM. The question is: "Which way do the eyes move if postprism light directs the eyes in one direction to remain stabilized while the semicircular canals of the inner ear direct the eyes to move in the other?" The answer is that the eyes move in the direction required by postprism light, essentially "overriding" the lifelong, reflex-like, vestibular connection that normally controls these CEMs. This effect has been anticipated by only one experimenter (viz., Ewert 1930, pp. 316, 349, 1937, p. 106).

Direct Observation: CEMs Are Reversed

The effect was apparently not directly observed until I did so unexpectedly in 1971. I was not consciously aware of this effect during the Prism Study. I first noticed the reversed CEM after observing the direction of another spectacle-wearer's EMs during active up–down HMs.[11] The eyes move downward whenever an observer moves his or her head down while fixating; with spectacles, they now pursue downward and jerk upward instead of the reverse. In 1973, I (Dolezal, unpublished data) secured additional confirmation for the reversed CEMs via electrooculographic recordings. The observers' task was continued foveation of a stationary place in a fully illuminated room as they turned their heads from right to left or from up to down at metronome rates up to 80 beats/minute per one-half oscillation. CEMs led the head in the direction of the ensuing HM. This effect was *immediate* (i.e., not dependent on a period of adaptation as a function of prior exposure to gazing through reversing prisms).

[11]This individual served as the first subject in a follow-up study at Cornell that was designed to probe the effectiveness of (rapid EM) sleep in inhibiting nausea and speeding adaptation in a wide variety of visuomotor tasks.

Measuring the Aftereffects of Reversed CEMs in the Dark

The aftereffects of this immediate consequence of wearing reversing spectacles were reported by Melvill Jones in 1971 and cited in Carpenter 1977, p. 35; Davies and Melvill Jones, 1976; Gonshor and Melvill Jones, 1973, 1976b; Melvill Jones, 1976; Melvill Jones and Davies, 1976; and Melvill Jones and Gonshor, 1972, 1975. Prolonged exposure of humans to optical right-left reversal brings about effective reversal of the slow phase of the VOR in the dark. Specifically, after 3 days of continuous wearing of a reversing prism, normal compensatory nystagmus, measured during passive angular oscillation in the dark, was substantially suppressed and quite variable; by the eighteenth day, however, the response was reorganized in the reversed direction (i.e., the eyes were almost 180° phase-reversed relative to their vestibularly controlled direction [Melvill Jones, 1976, p. 13]. Gonshor and Melvill Jones have thus demonstrated that the normal coordination between visual, vestibular, and haptic-kinesthetic control was altered and that the so-called *vestibulo-ocular reflex* in man is plastic and sensitive to previously integrated optical information, even when tested in the dark. Although the specific pathways that might carry visual information from the visual to the vestibular system are not entirely clear, indications are that the enhancement and suppression of appropriate and inappropriate vestibular CEMs is mediated through the accessory optic tract and the flocculus of the cerebellum (Cohen, 1974, p. 484). For example, visual suppression of vestibular nystagmus is lost or severely attenuated after destruction of the flocculus on both sides; also, compensatory vestibular movements are reduced after flocculus lesions, which suggests mediation through the flocculus of visual inhibition and suppression of vestibular control normally exerted on the oculomotor nuclei (Cohen, 1974, p. 521; also, cf. Brecha & Karten, 1979).

Optic and Vestibular Information in the Production of Nausea

In summary, the evidence suggests that the behavior of the so-called *vestibulo-ocular reflex* can be modified to concur with novel optical facts (reversal or inversion) and with visual experience to maintain foveal stabilization. This result may be interpreted as an optically controlled or light-dependent, central-nervous-system "driven," override of either the vestibular and/or neck-joint and neck-muscle commands. The two main control systems[12] for the production of compensatory

[12]The idea of a dual mode of control for head–eye coordinations, usually thought to be subserved by the so-called *vestibulo-ocular reflex*, has found other empirical confirmation and theoretical favor (e.g., Barnes, 1976; Carpenter, 1977).

movements of the eyes appear to be able to work either together or independently; moreover, they appear sufficiently flexible to yield control when necessitated by novel requirements for effective stabilization. For this flexibility, the user pays an affordable and temporary price: Nausea and vertigo.

Nausea Is Due to (Incomplete) Reversed CEMs and the Seesaw Effect

With up–down reversing prisms, nausea is maximal following rapid up–down HMs during which the observer succeeds in only partial fixation. Nausea is expected to be slight when complete ocular stabilization is achieved, even though the observer's CEMs are in the direction of the head. (Even slight magnification or minification by prisms leads to some initial modification of CEM [Gauthier & Robinson, 1975] and thus to queasiness.) During any up–down HM, information from semicircular canals as well as from neck-joint–neck-muscle innervation contradicts the retinal information that specifies and controls both the direction of the CEM and HM. It is enticing to suggest that the experiences of vertigo, disorientation, and nausea are partly due to the optical override (i.e., because the reversed CEMs perform their stabilizing function essentially adequately, counter in direction to the presumed vestibular and neck-muscle commands). I think, rather, that nausea is maximal when the conflict for control of CEMs is greatest: when light-compensation cannot keep pace with the demands rapid HMs place upon it and when vestibular mechanisms momentarily succeed in moving the eyes in what is now an anticompensatory direction—against the head.

Yet, I recognize that we still have no explanation of why nausea occurs (i.e., why the visceromotor neurons react as they do. Is it too farfetched to suggest that vestibular effects are "recruited in reverse" (i.e., via afferent optic information from reversed CEMs causing labyrinthine "stimulation," which in turn produces nausea)? This possibility is suggested by Gernandt (1964), who reports "In man, strong natural stimulation of the labyrinths (or their abrupt destruction) causes many dramatic disturbances such as nystagmus, past pointing, bodily lurching, widespread visceral responses, and a sense of vertigo. These disturbances may be accompanied by a fall in arterial pressure, tachycardia, salivation, sweating, nausea and vomiting [p. 224]." I experienced virtually all of these effects during all but extremely slow up–down HMs. Indeed, the autonomic symptoms of vertigo—which include nausea, vomiting, pallor, sweating, and tachycardia—have been attributed to either an increase in vestibular output or a loss in vestibular function (Alpern, 1969, p. 39).

Nausea occurs, in part, presumably because the afferent visual and vestibular information for the direction of CEMs contradict each other. The result is visually induced inhibition of the customarily vestibularly controlled EMs. This inhibition may stimulate either enhanced or attenuated vestibular output to drive CEMs in the usual way and induce nausea, until a steady state in visual–vestibular input–output relations is reached. Further, the uncommonly rapid seesaw effect, which is perceptually uncorrelated with the rate or direction of the observer's HMs, as well as his or her inability to perceive himself–herself as stable, may well contribute to the observer's experience of nausea.

The phenomenon of motion sickness, further discussed in Chapter 12, is startling because it is, at once, both quite familiar and complex. We know what motion sickness is and under what conditions it occurs, but hardly what precise mechanisms are responsible for it or how these mechanisms work. Motion sickness, including vomiting, has been reported in response to moving visual fields while the observer remained stationary (Witkin, 1949). The fact that labyrinthine-defective humans are not made sick by these experiences (Money, 1970, p. 14; Money & Myles, 1975, p. 371) implies that visual motion information can act via the vestibular apparatus to induce motion sickness. Indeed, optical motion information that conflicts with information from the vestibular and haptic–kinesthetic system exacerbates motion sickness (Money, 1970, p. 23). The Prism Study confirms that it is the *dynamic* motion stimulation that is the most effective information for motion sickness because it inaccurately specifies "observer movement" or "observer being moved" or "observer's head being moved." Such dynamic motion information specifies observer movement in a direction opposite or different from the observer's actual movement as given by any other detecting system. Part of the rule for what constitutes effective stimulation for motion sickness seems to be that the information cannot be too abrupt—its onset–offset character must be relatively gradual and its phasic duration must not be too brief: The undulating swaying atop a camel elicits motion sickness more readily than the abrupt rise and fall of a horse's back.

In summary, it appears that nausea in the spectacle-wearer can be produced by these factors: (*a*) The reversed CEMs, especially if the optical "override" over their typical vestibular control is incomplete or when the rate of HM exceeds the normal capacity for the slow phase of optokinetic nystagmus (OKN). The competition between vestibular (VOR) and optic (OKN) control over CEMs, sensitively a function of the rate of HM, initiates nausea most directly, I believe, because the vestibular signal to the eye muscles continues to be "move in the opposite direction as the head at twice the speed;" (*b*) the seen reversed direction of motion of the FV that appears to move with the head during HM; (*c*) the seen excessive rate of motion (revealing and concealing) of the contents and the whole of the FV during HMs; and (*d*) the apparent reversal of the direction of gravity for vertical EMs (Carpenter, 1977, p. 30).

Adaptation: Nausea Disappears after Sleep and Returns During Involuntary Head Movements

Why does the inclination to vomit cease? No one yet has an answer. The first likelihood is that the nervous system operates on the rule that a repeated conflict ceases to be a conflict. Thus, repeated, incompatible optical versus semicircular canal information for head rotation, when recurrently coupled with successful ocular stabilization, should be ignored by the system. Specifically, the postulated visual afferent information may, at first, "recruit" labyrinthine disturbances but later become the expected constant and thus modulate or attenuate labyrinthine disturbances. Second, the likely role of REM sleep should be explored since my nausea ceased after an initial 4-hour period of sleep.[13] Another example where sleep preceded the attenuation of symptoms of vertigo was reported by Sjöberg (1970) during the fourth (1968) symposium on the role of vestibular organs in space exploration. The experience of vertigo during sharp HMs was reported by two of the Russian cosmonauts (Yugarov and Feoktistov) during the zero-g phase of the Voskhod flight. After sleep, the *vestibular syndrome* was said to have improved so that the crew was able to carry out its program (Sjöberg, 1970, p. 22). We need not necessarily postulate either an increase in total REM sleep time or a decrease in REM latency (Zimmerman, Stoyva, & Reite, 1978) to suppose that active processing, restructuring, and integrating of information occurs during periods of sleep (cf., Dewan, 1970; Shapiro, 1967). All we need to hypothesize is that a different form of activity occurs during REM sleep following exposure to transforming spectacles or to other novel conditions that require radical adjustments. If sleep rather than rest from the perturbing visual-vestibular conflict can be shown to be critical in inhibiting nausea, then we need to discover just how the interactions among vestibular, visual, haptic-kinesthetic, cerebellar, and central nausea-producing factors are redefined during sleep. It may well be that particularly vestibular–cerebellar inhibition of nausea is organized during sleep. Chapter 12 treats this issue further.

In the Prism Study, 9 days or 119 waking hours after I had ceased to experience nausea, vivid nausea returned when I was passively trans-

[13]I also observed marked improvement in gross performatory capabilities, particularly walking. These effects will be discussed in Chapter 8.

ported in a car (see Appendix A, Table A7.3). As early as 1923, Dodge found that during passive head-body rotation, the coordinate compensatory contribution was absent from CEMs. They are then vestibularly controlled. Indeed, I suggest that light-dependent compensation again enters a period of conflict with vestibular compensation and that this conflict accounts for my nausea. Immediately after being driven, I drove the car myself. When I thus regained active control over moving my head in response to the jarring movements of the car—the head and body transport system—I experienced no hint of nausea. This result clearly suggests the considerable functional advantage the observer has when he or she can take an active role in reacting and *pre*acting to perturbations imposed upon him or her in efforts at orientation. The observer apparently anticipates and smoothly coordinates his or her own HMs with the upheavals initiated by the environment that threaten to disorient. The results also indicate that adaptation to the ill effects of HMs—whether processes going on during sleep have an active role in such adaptation or not—do not appear to extend to head and body movements when they are not under the observer's control. In this connection, Fukuda (1976) has suggested that experienced bus conductors avoid the motion sickness that passengers occasionally suffer by inclining the head and trunk in the direction of a turn. Conductors thus adjust their posture in the same direction as the driver, whereas the head and body of unwitting passengers can be seen to be tilted in the opposite direction (i.e., in the direction of the centrifugal force). Both the lack of opportunity to "anchor" the eyes to some visual horizon and the vibration applied to the occupants of a car are known to exacerbate car sickness. Two experiments reported by Lackner and Teixeira (1977) demonstrate the advantage of self-generated HMs in situations that can elicit motion sickness: Subjects who actively turned their heads from shoulder to shoulder experienced fewer and less severe symptoms of motion sickness while exposed to optokinetic stimulation than did those who sat passively.

The Joggle Effect

On the third day after I began wearing the reversing prisms, I became acutely aware of rapid, jerky motions of the contents of the FV during my own movements, making accurate recognition and perception of detail difficult or impossible. These joggling motions were experienced as vibrations and were particularly acute when I walked and ran, when I rode a bicycle over rough terrain, and when I water-skied over choppy ocean water. The effect was maximal during activity that sent vibrations through my body and set the helmet with the attached reversing prisms into vibration. Small tremor movements of the head may have contributed in small measure. At any rate, I was unable to compensate for the effect. (This fact is of some concern to those assessing visual acuity during space flight in capsules that undergo vibration [cf. Griffin, 1975; Snyder, 1965]). It might be argued that my noticing the small joggle movements indicates some measure of adaptation to the global upheaval of the FV due to my larger HMs. However, the argument may be reasonable only in the restricted sense that global field motions were so obtrusive for the first 30-odd hours that I was unable to pay attention to the then less troublesome consequences of vibrations of the prism spectacles relative to the head and eyes.

The phenomenon I experienced not only bears a striking resemblance to oscillopsia as described by Bender (1975, p. 452), but, more importantly, to what labyrinthectomized patients experienced when they were wheeled around postoperatively in a wheelchair: The vibration produced a loss of acuity that did not allow them to recognize familiar faces (Floyd & Neil, 1952, cited in Whitteridge, 1960, p. 1104). There also, CEMs did not nullify the small accelerations of the head. In the spectacle-case, joggle was experienced because CEMs cannot serve two masters: They cannot move in the direction of an observer-initiated HM to achieve stabilization and compensate for vibratory movements of the prisms that are out of phase with the direction of the vibration of the head. This is particularly evident during slower rates of shock, for example while walking.

During activities such as water-skiing, when the joggle effect was particularly fierce, an additional factor became superimposed: The rate of vibration may be too rapid for any CEM to handle. It is interesting to note that nausea did not return even when the joggle effect was most disconcerting. My stomach remained untouched by this austerely visual experience.[14] The possibility suggests itself that adapting (CEMs) to reversing or inverting spectacles is a method for warding off motion sickness in future situations, particularly if the conflict that brings motion sickness about is one of discrepant visual and vestibular information—as in altered-gravity environments such as space flight (treated in Chapter 12). The joggle effect is also reminiscent of a situation in which the vestibular system has been put out of business. Ford and Walsh (1936) describe several vertigo cases that required operative section of the ves-

[14]Lackner and Graybiel (1974) have shown that regional vibration to the head can produce motion sickness when combined with optical information from a rotating environment.

tibular component of the eighth nerve on one or both sides. Loss of ocular fixation during HMs resulted in all cases. During walking or riding in a car, objects appeared to "jump" or oscillate before the eyes and the patients had difficulty recognizing the faces of friends. Improvement within 3 months was reported. More recently, Steinman cites the report of a physician whose vestibular mechanism presumably became functionally destroyed through clinically administered streptomycin: "even the pulse beat in his head while reading made the letters on a page jump and blur, and . . . walking destroyed his ability to read signs and recognize faces [1976, p. 144]." These descriptions are strikingly similar to my own experiences.

It is generally asserted that motion sickness is an evolutionary anomaly and that there is no survival value in experiencing nausea (e.g., Money & Myles, 1975, p. 372). I would argue, on the contrary, that the noticing of motion sickness and feelings of nausea alert the affected creature to a state of extreme vulnerability—that of being destabilized and disoriented. The multiple perceptions that alert the observer to the imminent onset of motion sickness motivate postural stabilizing and orienting behaviors (visually "locking onto" the horizon, moving with or against the direction of upheaval, lying down, etc.) designed either to regain one's former control or to avoid or escape the offending circumstance.

SUMMARY

Visual stability is necessary for successful orientation, locomotion, and other visually guided actions. This stability can only be had if the observer achieves *visual position constancy,* which means that the observer experiences a stable visual world and is capable of perceiving the difference between his or her own movements and (apparent) movements of the visible environment. Using Stage 3 of the Prism Study as a paradigm, I describe in this chapter three immediate effects and their adaptation of body and head movements (HMs) that interfered with my visual stability during optical reversal. They are the apparent and exaggerated swaying of the visible environment accompanied by perceived bodily instability: the disorienting *seesaw effect; nausea;* and the *joggle effect* (the small amplitude vibratory tremors of the field of view (FV) that made recognition of detail during movement very difficult). These were first noticed on the third day of prism-wearing, and they persisted through the last day.

In this chapter I also describe one *immediate adapting requirement* for successfully foveating an object during HMs while wearing reversing prisms attached to the head: compensatory eye movements (CEMs) now *have to* move in the same direction as the head but twice as fast, and therefore they move ahead of the head. Thus, CEMs now behave quite opposite to normal CEMs: They are reversed in direction. Far from being reflexive, these reversed CEMs are directed by the reversed postprism light that "overrides" their normal vestibular and neck-muscle control. These reversed CEMs may therefore be called *light-dependent stabilization,* reflecting the dominance of visual information. It seems the behavior of the so-called *vestibulo-ocular reflex* can be modified to concur with visual experience.

The adaptation of the seesaw effect was preceded by the disappearance of nausea after my first period of sleeping in the Prism Study. A fuller investigation into the possible role of (REM) sleep in the amelioration of nausea is suggested by this finding, particularly since the swaying of the visible environment persisted for 7 days. Adaptation consisted of my visually perceiving that my own HMs caused the seen upheaval. Concurrently, I no longer perceived that the phenomenal motions were responsible for inducing my instability. Thus, I came to understand the new relationship between the exaggerated *rate, wrong direction,* and *extent* of HMs and FV motions. At that time, I also experienced a decrease in the rate of seen FV motion. I argue that the information responsible for the seesaw effect and its adaptation is optical. For example, to be clear about the true *direction* of his or her own HM, the observer must attend to an optical constant, which tells him or her that the head moved downward during such a movement, rather than to the new optically reversed motions of the FV, which make it appear as if the observer is moving the head upward. Once shoes become visible, the observer knows beyond doubt in what direction he or she moved the head. Hence to adapt to the misleading directional characteristics of the motion of the FV, the observer solves a conflict between two types of optical information: that perceived *during* the HM and that gained after its completion. The resolution of this conflict is a change in the *visual meaning* of the direction of the optical motions experienced during a HM and hence supplies knowledge of the true direction of his or her own movements. A similar analysis is described for the optically doubled rate characteristics of the motions of the FV.

Nausea during HMs may be attributed to two influences. First, there is the conflict between optically controlled, reversed CEMs and the near simultaneous vestibular and neck-joint–neck-muscle innervations that tend to "drive" the eyes in the other direction as an up–down HM begins. Second, the seesaw effect also accounts for some portion of the observer's initial nausea.

8

Action in a World Transformed

The picture of the spectacle-wearer in his or her natural ecology must now be expanded to include all forms of visually guided actions. A *visually guided* action is dependent on direct optical information. You can see where the handle of the morning cup of tea is, and your eyes guide your hand to reach for it. This is unlike a *vision-based* action, which depends on a visual–cognitive memory—an internal representation or schema. You enter your dark office and, remembering where the light switch is located relative to the door and relative to yourself in relation to the door, you find it again.

This chapter serves three functions. First, in it I consider three phenomena essential to understanding successful visually guided action and its adaptation: (*a*) The mutually dependent relationship between perceiving and acting; (*b*) the constancy of visual direction: Mona Lisa's right eye does not "jump" or move as you shift your gaze from her right eye to her mouth; (*c*) the need for the observer to know the position of his or her eyes and other body parts that he or she will use in visually guided action: You must know where your eyes are in your head and where your arm and hand are before you can direct them to grasp a pen. Second, I introduce and discuss in this chapter those results of Stage 3 of the Prism Study that illustrate the intricate relationship between perceiving and acting. Third, armed with the data, I describe the information that makes these observed adaptations possible in the discussion section.

THE INFORMATION FOR VISUAL STABILITY AND DIRECTION

Perceiving and Acting: Concomitant, Synchronous, and Reciprocal Activities

The cliche, "you learn from experience," is an explanatory white elephant unless we can detail what kind of experience is at work and how the doer profits from it. Surely, attentive perceptual guidance of action is part of the experience that improves competence, and I will comment briefly on it. Most interesting human actions proceed from and imply an intention. Intentions direct our *attention* to and keep it on what we want to accomplish. Your intention is to serve a tennis ball over the net. You see yourself throw the ball into the air while you raise your other arm with the racket to intercept and strike it with a speed, force, and at an angle that will propel the ball over the net. Now you are informed about what and how to repeat or not repeat what you saw yourself doing in order to equal or improve the last serve. Attending to the felt aspects of differently postured and moving body parts before and during the swing and attending to relevant sounds, such as the unique cracking sound of a well-hit ball, can also tell you something about how to proceed in the future. But the observer must relate such perceptions to the seen consequences of these movements to reap the benefits. The observer profits "from experience," then, because perceiving and acting are the counterparts of a reciprocal cycle of action in which perceiving furnishes the observer with information about the opportunities as well as the limitations for action. In turn, acting makes available new afferent information to be used in perceptual exploration that directs future action.

Information, therefore, potentially contains meanings in the sense of apprising the observer as to what he or she can do, what he or she cannot do, and sometimes as to what he or she must do. Thus, at least three kinds of links between perceiving meaning and acting may be listed. First, perceiving meaning *provides* the observer with possibilities for action: The color and odor of fruit hanging just above head level may manifest edibility and hence invite reaching and ingestion. Second, perceiving meaning may also *prevent* specific action. The visual, haptic, or auditory perception of a dropping-off place signifies danger and literally paralyzes action by inhibiting further locomotion in the direction of a cliff (Gibson & Walk, 1960). Third, perceiving meaning may also *demand* specific action. The perception of visual or *acoustic looming* portends imminent collision and literally necessitates situationally appropriate action such as jumping out of the way of an oncoming, ever more loudly roaring truck (cf. Schiff, Caviness, & Gibson's 1962 descriptions of visual looming).

Information that has its origin in the environment takes on meaning, usefulness, and adaptive significance only relative to information the observer has about his or her own characteristics and abilities. Thus the import of a windstorm is considerably different to an elephant and to a young bird, and a 6-foot man will duck just before going through a 5-foot doorway if he notices the doorway. If he does duck, he has demonstrated that he perceived the height of the doorway relative to his own height rather than some "absolute" or nonself-related value.

The world of perception and the world of action are thus well synchronized. The first time a person attempts to lift a large piece of styrofoam, he or she will usually apply more effort than necessary and the hand will shoot up beyond the intended stopping point. Surprise accompanies such an action, and we say that we misjudged the object's weight. But we did more than that. The fact that misjudgments of this sort are a relatively rare occurrence underscores the assertion that perception regulates action and that misinformed perception directs incompetent action. Not surprisingly, *how* the spectacle-wearer's own movements look to him or her *during* action defeats this synchrony and greatly increases incompetent action. The fact that some veridical information remains for perception despite the optical transformation is largely responsible for the observer eventually achieving competence.

Therefore, we can say that "learning from experience" is dependent on witnessing and coordinating information from two sources: the environment and the self. When our actions become competent, we have adapted; we have overcome the obstacles in our visual environment that interfere with what we want to do. When an observer dons spectacles, his or her perceptions of the environment and himself-herself are reshaped; actions that are based on these perceptions are also changed. Only after visually guided actions in this transformed world are performed and perceived by the observer's visual system and performed again will adaptation to this "new" world begin to occur.

Visually Guided and Vision-based Action Depend on Optical Information for Body Parts

In what follows, my main intent is to show that the perceiver-performer has direct optical information about himself-herself from himself-herself and from the environment. Since the observer is obviously part of his or her optical environment, I contend that he or she has direct optical information for the location and orientation of all body parts that are in the field of view (FV), including the position of the eyes in the head, the head on the shoulders, and the shoulders, arms, legs, etc. Specifically, I argue that the information for eye posture and for egocentric visual direction is optically given and directly seen. Egocentric direction refers to where objects, places, and events are judged to be located relative to oneself. You may readily accept that you have visual information for body parts that you can look at directly. When it comes to the head, you may already need some convincing. But to hear it argued that you have direct, *optical* information for the position of the eyes in your head may appear to be going too far. It is not.

The old puzzle about how eye position is registered by motor outflow or so-called *proprioceptive inflow* signals has a more direct solution: I contend that by far the most precise and reliable information for eye position, as well as for having moved the eyes from one fixation to another, can be had for the looking. To convince yourself of the viability of this proposal you need to become consciously aware of the kind of information that is available to you whenever you move and reposition your eyes in a lighted environment. Close your right eye. Turn your head to your left and cast your gaze to your extreme right. You will now become aware of the optical information that is available to your left eye whenever it is in that position in the head. The left ridge of your nose extending upward to the orbit of the eye with its overhanging eyebrow describes an oval that hides part of the environment, and so it is for your right eye when you look toward your left. Shifting your gaze downward reveals more nose and maybe a mustache, while the eyebrow goes out of sight. Your eyebrow comes into sight as you shift your gaze upward and less of your nose is visible, or it disappears altogether. Shifting your gaze toward the primary or center position within the head decreases the total area of the nose that is retinally available while increasing and bringing into focus light reflected from environmental surfaces. Indeed, the primary position is especially clearly signaled: Each retina has access to bilaterally symmetrical portions of your nose;[1] concurrently, when an object appears distinctly in the center of the FV and thus bisects it, the observer knows tacitly that the eyes are centered in the head. The primary position functions as a "resting" position and as such, may also function as a "crosshair sight," a reference point of egocentric orientation (Trowbridge, 1913), a functional zero position with respect to which

[1]The idea that the nose may provide an important cue for visual direction, particularly for the straight ahead, was suggested by Bower (1974, p. 54) but was not taken far enough.

other eye positions can be calibrated and eye movements (EMs) are most readily and most accurately guided and executed.

No matter which way an observer moves his or her eyes, places in the environment and parts of the body that were not in the FV of the eyes become visible and distinct, and other parts of the body and of the environment go out of sight. The point is, maintaining any eye posture, as well as any change in eye posture, yields an *invariant relationship* between where the observer is directing his or her gaze and what optic information he or she has about himself–herself as a consequence: Each eye posture optically reveals to *each eye* a unique (perspectival) view of particular parts of the observer's anatomy that is peculiar to assuming that eye posture. For example, when an observer gazes to the extreme left while the head is in the primary position, a particular portion of the right side of the nose and eyebrows are optically revealed to the right eye; concurrently, none of the light reflected from the left side of the nose may be available to the left eye; instead, a particular view of the left shoulder is afforded the left eye. Finally, the portion of the head and body represented *binocularly* is also unique for any given eye posture. If the observer now gazes to the extreme right, the optical information specifying the location of various body parts relative to the environment is drastically changed. It is this sort of optical information that specifies eye posture relative to head posture, relative to body posture, and relative to visible places in the environment. *Conscious awareness* of these facts is not a necessary prerequisite to making effective use of that information for redirecting the eyes correctly, or for directing the head or arms, for that matter.

To direct his or her gaze to a place of interest within the FV, and to subsequently reach for the desired object, the observer must know (*a*) his or her point of observation; (*b*) the direction and distance of the new target from the object currently foveated; and (*c*) where the reaching arm is positioned. Knowing (*a*) and (*b*) entails knowing where the observer is looking before the gaze is shifted. Knowing where the eyes are in the head per se is not necessary since information about where the eyes are foveating is effectively information about the posture of the eyes in the head. Knowing where the observer "parked" the eyes requires having information about *having moved* the eyes rather than keeping track of information for eye posture *during* an EM. The information that enables an observer to know *that* he or she has moved the eyes is most obvious: The observer can *see* that now, during the new fixation, he or she is looking at something different in a different place in the world and hence in a different direction. I also argue that the observer is not only directly cognizant of the visual self, but that he or she can direct all manner of movements in the dark. Such vision-based action is contingent on the observer having stored in memory, visual–cognitive representations or schemas of the layout of the body within a context of many familiar environments.

The observer's highly textured ecology supplies a rich optical context, which specifies many relations between the seen self and the seen environment. Consequently, his or her egocentric coordinate map is optically available to be cognitively stored and preserved. This rich optical self–environment context enables the observer to execute motor commands that accurately direct the entire hierarchy of articulators in action: the eyes; the head; the limbs; and the body. Finally, even though the observer may be capable of using both efferent and extravisual afferent information to guide action and to confirm, negate, or supplement direct optical information, I believe that optical information is the basis for issuing efferent commands, for modifying them, and for apprising the observer of the result of having repositioned any body part.

The Constancy of Visual Direction

To understand competent action and its adaptation, we need to know how moving the eyes saccadically affects the seen position of objects in the visual world both during and after such EMs because my evidence shows that performatory adaptation is a function of the kind of EM used to carry out a given activity.

Strictly speaking, visual direction constancy (VDC) consists of two phenomena: (*a*) Experiencing a stable visual world *during* EMs while the head is stationary and (*b*) the observation that seen objects remain in an apparent constant direction relative to the observer's head and–or body midline *after* he or she has moved the eyes to a new position in the head and the foveated object is now imaged on a different location on the retina (e.g., you judge the nose of the Mona Lisa to still be where it was before you shifted your gaze to the frame of the painting, even though her nose is no longer in the center of your FV).

Optical Information for a Stable World during Eye Movements

When you look at an immobile object while your head is stationary, the object does not change its position. If you then move your eyes without moving your head, the object still does not appear to move. The light from the object is *presumed* to move across the moving retina both *during* the EM and when the object actually moves while you do not move your eyes. Therefore, the question arises, "Why does not an immobile object seem to move as did the moving object, given that they both have moved with respect to the retina?" The generally agreed upon answer is that in order to differentiate the two events, the observer somehow knows he or she has moved his or her eyes, somehow "cancels" or "discounts" his or her own EMs. The disagreement is about the means and mechanism used by the system to tell the difference.

I believe, rather, that the answer is as follows: The optical image of a stationary object does not "move across the retina"; it is the retina that moves relative to the unchanging optical image.[2] Optical motions occur only during environmental events—when the object moves. Yet, whether the eye moves or the object moves, relative motion occurs. How can an observer tell them apart? The answer may be quite simple: Objects in the FV do not appear to move *during* an EM because they do not and because the observer can *see* that they do not; moreover, the observer can *see* that he or she is moving the eyes as he or she does so; the observer can also see that he or she *has moved* the eyes as soon as he or she has done so. This answer is a logical extension of Gibson's (1968) view that the observer can differentiate objective motion from self-generated motion because the optical information is distinctively different in each of these situations. The simplest explanation for VDC is that the visual system is built to make optimal use of optical information—not *during* saccades, when the retina is in rapid motion, but while the retina is at rest, during its relatively long periods of fixation of stationary objects and during pursuit movements of events. It would be most surprising if the visual system that is capable of so many specialized and precise discriminations were incapable of the rather gross distinction between optical motions generated by an environmental event and changes in the line of fixation—the discrimination of having shifted the fovea to a new and easily discriminable object of interest. When nothing moves, retinal cells register an afferent optical context of "no optical motion" before the initiation and after the conclusion of the saccade. The visual system also registers the fact that no displacement-motion occurred "on" the retina, independent of the rapid sweeping of the retina over a static optic array. Consequently, a veridical judgment of *having moved* the eyes is rendered: The observer experiences no optical *event* that he could ascribe to the motion of any object in the FV. An attractive corollary is Howard's (1970, p. 339, 1973, p. 400, 1974, p. 304) suggestion that visual attention may simply not be invested or recruited in as shortlived an event as a saccade, which lasts about one-fifth second. This suggestion makes good sense when we

[2]See Footnote 3 in Chapter 1 (p. 8).

consider that the interruption of vision during a normal blink is approximately 300 msec (Miles, 1931), and, though longer than most saccades, the blink is neither noticed nor does it interfere with one's ability to perceive a perfectly stable and temporally persistent visual environment. Moreover, fine discriminations and spatial resolution during saccadic EM—temporal resolution—appear not to be a necessary feature of the visual system when we consider these facts:

1. Proportionately, the greatest amount of time is spent in holding the eyes stationary (Boynton, 1960; Hochberg, 1978), and during fixation, the discriminations made are sufficiently precise to direct future adjustments leading to a new fixation.
2. Two to three saccadic EMs per second are not uncommon (Hochberg, 1978), particularly while looking at Mona Lisas or while reading a good novel; and processing information *during* these many movements would be uneconomical in view of the fact that any information picked up during the saccade was already available up to approximately 50 msec before and will again be available approximately 100 msec after its initiation (Volkman, Schick, & Riggs, 1969).
3. The visual system is exceedingly good at picking up any optical event information, and virtually any natural event—even a lightning flash—persists for longer than 150 msec.

Ecologically valid (Brunswik, 1952) events are therefore sure to be noticed even though EMs occur. Motion perception during a saccade is thus not of crucial importance. Indeed, if optical information were obtrusively noticeable during an EM, masking of information gained during fixation might well occur. An unqualified conclusion is premature, however, because some evidence suggests that an observer can make use of optical information during a saccade to direct the next saccade accurately: Hallet and Lightstone (1973, 1976) reported that if a target is shifted to a new position during a saccade and extinguished before the saccade is terminated, the next corrective saccade places the fovea accurately on the new position.

My interpretation challenges the widespread assumption that optical information is not enough to explain why the observer's world remains immobile during EMs and that so-called *extraretinal* information is necessary to somehow discount the fact that the observer moved the eyes. The following assertion exemplifies that position: "Clearly in interpreting our retinal impressions allowance is made in some [*extraretinal*] way for the movements of the eyes in the head, otherwise the movement of the image over the retina would be bound to give a sensation of movement of the objects in the external world [Merton, 1964, p. 315]."

Three other explanations for VDC during saccades are frequently cited: (*a*) The visual system somehow "suppresses" vision; (*b*) the visual system has to take account of its own "effort of will"; (*c*) initiating, storing, and canceling the motor commands issued to the eye muscles is required to differentiate environmental and retinal motion during a saccade. Explanations (*b*) and (*c*) are also considered as evidence for the proposition that the information the observer has for the position of the eyes in their orbits is efferent outflow information and are also discussed under that heading.

Saccadic Suppression

Saccadic suppression is a sizable reduction in clarity and recognizability of objects that has been observed during saccadic EMs (Carpenter, 1977, Chapter 11; Dodge, 1900, 1905; Woodworth, 1938, pp. 591-594; Yarbus, 1967, pp. 144-145). It occurs either when the retina moves very rapidly behind an optic array, as it does during saccades, or when a portion of the optic array moves equally rapidly across the stationary retina. Try it. Move the eyes rapidly from the left margin of this page to the right or move your index finger in front of your face as fast as you can. The result is similar: You cannot make out detail until either your eyes or your finger come to rest. But why? The postulate that suppression is a central nervous system phenomenon that works for the sake of suppression of vision during a quick EM should be distinguished from the fact that a functional attenuation occurs in the observer's ability to see things in the stationary environment while the retina sweeps rapidly across it.

So-called *saccadic suppression* may turn out to be an inaccurately inferred phenomenon based on this fact: The visual system is not only poor at extracting usable (shape) information during rapid, relative motion of the image and retina (Dodge, 1900; Gresty, Trinder, & Leech, 1976), it is also poor at identifying blurred information (letters) presented at progressively briefer durations (Dolezal, 1968). Blur during relative motion of the eye or of the optical image and a stationary but blurred image presented at brief exposures to a fixated eye may be neurologically equivalent events. That suppression is not a central phenomenon may also follow from the finding that observers can see perfectly well during a saccade, provided that the object looked at moves at about the same velocity as the eye (MacKay, 1973; Woodworth, 1906). When I was a boy, I recall standing on the rear platform of a rapidly moving train and looking down onto the track. Every detail was clear for a moment while I quickly moved my eyes from just under the train out to the horizon but not while I tried to stare at one spot. This observation can be easily confirmed from any rapidly moving conveyance. Indeed, the only time the observer should be *confused* about whether he or she moved the eyes or whether motion occurred in the environment is when the optic array is (experimentally) shifted by *approximately* the same rate and extent as the actual EM.[3] Note that in this situation, pursuit conditions during a saccade can be experimentally arranged (cf., Dodge, 1900; Festinger & Holtzman, 1978). Accordingly, such an experiment could provide information about the existence of a central registry, the length of time the information is stored, and how precise the output parameters are that enable an observer to distinguish retinal movement from optical image motion—movements of the eyes from object motion. I believe that during successive fixations, the visual system also affects a comparison between the optic array before and after the EM. What may suffice to account for the observer's experience of a stable world during saccades is the directly visible fact that an EM has been made because the observer can see that he or she is now looking at a different place or object.

VDC and Knowledge of Eye Position

It has been widely accepted, at least since Helmholtz (1867, Vol. I, pp. 601–602), that some kind of knowledge of eye posture relative to the head is a necessary condition for the accurate production of at least saccadic EMs (e.g., Gyr, 1972; MacKay, 1972) as well as for executing accurate visually guided movements. Yet, a puzzle remains in our understanding: How does the observer know where the eyes are located in the head and where they are relative to the location of objects in the environment? Two basic answers, still surrounded by controversy, have been proposed.

First, *inflow theory*, Sherrington's (1918) hypothesis, supposes that directing EMs in the dark can be attributed to (a conscious appreciation of) the "muscular sense," derived from the stretch receptors of the extraocular muscles. This proposal has been disconfirmed—at least in its strict form—by Brindley and Merton (1960). Similarly, Carpenter's analysis of the role of proprioceptive input in determining knowledge of eye position led him to conclude that "information about the position of the eyes is essentially derived from knowledge of the commands that are sent to the eyes rather than from sensory information from the muscles themselves. . . . this source of information is too slight to be of practical

[3]The exact rate and extent of image displacement amounts to "stabilizing" the optical shift relative to retinal movement; no relative movement between image and retina takes place, and the image should disappear (Ditchburn & Ginsborg, 1952).

use under natural conditions [1977, p. 262]." Others believe that proprioceptive inflow signals do provide significant information to register eye position; moreover, they are not persuaded that outflow information is a direct source of registered eye position (Matin, 1972; Shebilske, 1977). Indeed, inflow theory, thought to be thoroughly discredited by most, is experiencing a revival under the creative baton of Matin (1972). (See Shebilske, 1977, for a review of these developments.)

Second, there is *outflow theory,* Helmholtz's (1867) hypothesis that, in the absence of conscious position sense, the observer knows how far he or she has moved the eyes in the dark by judging the intensity of the effort of will exerted to move them. Helmholtz believed, in short, that the system must monitor its own output of energy to assess its eye position. Helmholtz's notion leads to the prediction that if the eye could be arrested from actually moving while the observer applied effort to move the eye, the FV should appear to "jump" or be displaced in the direction of the intended EM. Experimenters who have *partially* paralyzed the eyes of observers with curare or procaine confirmed this prediction (e.g., Brindley & Merton, 1960; Kornmueller, 1930; Stevens, Emerson, Gerstein, Kallos, Neufeld, Nichols, & Rosenquist, 1976). However, when total extraocular paralysis is achieved, no FV displacement during a saccade is reported (Brindley, Goodwin, Kolikowski, & Leighton, 1976; Stevens *et al.*, 1976). Nonetheless, Stevens, the heroic subject, did report "nonvisual" displacement, described as "the feeling that if you wanted to touch a given [straight ahead] object you would have to reach to the right, left, up or down, etc. [1976, p. 97]."

Shebilske suggests that the extreme effort used by Stevens to turn the paralyzed eyes induced a change in the registered head position (1977, p. 43). I repeated Shebilske's suggested observations and my introspections support his in that turning the eyes to an extreme position with closed eyes leads to an experience of having turned the head also. There are, however, very important differences between Stevens' and Shebilske's observations: Stevens had direct optical information for the layout, for head posture, and for the fact that he had not actually moved either head or eyes. Stevens did not have inflow information from the eyelids that the eyes had moved relative to them. Helmholtz's prediction is certainly not confirmed for attempted saccades, which suggests that in the absence of direct optical information for a change in eye position, motor commands are not a sufficient condition for judging whether the eyes have moved. Do the partial (curare or procaine) paralysis results then confirm outflow theory? I think not because if outflow information were sufficient to tell the observer that he or she had moved the eyes, the observer should be able to discern having done so. Yet, Stevens was unable to say whether his eye had moved or not, even though some EM was present (Stevens *et al.*, 1976, p. 96). This failure of efference, together with the fact that the partially paralyzed eye does undergo some movement, makes another interpretation likely: In the partially immobilized eye, distinctive retinal image motion specifies a curious "motion" of details in the FV, and it is this optical inflow information that specifies EM or having moved the eye.

In summary, I believe that the evidence considered does not allow the *unequivocal* conclusion that registering efferent outflow information is necessary to experiencing VDC during EMs or that efference specifies eye position, nor does the evidence contradict the more parsimonious idea that the afferent optical information available to the observer suffices to distinguish environment- and EM-generated seen motion. At best, the evidence can be construed to suggest that the visual system can register a motoric intention or the actually generated EM; also, an extreme effort to move the eyes can become consciously available. However, this efference typically occurs in an afferent optical context of "no optical motion" before initiation and after the conclusion of saccades. This "before"–"after" context provides information as to whether the observer has or has not shifted the gaze.

VDC and Mechanical Vibration of the Eye. The method of lightly pushing against the eyeball with one's finger to displace the retina relative to an optical image yields the report that external objects appear to be jumping about. Such observations have been interpreted as supporting a motor outflow theory (Merton, 1964, p. 315). The logic is this: Since the world appears stable even though the retina moves during voluntary saccades, efference must somehow account for the retinal motion. If the world appears to move while the retina also moves, but by passive means rather than by efferent command, it is thought that efference must indeed be responsible for discounting retinal motion.

My own phenomenology and description of what I see whenever I jiggle one or both eyes is this.[4] I am never fooled into *perceiving,* let alone believing, that my visual world or even an object in my FV is moving normally. I do notice uncommon rubbery transformations. Objects do joggle about in a queer sort of way and my visual field is agitated and jerks about, but through it all, the visual world and its furniture remain "fixed," though I see them unnaturally shaken. As I walk, I find the *world* stationary and safe to walk in. Superimposed on these movement-like perturbations is the blur produced by mechanically distorting the shape of the eyeball. There is nothing passive about pushing against your own eyeball. Occasionally, I experience a queasy stomach.

[4]I recommend against this procedure, except if conditions of safety are assured. Contact-lens-wearers are urged NOT to displace their eyeballs by any mechanical means.

When I held an electric toothbrush against the side of one eye (with the other occluded), the visually witnessed vibrations were fierce, blurring, and mildly disconcerting, both visually and gastrically. Yet, I had no difficulty discerning the facts. Finally, my interpretation is this: I do not believe that observations of this kind allow any conclusive inference about outflow or inflow theory. First, the parameters of these mechanical EMs are vastly different from normal saccades. Second, the likelihood is high that the observer engages in saccades during the finger-pushing either with or counter in direction. Third, the observer has clear optical information that he or she has moved the eye at an unaccustomed rate and that the eye has been actively moved by a seen foreign agent—the hand; not surprisingly, the observer's perception is correspondingly different.[5]

The Reafference Principle: Visual Stability During Saccades

The reafference principle was intended to account for an animal's ability to distinguish between its own movements and motions originating in the environment (von Holst, 1954; von Holst & Mittelstaedt, 1950). It postulates, after Helmholtz, that a motor command directing the eye is issued. A copy of this command—the efference copy—is retained and stored. This idea, too, is foreshadowed by Helmholtz (especially 1910, Vol. III, p. 205) and clearly anticipated by James (1890, Vol. II, p. 492). Next, the retinal image motion produced by the EM—the

[5]In February, 1979, I applied an extremely rapidly oscillating battery-powered vibrator to one uncovered eyeball. I experienced no visual effect, provided I was careful not to make contact with the bony orbit. This suggests that applying a pulse that is within the range of typical frequencies of saccades should prove more instructive than pushing with the finger against the eyeball. If experimental confirmation is found, the implication would be hard to avoid that so-called *saccadic suppression* is not an active process. One would suppose, rather, that when the retina moves or is moved at speeds comparable to normal saccades, the visual system simply has insufficient time—due to backward masking or not—to identify the information. Given such results, the solidity of outflow theory would suffer.

The following phenomenon has special relevance to the three often cited explanations for visual direction constancy, discussed earlier in this chapter: During June and July of 1981, I repeatedly observed an 18-year-old female, M.B., voluntarily "vibrate" her eyes from left to right at rates ranging between 6–15 times per second for durations of 1–5 seconds at a time. The extent of these movements ranged between 1.3–4.0 degrees. M.B. reports that *during* these consciously self-initiated rapid oscillations, letters or objects appear to jump laterally and become a blur; while the regarded portion of the environment appears to be moving, M.B. perceives herself (head, shoulders, etc.) to remain stationary even if she is walking at the time. While a passenger in a car, on the other hand, M.B. sees exaggerated movement, akin to swaying in a boat. M.B. reports that if she "holds on" for five or more seconds the rate of EMs decreases; she begins to feel faint, and her ability to concentrate afterward decreases. Following prolonged and repeated oscillations, M.B. sees a slight and slow movement aftereffect. M.B. first noticed this phenomenon she aptly calls "buzzing" at age 8. According to M.B., her brother, then 16, was also able to "buzz."

reafference—is compared to the efference copy. If the two correspond, the reafference is "canceled," and therefore the visual scene is judged stationary. If a discrepancy exists between efference and reafference, then the scene is seen to move. Much of the evidence described above is supposed to support the cancellation hypothesis. However, it can be readily computed that the scheme could only work for a very limited domain of saccades (von Holst and Mittelstaedt acknowledge this limitation [1950, p. 469]). Visual direction constancy *during* saccades is too burdensome for the system. A continual and much-too-rapid sequence of initiating motor commands, storing copies of commands, carrying them out, comparing them, and canceling or not canceling them would be required. Given the great frequency and rapidity of individual saccades and the short latency between them (Hochberg, 1978), the scheme does not seem biologically viable. Moreover, it is quite unclear how copies are produced or stored or how interference from "uncanceled" copies of motor commands is avoided during the following saccade. My argument is an extension of Howard's (1974, p. 303). An elaborate version appears in Matin (1976). The one cognate notion that seems to have survived as almost unavoidably useful is Sperry's (1950) concept of a corollary discharge: The motor system executes the command while concurrently signaling to the relevant sensory system what the motor system is about to do.

Apparent Direction Constancy for Successive Fixations

Why does an immobile object seem not to have moved, as does the object that actually moved, given that they both now occupy a different position on the retina? I believe general agreement exists that VDC is guaranteed, provided that two sources of information are registered and integrated by the visual system: (*a*) The retinal locations of objects invariantly specify their phenomenal locations relative to one another (Hering's concept of retinal local signs) and (*b*) the observer has accurate (extra-retinal) information about the position of the eyes in the head (Rock, 1975; Skavenski, 1976). An impressive array of evidence has been mustered to support the first source (e.g., Rock, 1966; Walls, 1951). Although I agree that two sources are required to guarantee VDC, I disagree that either nonretinal inflow or outflow information is *necessary* to specify either the invariant direction of objects relative to the observer or the position of the eyes in the head. At least three covarying forms of optical information specify egocentric visual direction. First, the observer has optical information that the array filling this FV has remained stationary: If he or she moves the eyes back to the primary position, the fixated object will still be *there* and will not appear displaced to the other side. Second, once the second fixation commences, the observer sees that the relative position of objects visible during the first fixation remained unchanged. Third, some objects and body parts visible during the first fixation disappear from sight, and some that were not visible come into view: As the observer looks to the right, the left shoulder disappears and the right shoulder comes into his or her FV.

The Information for Eye Position and Other Body Parts Is Optical

Information for eye position is thought to provide information for *egocentric localization,* which has also been called *radial direction* (Rock, 1966, 1975). Howard summarizes the notion neatly. "The object of attention is normally imaged on the fovea and the task of judging the visual direction of an object in relation to the head therefore boils down to knowing' the position of the eyes in the head [1974, p. 303]." Normally, the motor program for how far to move the eyes and limbs and in what direction to move them derives from the *relational* optical context provided by a rich and varied optical environment that includes direct information for the observer's body parts. Specifically, the *direction* and *distance* from the observer's fixation point to an object about to be foveated is given by the spatial relationship of the peripherally visible objects in relation to the foveated object. Thus, the observer has an optical frame of reference—a *functional* local sign system (after Lotze) that assures that the relationships in the array remain invariant despite EMs. The *extent* of an EM could well be signaled by this invariant: How much of the eye's bony orbit, the nose, head, and other body parts become visible as the observer shifts his or her gaze; also, the observer can see how far apart places in the environment are that he or she successively fixates. Moreover, when an EM starts from the primary position—the observer's most frequently used prinicpal visual direction (after Hering)—the EM should be most precise; also, the egocentric judgment of the direction of an object should be most precise when fixated from the primary position. Paap (1976) found, indeed, that asymmetrical position of the eyes leads to misinterpretation of the observer's subjective straight ahead.

If the afferent optical information just described specifies eye position, as I contend it does, then the observer should be much poorer at judging the direction of his or her gaze and at pointing the eyes at any object when looking "into" a Ganzfeld—an environment of homogeneous optical structure (Metzger, 1930). Moreover, he or she should be somewhat poorer at these tasks in the dark. Indeed, subjects exposed to a visual Ganzfeld by Cohen did report uncertainty as to whether or not their eyes were open. They were also incapable of voluntarily controlling their EMs. After 10–20-minute exposure, subjects reported a "complete absence of seeing [1960, p. 110]." (The Ganzfeld is a fine tool to analyze both outflow and inflow theory because the observer continues to make attempts at fixation and the accommodation mechanism "hunts" for a resting position [Gibson, 1966; Gibson & Waddell, 1952; Leibowitz & Hennessy, 1975]. Yet, the reafferent optical information the observer gets does not contain corresponding changes that allow him or her to redirect the eyes. The observer thus has to rely on nonoptic efferent and afferent information to monitor eye position and to direct the eyes.) Similarly, the finding by Merton (1961) and by Matin, Pearce, Matin, & Kibler, (1966) that judgments of eye position are poorer in the dark than in an illuminated environment strengthens my contention that eye position is monitored and that EMs are directed by assessing the location of the eye relative to a structured array in the observer's FV. More dramatically, placing an opaque cap over an observer's cornea (Brindley & Merton, 1960) severely impairs knowledge of eye position: Even when the anesthetized rectus eye muscle was pulled with forceps through 20° or more, the observer was unaware that the eye was being moved. This finding is frequently quoted in support of Helmholtz's outflow theory and as disconfirming Sherington's inflow theory. What it shows most clearly, however, is the effect of depriving the observer of direct optical information for eye position and for having the eyes moved by external force. Furthermore, Sandstroem (1951) has shown that the observer cannot point accurately to one point of light in a dark room: Efference does not appear to specify eye position precisely and is insufficient to inhibit the autokinetic effect.

The Primary Position and Compensatory Eye Movements Provide Information about Eye Posture in the Light and the Dark

The information about when the eyes and–or the head have achieved the primary position is also available in the array by virtue of direct optic information about what is being foveated and what portions of the observer's anatomy are optically represented. Thus, the bilateral symmetry of the nose and other body parts, including the shoulders, provides a convenient optical reference index for the system by which to judge eye posture relative to head posture and these relative to body posture. Moreover, the correct execution of any EM from this reference posture to another, peripherally visible, place should thereby be possible (cf. Craske & Crawshaw, 1979). The optical specification of eye posture relative to the head is sufficiently guaranteed by the fixed position of the nose relative to the head. The visual system may have simple "rules" for such knowledge of eye posture. For example, whenever the nose is optically "balanced" on the two retinas, the eyes are in the primary position. Moreover, both in the light or dark, the return of the head to its primary position guarantees a compensatory return of the eyes to their primary position: The visual nervous system registers where the observer "parked" the eyes and faithfully returns the eyes to their "reserved parking position" after use.

In the normal environment, eye-posture information may also be provided during and following light-dependent compensatory EMs and in the dark, by vestibular and neck-muscle-neck-joint compensation. Both guarantee an invariant dynamic relationship between head movements and the angular rotation of the eyes. Thus, if the head and eyes are in the primary position and if the observer turns the head 30° as he or she fixates, light-dependent compensation necessarily reveals that the head is pointing in a new direction and that the line of foveation continues to coincide with the body midline—that the eyes are turned in the head.

RESULTS OF THE PRISM STUDY

Immediate Effects: Disorientation and Incompetent Action

1. Disorientation was characterized by my initial inability to walk without danger of falling; my inability to sit on a chair without sitting next to it or trying to sit in it head first; my incompetent reaching and pointing; my inability to visually guide my eating, drinking, and pouring; my errors in dressing myself; and so on (see Appendix A, Tables A8.1–A8.12).
2. Reaching and pointing geographically upward was visually and performatorily confused with reaching and pointing downward, and vice versa; reaching, pouring, pushing, and pulling away from my midsection was confused with moving toward it, and vice versa; twisting the hand clockwise was confused with twisting counterclockwise, and vice versa.
3. Other immediate effects included committing errors in the direction in which I moved my head while engaging in eye–head pursuit of a moving target (event). For example, I lowered my head in an attempt to follow the skyward flight of a flock of doves.
4. Nosmic "capture" was also observed: I smelled aromas where I *saw* their source, not where they were actually located.

Gradual Modifications and Final Accomplishments: Perceptual Understanding and Competent Action

Adaptations to watching myself act proceeded from a stage of confusion and surprise to a perceptually gained conviction that actions were

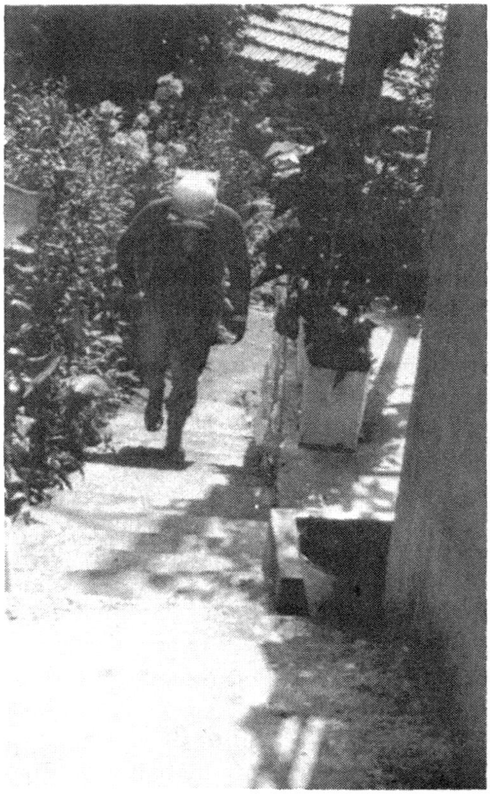

a

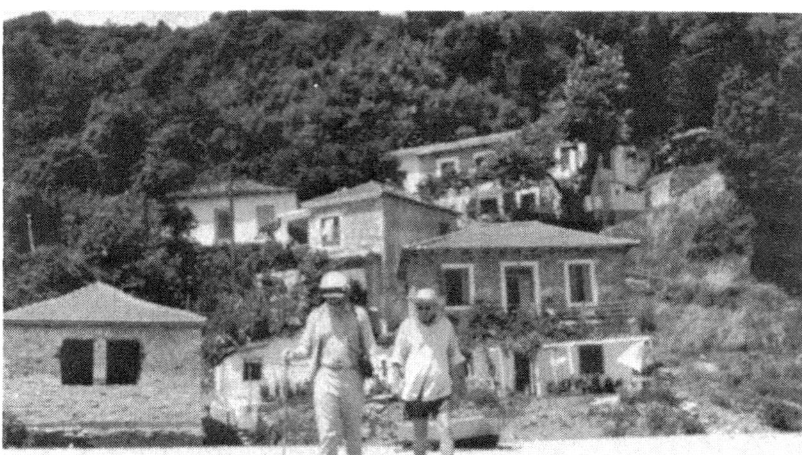

b

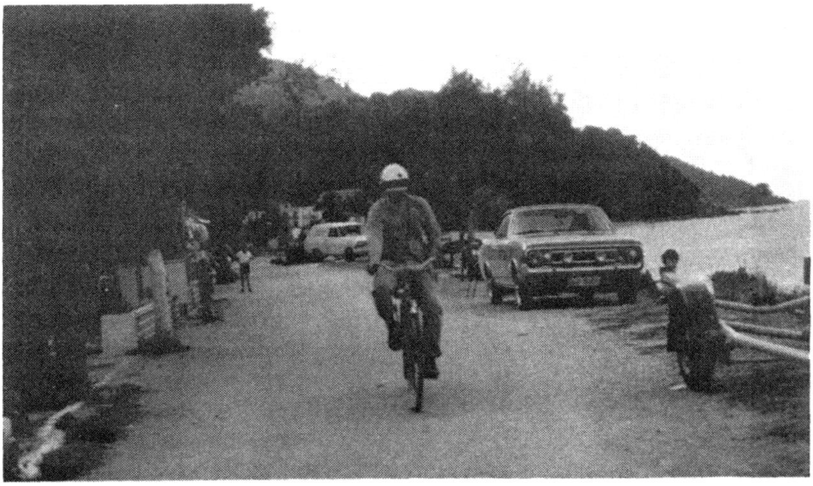

c

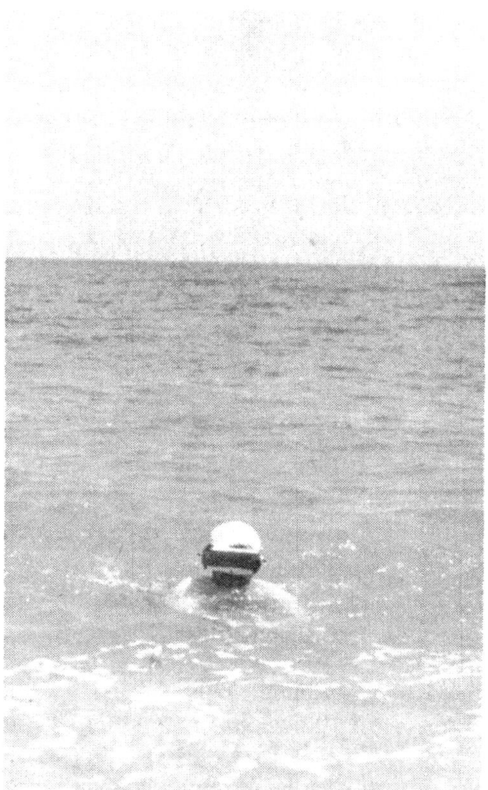

d

FIGURE 8.1. Walking (a and b), riding a bicycle (c), and swimming (d), with up–down reversing prisms before my eyes during Stage 3 of the Prism Study.

competent though they were actually incompetent to a final stage of perceptual-performatory consistency, lack of surprises, and an understanding of the perceptual meaning of actions. Performatory adaptations proceeded from a state of massive disorientation, incompetence, and variability (including engaging in hybrid actions) to a stage of consistency and competence. Gross motor actions like swimming, walking, and bike riding (Figure 8.1) were accomplished most readily. Certain visually guided actions like drinking, eating, reaching, and getting dressed took more time and more concentrated effort to perform competently; others, which required precise and coordinated eye, head, arm, finger movements toward and away from me and upward and downward as well as clockwise and counterclockwise twists presented the greatest difficulty and were most refractory. Examples include inserting batteries into a portable tape recorder and finding and operating tools such as a screwdriver. Some visually guided actions such as those requiring the rapid coordination of eye-head-arm pursuit sequences were never executed satisfactorily in spite of 15 days of practice. Thus, I was totally unable to *consistently* grasp or catch a ball. Finally, some tasks were performed smoothly following some intervening period of not using the relevant limb or not practicing that task at all. Such near flawless actions were obtained even though I was at first quite awkward or incapable of executing the desired task. Specifically, eating with the left hand, which had not been used for that purpose for 12 days, suddenly proceeded smoothly. Writing, too, was smooth, although I did not touch a pen for the first 128 hours of Stage 3.

Observer's Direct Report

Visually Guided Pointing and Reaching for Stationary Objects.

The difficulty I was to experience in reaching for and pointing at stationary objects was foreshadowed in one of the earliest observations (1/0.5–1/0.5)[6]:

> *Suddenly my hand came into the FV and it was an entirely odd* object.

I initially made gross errors in pointing (1/2.5–1/2.5):

> *I am lying on my back on the beach, trying to point at a person standing at my feet. I close my eyes before I make the arm movement to avoid introducing a correc-*

[6]See Footnote 1 in Chapter 7 for an interpretation of the time code. This particular observation was recorded for the first and last time on Day 1 of Stage 3 and within one-half hour of donning the spectacles.

tion during the movement. In pointing at him, I actually point back over my head, as if I were pointing at a person standing behind my head.

I describe gross changes in the normal relationship between the perceived self, the perceived world, and the world of factual demands (1/2.5–7/87):

> *Whenever I point at, or reach for, anything actually above eye level, I point toward my legs, and whenever I point at anything below eye level, I point toward the sky. Whenever I point at anything directly at eye level, I point correctly. This is true if I gaze at the object, close my eyes, and then point. If I keep my eyes open, I can introduce corrections during the pointing movement. The directions which all of these arm* movements *take looks to be correct, and the final position of my arm looks to be correct until I begin comparing the location of the viewed object and that of my hand and finger relative to the object. It is this* discrepancy *which tells me that I've pointed incorrectly, but this discrepancy information does not alter the report that the direction I'm pointing in is the direction I intended to point in. Moreover, phenomenally, there is nothing amiss haptically. Pointing toward the ground as I'm inspecting a fly on the ceiling does not feel strange. On the other hand, if I point, using a laborious and error-prone technique of lining up my finger with the object I'm looking at, I am aware of having my arm and finger lined up with the object of interest. However, simultaneously, I judge my arm to be pointing in the wrong direction, visually speaking. Moreover, haptically the arm position feels wholly unfamiliar or "wrong."*

A comparison between the haptic experience of reaching with and without visual guidance resulted in this report (1/4–2/14):

> *There is a clear difference between the haptic appreciation (the "feel") of actions like reaching and grasping when I close my eyes (or operate outside the FV) and the haptic perception of such actions under visual guidance. The "feel" of actions outside the FV and the actions themselves are stable, secure, and unhesitating, whereas under visual guidance, a great deal of concentration is required, and yet I experience a great deal of hesitation and frustration and my performance is incompetent.*

(1/8–2/20.5):

> *Reaching with visual guidance: As a rule, while reaching for doorknobs, for example, I reached far above them at first and sometimes kept "searching" to find them. After noticing the discrepancy between the final position of my hand and the doorknob, I reached again, determined to open the door. The second reach, intended to "correct" the first, was generally even further above the doorknob than the first reach. Visually, this was the correct arm movement to carry out, of course, because reaching geographically upward looks like (visually* means*) reaching geograph-*

> *ically downward. If I moved my arm very slowly under visual guidance, my arm would start off as before, be stopped, and then continue on in snake-movement fashion, discontinuously veering toward and away from the doorknob.*

The haptic appreciation of these arm movements was unique. The fact that the point of entry of the hand into the FV appeared to be reversed engendered considerable and persistent difficulty (1/13.5–4/48):

> *Reaching down visually means reaching up, and vice versa: The reaching problem is evidently engendered by the fact that as I reach geographically upward, my arms appear to enter the FV* from above *rather than from below as used to be the case, and when I reach geographically down, my arm is seen to enter the FV from below, continuing upward. Hence, I have repeatedly reached* down *in order to hang clothes on a line above head level.*

On the second day of Stage 3, I began to develop a strategy to increase pointing accuracy (2/14–11/143):

> *A moment ago I regarded a ball at my feet, closed my eyes, and tried to point to it. I pointed toward the sky (I found out after opening my eyes) but was haptically quite convinced that I was pointing down into the sand. Only when I gain knowledge of results by opening my eyes after having pointed incorrectly and then pay careful attention to shoulder and elbow joint information on the next trial, do I assess the direction of the pointing arm correctly. Moreover, if my pointing arm or finger makes accidental contact with some object as I'm performing the pointing movement (eyes are closed), I immediately know not only the true arm position at that moment but also roughly how far off the true mark I shall be on completing the ongoing movement. Paying attention to haptic information for arm position during the movement leads to greater pointing accuracy.*

(2/14–2/14):

> *Competent reaching is visually judged to be correct: This morning my first attempt to reach slowly for the doorknob was successful. Most importantly, my hand came into the FV and* appeared to be moving in the right direction. *Yesterday (Day 1) I visually judged that arm movement to be geographically up when, in fact, it is away from the midsection and slightly downward. Subsequent reaches today, particularly if I closed my eyes just before the reach, were again substantially above the doorknob.*

(2/25–4/42):

> *Competent reaching is visually and haptically judged to be correct: My toe is exactly 2 feet from the closed bedroom door. The doorhandle is visually perceived to be far down, and once I reach it is also haptically judged to be far off. When I reach for the*

doorhandle, I visually appear to reach from "up here" to "down there"—in the direction of the top of my phenomenal head, that is, geographically down.

In spite of performatory competence, I experienced perceptual inconsistencies (2/26.5–2/26.5):

I lay in bed in the supine position with the helmet off, and I was wearing my light-occluding mask. I reached and successfully grasped my head between my hands as I had intended to. Yet, haptically, I was convinced that I had reached geographically down, *toward my knees.*

(4/48.5–4/48.5):

The rate of success of reaching for things that are clearly located up or down in the vertical plane is considerably greater than when these objects are in odd positions, off to my right or left on the diagonal.

(4/51–4/51):

Head-eye posture and the motoric up and down: It appears that a new correlation is being established between a given head-eye posture and what is now visually regarded as correct up and down reaching. Ostensibly, as concerns me as an observer of my own actions, *head posture has become an indicator of up and down reaching. This is so because I have no (haptic, so-called* proprioceptive*) information for eye posture unless the eye movements are consciously initiated after a particular head posture has been established. With the head down (in the chin-to-chest position) reaching down is now beginning to be regarded as reaching down; and with the head in the up position, reaching up is beginning to be regarded as just that.*

(6/73–6/73):

I'm beginning to feel at home with these prisms. Reaching is accurate for at least the most familiar and practical tasks, say reaching for particular doorhandles.

Eye-Head-Arm Pursuit and Errors in Head Movements (HMs)

Several of the direct observations about moving my head in the wrong direction while trying to track a moving object in the up-down plane were already presented in Chapter 2. On the second day, I additionally noted (2/13.5–2/13.5):

The observation that my head *is somehow visually controlled and guided* in much the same way *that my arms (and limbs) are during a reaching or grasping movement, is inescapable. It is as if my head were another appendage following the "commands" of the visual system!*

Although my awareness of, and conscious control over, these errors increased, they continued to occur, especially when a coordinated movement sequence was suddenly required (5/60–5/60):

> *In trying to catch a ball, my HMs (as were my arm movements) were frequently in the direction opposite to that necessary to keep the ball in the FV. These HMs preceded any arm movements.*

Figure 8.2 gives some indication of the difficulty I experienced in handshaking—in ballistically reaching for a normally extending hand—even when I kept my head stationary and consequently reached only in accordance with my pursuit EMs. Performance worsened considerably when the head was free to move also, thus introducing compensatory

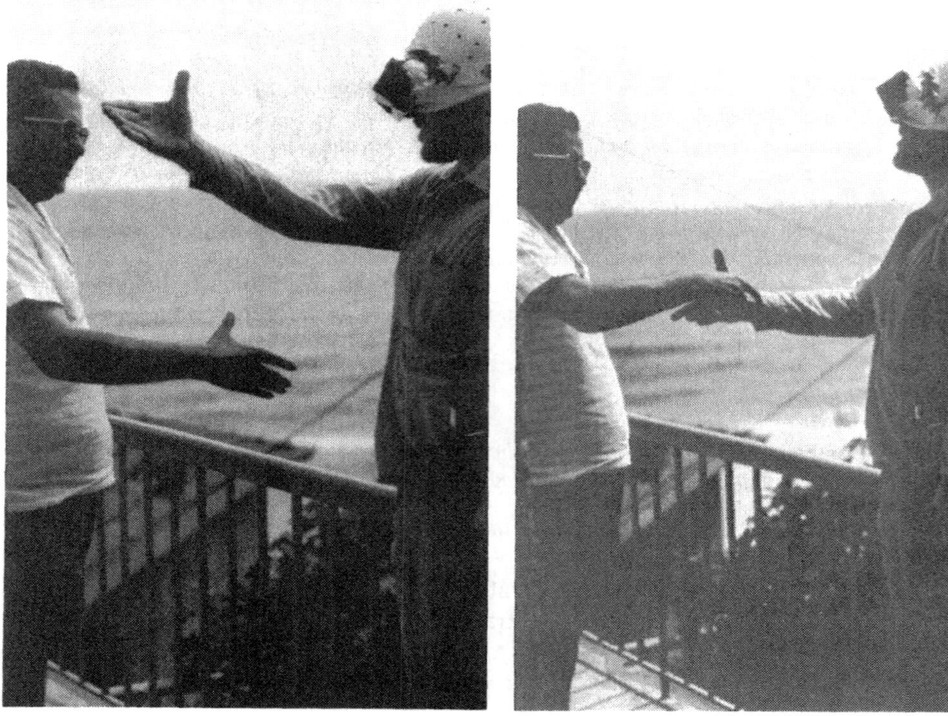

a b

FIGURE 8.2. (*a*) Attempting to shake hands wearing up–down reversing prisms; (*b*) success is finally achieved by assuming a novel head position, which keeps the reaching arm–hand in the field of view. (Stage 3 of the Prism Study.)

EMs as well. Figure 8.2b also shows the novel head posture I had to maintain to have the reaching arm-hand in my FV.

Tracking and intercepting any moving object, particularly when rapid, coordinated eye-head-arm pursuit was required, proved to be the most unmanageable visually guided action, as these observations of ball-catching in shallow water indicate (2/20–12/200):

> *Ball-throwing accurate, ball-catching totally impossible: Whenever I attempt to catch a ball thrown at me, I invariably misreach. This is true regardless of the accuracy of the throw and regardless of the consistency in the number of repetitions of a particular trajectory of the oncoming ball. One hundred throws in a session yielded 100 misreaches. When the ball comes at head level, I reach downward; when it comes at belt level, I reach skyward [see Figure 8.3a for an example on land]. After 60 hours of prism-wearing, I played ball in the water. Not once was I able to make effective contact with the ball before it hit the water surface or me. Neither did I have any idea where the ball was once it landed. Most of the time I was able to follow its trajectory, but frequently my HMs were inappropriate to that trajectory—I did the exact opposite of what I needed to do to successfully track the ball and to keep it in my FV. For example, the ball left a partner's hand going up and, in response, my head went down, filling my FV with water. As a rule, I was temporally way ahead in my (upward) hand movement in an attempt to catch the ball. Even if I managed to keep the ball in my FV at all times, I was unable to catch it once in 50 trials. . . . After 75 hours of prism-wearing: Today in some 100 trials my arms shot up into the air considerably prior in time to ball-landing, and the best I've been able to do in the last 20 trials is to keep my arms to the side of my body until the ball has hit the water. Not to reach up was literally a painful experience. Keeping my hands to my sides was difficult to accomplish because the instant I would throw my head back to visually pursue the ball, my arms would shoot up as if there were a direct coupling between the two movements. To inhibit these apparently sequentially head-yoked arm movements took some 60 trials today, and total success is not insured unless I concentrate greatly. Knowing what I must do to catch the ball seems about as irrelevant as can be to what I actually do.*

(3/30–3/30):

> *I stood on a concrete floor and threw a rubber ball (size of a cantaloupe) to the ground and tried to catch it when it bounced back. All throws were well directed and controlled. I consistently misreached the ball on its return. What I am apparently lacking is the complex coordination of judging the velocity and direction, at any point in time, of the moving ball and synchronizing this judgment with the requisite eye-head-arm movements.*

(4/51–4/51):

> *I attempted to play a tennis-like game. The only difference between this game and tennis is that the racket is of heavy wood and the size of a Ping-Pong racket. When I*

attempted to deliver the ball (overhand serve), I hit at the ball much too early and hence missed it. On the return, on the other hand, I was much too late in trying to hit it. Only after being given extensive and detailed knowledge of results—I could not figure out what I was doing wrong by myself—was I able to hit the ball while delivering it to my partner. However, even following extensive practice (40 attempts or so), my rate of success in hitting the ball for delivery was about 40%. I was unable to hit the ball even once when my partner had delivered it and it came flying toward me. Being coached as to what I was doing wrong and what I should do was of no avail in intercepting.

(11/146–15/200):

Ball-heading and -catching still virtually impossible: In about 200 throws and attempted catches, 10 were successful [see Figure 8.3]. Self-partner distance: at first, 10 feet. Throwing accurate; catching impossible. New self-partner distance: 4 feet. Caught 10 of 170. Following this lack of success, my partner began handing *me the ball—she never released it. Even so, I would clasp my hands underneath hers in order to receive the ball. Visually, what appears to be happening is quite confusing: First the ball takes a dip toward the ground and then rises toward the sky; the reverse happens, in fact. Perceiving a ball handed to me required very tiring concentration, to say nothing of ball-catching. After 10–15 minutes I'm exhausted.*

Manipulation and Hybrid Actions[7]

The immediate effects and adaptations of optical up-down reversal are exemplified by these observations on lifting, pushing, and pulling in the vertical plane (1/0–1/0):

Lifting the portable tape recorder from the table has an entirely absurd "feel," not just look; it's as if it were floating up toward me, very little effort being necessary on my part.

(1/6–7/87):

Pushing geographically down visually means (affords) lifting up, and vice versa: One of the persistent sources of frustration is that whenever I attempt to lift or pick up something, I proceed, under visual guidance, to push it down, and vice versa.

[7]During adaptation, I frequently engaged in highly atypical or "hybrid" actions, reorganizing totally what I did, not just what I visually perceived or judged myself to be doing. For example, using direct visual guidance, I twisted my right hand approximately 200° counterclockwise as I reached for a glass of juice.

FIGURE 8.3. Attempting to catch a volleyball with up–down reversing prisms. I was successful in 10 of 170 trials at a distance of 4 feet. My hand clasp is ahead of the arrival of the ball and uncommonly stiff. (Stage 3 of the Prism Study.)

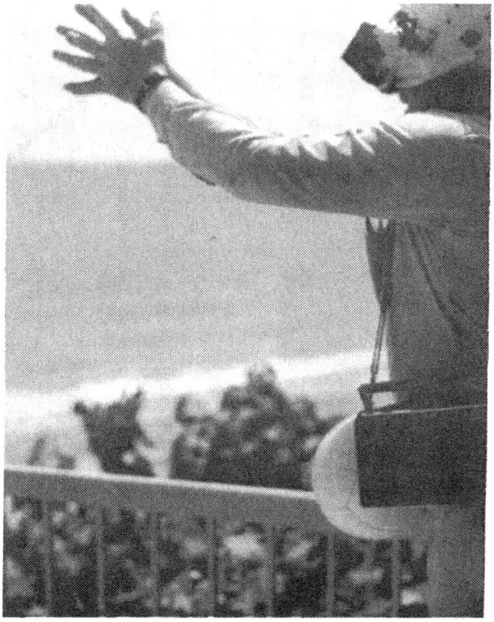

a

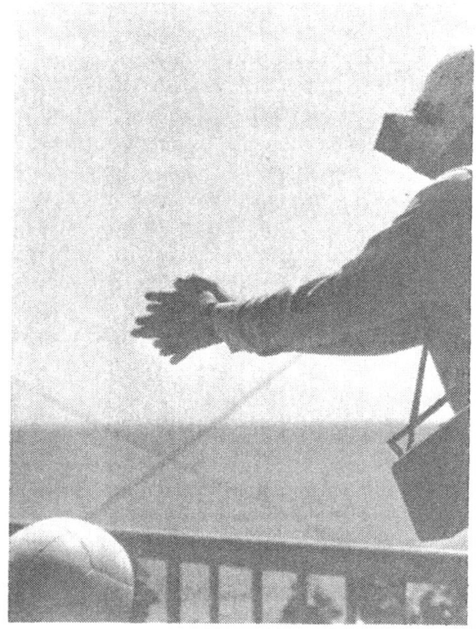

b

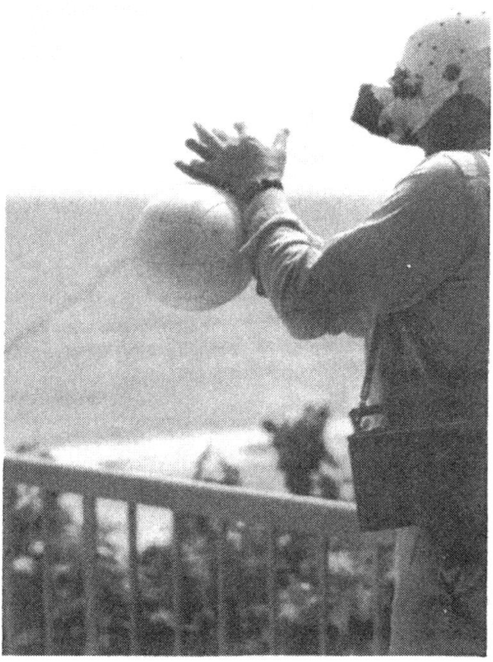

c

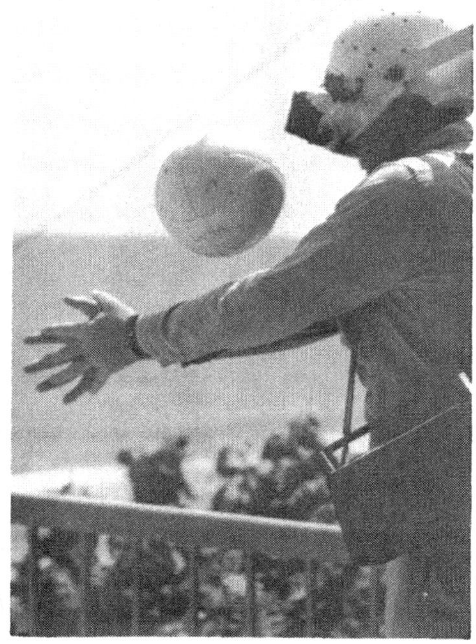

d

> *For example, I have a piece of meat on my fork which I desire to raise to my mouth. Yet I continue to push the fork* into *the plate because* visually *the* meaning *of that pushing action is the correct way to* raise *the fork. This leads to the strange haptic perception that as I am laboring to lift the fork off the plate, some hidden magnet is holding me down and preventing me from doing so. Once I manage to raise my arm off the plate—often by briefly closing my eyes or looking away—upon looking again at this arm movement I judge it to be wrong and incongruous because the visual meaning of that movement is: "You're pushing the fork* away *from you, toward the plate." Knowledge, divorced from the immediacy of perception—call it "intellectual" knowledge—is of no help in resolving these difficulties. There seems to be no immediate way of "translating" such knowledge into competing, competent performance.*

(3/38–4/48.5):

> *Pulling down is visually confused with lifting up, and vice versa: The problems with hanging or removing some clothing article from a hook are unbelievable. Visually, a hook's open (receiving) part appears to be pointing toward the ground so that anything that one might hang on it would immediately drop to the ground. Also, the visual meaning of the correct hand movement which needs to be executed to hang something on a hook—the one I have been using for years—is that it is incorrect or awkward. Thus, under visual guidance, this hand movement is "corrected." Hence, in order to take something off the hook, I have been pulling wildly, almost taking the hook with me. This action was invariably accompanied by surprise, then disbelief (that the shirt wasn't doing what a shirt in that situation should be doing visually), and finally, frustration. It took me* minutes *of pulling to convince myself that I needed to lift the shirt in order to get it down in one piece. This "convincing" required engaging in an arm movement, the visual meaning of which is contrary to its actual effect. Lifting, of course,* looks *like (visually affords) pulling, and pulling looks like lifting. Ten hours after this initial encounter, I'm not so sure anymore. If nothing else, my "hook" behavior is more appropriate on Day 4 to what hooks require as well as afford. It must be noted that the gains made in this task are virtually wiped out unless I stand directly in front of the hook; when I'm off to the side—when the hook is no longer in the sagittal plane (i.e., directly in front of my body)—the old problems spring up.*

Less expected, perhaps, are the results of near–far reaching, grasping, pushing, and pulling—of the optical reversal in the horizontal plane (1/4–2/20):

> *Reaching, grasping, and cutting: The handle of the knife on the table was actually pointing away from me (i.e., appropriate for someone sitting opposite me). When I reached for the handle of the knife, I didn't reach nearly far enough and grasped the knife by its cutting edge. Visually, this action was (looked) correct, that is, I was visually convinced that I had reached far enough to grasp the handle* until *I made the* simultaneous *comparison between the final position (location) of my hand*

relative to that of the knife handle. Cutting some meat on my plate required great concentration. At first, I attempted to "cut" the meat using the dull edge rather than the cutting edge. On first view, the orientation of the knife—cutting edge pointing toward the sky—was phenomenally the correct one to use.

(1/6–6/73):

Whenever I attempt to pull something toward me under visual guidance, I promptly proceed to push it away, and vice versa.

(4/42–4/50):

Reaching close to my body and under an obstacle, visually means reaching far away and over it: Reaching movements are still frustrating and error prone. This is particularly true of actions like reaching over a teacup to get at a slice of toast. Unless I guided my hand very slowly—which looked and felt like guiding a "phantom limb" with intentions of its own—I invariably reached short of the goal and below the cup, thereby upsetting it. I still reverse the amount of distance along a surface like a table top in reaching for a desired object. One close to my body will be reached for by extending my arm fully and one at arm's length will be reached for by hardly extending my arm. Visually, of course, the nearby object (along some surface) is way off, so that visually I'm doing the "correct" thing.

(4/48.5–4/48.5):

Reaching away from my midsection for partially occluded objects, or for objects in full view but further away or underneath others, is most difficult and least successful. During the latter reaching movement, I'm experiencing as much frustration as on Day 1 because in reaching for something on a table, I still stub my fingers on the table edge or knock over objects over which I intend to reach.

(6/77–6/77):

Day 6: This afternoon I almost pushed my son off the bed, visually convinced I was saving him from falling off the bed. Both my 1-year-old son and I were sitting on the bed. He appeared to be crawling away from me toward the edge of the bed. Actually, he was coming toward me. In order to save him from crawling off the bed, I pushed him off. It was only at the last instant—as he was going over the edge—that I realized that I was pushing rather than pulling him. This realization was a function of multiple information. Suddenly, I was leaning over the edge of the bed looking at the floor with my son going over the edge toward that floor. Yet my action again was a hybrid action, *which is so common to the adaptational limbo. . . . You see, I* grasped hold *of his clothing, yet pushed him. One does not grasp someone's clothing when the intention is to push—one uses one's unclenched palm. This was the sole reason why I was able to pull him back over the edge of the bed. If I had merely pushed him, he would have fallen. So this visually guided action was neither a clear push nor pull. It was a strange package of haptic-motoric intentions and visually guided and commanded action—a hybrid.*

(6/77–13/166):

Pushing away from me under visual guidance still confused with pulling toward me.

And finally (13/175–13/175):

Reaching movements *close to my body are still visually judged to be at arm's length, and those extending fully are visually judged to be close to my body. Examples: Washing out my bathing suit and holding a desired part of it under the running water is among one set of actions* [*that is*] *still devilishly difficult to carry out. Putting the tape recorder on a chair standing 2½ feet from my midsection is another; instead of extending my arm, I pull it close to myself (all this under visual guidance) and drop the recorder in the space between myself and the sitting surface of the chair. This error of "visually it's toward me but actually it's away from me" is really hard to overcome. I need to repeat a particular action many times to perform it competently and then to perform repeatedly this competently executed action; but this in no way insures that another task, involving the same push-pull problem, will be performed effectively. This rule has been substantiated throughout this study, time and again (e.g., learning to place the recorder correctly on the chair 2½ feet away from me will not insure putting the bathing suit under running water 2½ feet away from me, though both involve the rule: Don't pull but push your arms out.*

The apparent direction of motion and observer-directed clockwise–counterclockwise twisting was also reversed. Consistent with the observations above, adaptation occurred in certain familiar tasks but persisted in novel situations (1/12–6/73):

Twisting counterclockwise visually means twisting clockwise, and vice versa: My initial attempts to open the water spigot to wash up met with failure. I busily tightened the spigot by twisting counterclockwise. Visually, that was the correct movement for clockwise action. I didn't have the faintest idea of what was wrong, accusing others of tightening the thing to a point where I couldn't open it. After several minutes of experimenting, I managed to get water flowing. Later, instead of shutting the water down (requiring a counterclockwise turn), I flooded the kitchen. In spite of knowing what the problem was now, I was unable, under visual guidance, to turn off the water. The haptic perception of performing a clockwise turn which visually is a counterclockwise turn is totally incongruous.

(6/73–6/73):

Turning the tap on and off no longer presents the difficulties it did. Motorically, the performance of this task is smooth. Moreover, I don't recall noticing any discrepancy or contradiction between visual–haptic system information with this particular *task.*

(11/152–11/152):

Clockwise twisting movements in novel *situations are visually judged to be counterclockwise movements, and vice versa: We overloaded a fuse, and I tried to exchange it standing on a chair, fuse above my head. Knowing full well that one needs to unscrew a fuse counterclockwise, I twisted the fuse clockwise under visual guidance. This continued for* minutes. *I finally closed my eyes in utter frustration in order to succeed. On inserting the new fuse, I now screwed the fuse counterclockwise. Visually, the meaning of the hand movement was that I was twisting clockwise and hence correctly for successful completion of the task. I persisted.*

Adaptation was more readily accomplished for such everyday visually guided tasks as drinking, pouring, and eating, which require combinations of up–down, near–far, and clockwise–counterclockwise hand movements (1/2.5–2/20):

I reached for a glass of juice under visual guidance. I twisted my right hand about 200° counterclockwise so that my palm was pointing toward the sky, yet I was visually convinced that I had reached for the glass in the usual and appropriate fashion—I thought my palm was facing toward the ground. I was convinced in spite of the fact that the haptic information was that I was engaging in a unique and awkward action. When I again reached for the glass, this time palm pointing toward the table top, I was convinced, based on visual information, that my palm was facing the sky and that I would not succeed in grasping the glass. I grasped the glass and then tilted it away from me, pouring its contents on the table. The visual information was that I was tilting the glass toward myself. When I close my eyes, or the instant my hand is outside the FV, I manage to drink without complication.

(1/4–4/55):

I am trying to pour water from a glass into another glass containing lemon juice. I am holding both glasses. As one hand begins to tilt its glass to the left, so does the other. The hand which initiates the action is being "followed" by the other—as if my hands were coupled or yoked in that sequential-action fashion. [This phenomenon is reminiscent of the apparent head–leg movement yoke reported in Table A8.1, Appendix A.] That way I am, of course, simply unable to pour water into the lemon juice, or vice versa. Without success, I have tried to overcome this "magical connection" between my arms. I practiced twice, for 10 minutes each, separated by 4 hours of other activity. However, if I touch the rim of one glass to the other or if one glass remains standing on the table, I can successfully pour.

(3/40–3/40):

On several occasions today I grasped a glass and inverted it in order to drink, emptying its contents on myself.

(4/55–4/55):

I can now pour liquid successfully from a bottle into a glass provided the glass remains standing on the table.

(7/87–7/87):

No problem with any kind of pouring of liquid from one glass to another. Drinking behavior is quite smooth and error free.

Eating, too, became relatively easy, though only after a long, frustrating beginning (1/4–4/46.5):

On numerous occasions now I have lifted the fork (after finally managing to rake up some food) and noticed that the fork was facing "wrong way 'round.'" I promptly "corrected" this by twisting my hand. Now the concave part of the fork was facing the plate, and this was visually correct, in spite of the fact that I now also noticed that all the food had dropped back onto the plate. On another occasion, my visual attention was elsewhere, and I didn't notice that the fork was "wrong way 'round'" until it was halfway to my mouth. Never mind that I knew *(in the sense of being able to draw the correct conclusion) or could have deduced that the fork must be oriented correctly since it was loaded with food. As soon as I visually discovered this "error," one quick 60° counterclockwise twist of the wrist and all was well—on my trousers.*

(4/55–4/55):

Meaning change in the orientation of the fork. A clever dinner companion fed me a fork full of food, but that fork was inverted, the concave portion pointing toward the table top. The food had been speared and wound around the fork so that no food could fall off. As the fork was coming toward my face, I immediately noticed that there was something wrong with it. I reached out, took hold of the fork, and twisted it around correctly.

(6/75–6/75):

Reaching and spearing food pretty well errorless now, but increasing the speed of arm movements causes a corresponding increase in "accidents": food falling off the fork, knocking over glasses, and so on.

(7/87–7/87):

> *Eating behavior is quite smooth and error-free now, even for normally difficult tasks such as spearing olives.*

(10/138–10/138):

> *Eating behavior practically back to normal: The only difficulty which remains seems to be due to the new optically produced effective point (location) of observation at which I seem to find myself. I'm talking about the apparently novel way in which objects in the line of sight occlude other objects and events. Perhaps the problem is that particular portions of* familiar *objects and events (usually found on tables), which have never been occluded before, are now hidden by particular portions of other objects. Part of the problem seems to be that in order to see and effectively reach for these hidden objects, I must engage in a great many novel exploratory HMs. In addition, seemingly novel reaching movements are sometimes required to make contact with a particular hidden object, knocking the occluding object over.*

I adapted sufficiently to write legibly with very little practice after initial failure (2/25–2/25):

> *Writing with visual guidance a total failure: Any 6-year-old could have done better. Both visually and haptically all attempts at writing were judged to be inappropriate, awkward, and unique.*

Though far from normal, writing was reasonably legible 5 days later (8/100–14/182):

> *Writing under visual guidance is suddenly surprisingly smooth and legible, yet I have not touched a pen or pencil during the past 128 hours (75 waking hours). It appears as if somehow I have "learned" how to write again during the past 5 days. My writing movements are visually inappropriate (it "looks wrong") and haptically totally unfamiliar and awkward (it "feels wrong"). In spite of that, writing is competent and legible both to me and others [Figure 8.4].*

DISCUSSION: THE INFORMATION FOR VISUALLY GUIDED ACTIONS

Following a brief historical survey, three examples from the above data are analyzed in detail: (*a*) Vision-based pointing and visually guided reaching; (*b*) reaching for moving objects (which entails eye–head–arm pursuit and produced errors in the direction in which I moved my head); (*c*) manipulating objects, which resulted in novel or hybrid actions. The

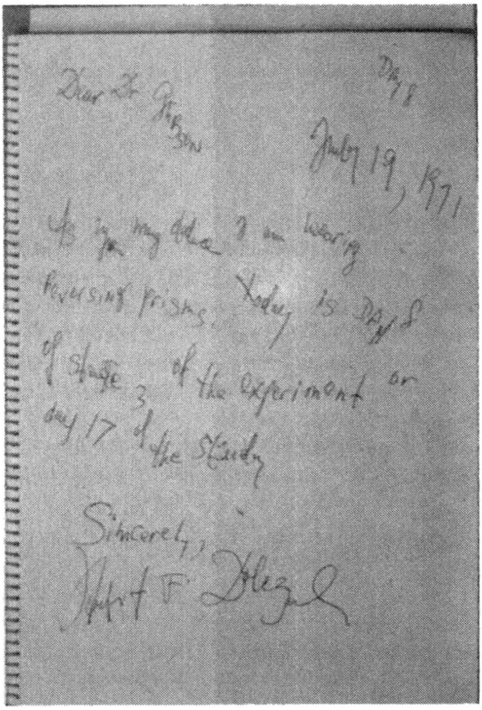

Dear Dr. Gibson Day 8

July 19, 1971

As you may know I am wearing reversing prisms. Today is Day 8 of stage 3 of the experiment or day 17 of the study

Sincerely,

Robert F. Dolezal

FIGURE 8.4. A letter written while wearing up–down reversing prisms after 8 days. My writing was legible although I had attempted to write only once prior to this on the second day of Stage 3 of the Prism Study.

principles proposed there may be fruitfully extended to many other forms of visually guided action found in the protocol and described in Tables A8.1–A8.12 in Appendix A. It will be recalled from Chapter 3 that when an observer dons the spectacles, he or she faces a new set of adapting requirements for successful looking and competent action: He or she must respond to the unchanged facts of the environment, even though where things and parts of himself-herself appear to be and where they actually are do not correspond. The data also present an opportunity to describe the information the observer uses to adapt.

Historical Precedents

Stratton: Touch–Vision Reciprocity

Helmholtz was the first to describe and analyze reaching behavior (1867, Vol. I, pp. 601–602). He fixed his gaze on the object through displacing prisms[8] and then closed his eyes during the reach. Stratton's observations on misreaching while using inverting lenses are more relevant, however, because they were the first involving an up-down reversal transformation and because his spectacles necessitated the kind of unique adapting requirements for eye-head-arm movements that are also requisite for visually guided actions in my Prism Study. Stratton's observations make clear that his visually guided movements were more than simple errors in their direction: "All movements of the body at this time were awkward, uncertain, and full of surprises . . . the movement was a series of errors and attempts at correction, until the limb was finally brought into the desired position in the visual field [1896, p. 614]." Similarly, on the first day of his 87-hour study, Stratton reports: "Almost all movements performed under the direct guidance of sight were laborious and embarrassed. Inappropriate movements were constantly made [1897b, p. 344]." And on the fourth day: "But the more common form of inappropriate reaction now was a movement of one hand when the circumstances really required a movement of the other; as when I reached with my right hand to pick up a book on the floor to my left [1897b, p. 352]." Stratton's analysis also challenges the oversimplified conclusion that sight "teaches" touch or that the latter simply accommodates itself to the former. He says: "during my experiment the translations of touch-perceptions into terms of sight continued so long in contradiction to the actual visual experience; and . . . on the other hand, the visual perceptions so long suggested tactual or motor images not in accord with the tactual or motor perceptions [1897b, p. 473]." Rather, his analysis suggests a reciprocal relationship between visual and kinesthetic-haptic perceptions. He writes: "When touch and sight agree, it means that the perceptions of sight are spatially identical with the visual suggestions produced by touch, and that the perceptions of touch are spatially identical with the tactual suggestions produced by sight [1897b, p. 481]." Finally, Stratton's descriptions of visually guided movements, although not as detailed as those offered in the present study, are congruent with the observations that I have called *hybrid* actions. Furthermore, Stratton's interpretation demonstrates an awareness that a complex relationship exists over time among the visual and haptic perceptions during the course of adaptation. I attempt to describe that complex metamorphosis.

[8]Helmholtz's method has undergone refinements culminating in an ingenious apparatus that makes it possible to displace the visual and haptic loci toward which an observer might point independently, or simultaneously, by any desired amount with or without sight of the pointing arm (Lackner, 1973, 1974). A technique for increasing the precision in measuring and recording the pointing responses of a spectacle-wearing observer has also been developed (Bauer, Woods, & Held, 1969).

Ewert: Turning the Head the Wrong Way

Stratton did not report moving his head in the unintended direction. At least two reasons may account for this fact. First, as I have shown, with a severely restricted FV, the observer has much less, and likely inadequate, optical information available that specifies head posture and is therefore less likely to notice errors in HM. Second, since Stratton's FV was considerably smaller than the one used in my study, he had considerably fewer opportunities to commit such errors on the assumption that pursuit EMs dictate the direction of pursuit-like HMs. Chances to initiate an eye-head pursuit sequence were limited with his severely restricted FV because much less time is available for coordinated action before a moving object has passed out of a small FV.

Ewert was the first investigator to notice that subjects wearing inverting spectacles often turned their heads in the wrong direction and then quickly moved in the desired direction (1930, pp. 349–350). In both instances (his "orientation" and cardsorting tasks), optical event information was available that most likely elicted pursuit EMs. Ewert did not realize, however, that errors in the direction in which the observer moves the head are closely linked to eye-pursuit movements. The observations of the Prism Study, which indicate that eye pursuit most typically precedes and apparently directs (inappropriate) head-pursuit movements, are detailed and analyzed below.

Vision-Based Pointing and Visually Guided Reaching

The psychological literature on reaching and pointing with a transformed FV is extensive and almost exclusively devoted to an analysis of the effects of lateral displacement on pointing accuracy with the dominant hand (e.g., Cohen, 1967; Harris, 1963b; Hay & Pick, 1966; Held & Hein, 1958; Helmholtz, 1867; Lackner, 1977; McCarter & Mikaelian, 1978; Melamed, Wallace, & Seyfried, 1979; Scholl, 1925, 1926; Sekuler & Bauer, 1966; Thurner, 1967; Warren & Platt, 1974, 1975; Welch, 1971; Wooster, 1923).

A Test of Vision-based Pointing Accuracy

Problem and Procedure

To my knowledge, the method of Helmholtz's pointing experiment has never been applied to an observer wearing reversing or inverting spectacles. Pointing accuracy was assessed during the Prism Study using a test modeled after Helmholtz. Three main head and eye pos-

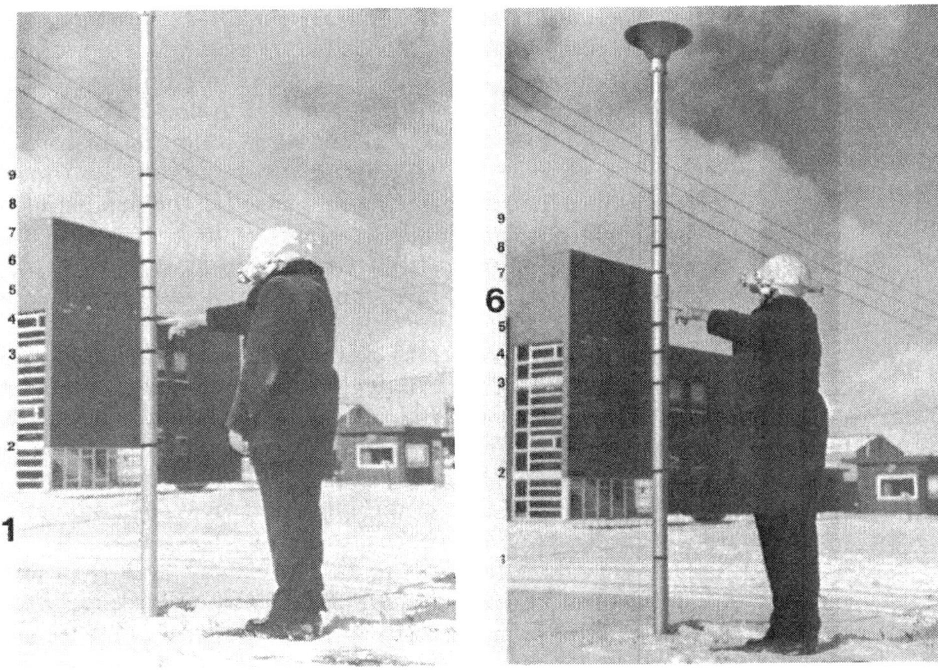

a b

FIGURE 8.5. Inaccurate pointing, with eyes closed, to the light colored tape—indicated by the bold faced letter—which I had foveated the moment before while wearing up–down reversing prisms and holding my head and eyes as follows: (*a*) Head down–eyes up; (*b*) head center–eyes down. The results of this experiment are shown in Figure 8.6. (Photos staged to depict actual results and shot at Cornell University during the winter following the taking of the actual results.)

tures, for a total of nine combinations, were used. Each head-eye posture combination corresponded to a particular location marked by black masking tape on a tall pole, which I necessarily foveated when assuming a given head–eye posture (Figure 8.5: simulation). For example, whenever I assumed the head-down–eyes-up posture prior to pointing, I foveated pole position 1, 36 cm from the ground (shown in Figure 8.5a; see also Figure 8.7 for other combinations).[9] My shoe tip to pole distance was 44.5 cm and indicated by a marker on level ground. The marker tapes on the pole were originally placed so that when I stood at this

[9]The pole in the actual study was thinner, the same color, and pieces of black masking tape were originally used as position markers. Means are represented, consisting of a total of 21 pointing responses over 7 consecutive days of spectacle-wearing during which readings were taken.

constant distance and assumed one of the nine head–eye posture combinations, the appropriate tape became visible. I began the daily session of pointing trials by stepping up to the marker on the ground and positioning my head and eyes in the primary position; to do so, I could rely on Pole Position Number 5[10] as a visual marker. I followed this procedure prior to each new pointing trial. Then a companion, who stood outside my FV and recorded all pointing responses to the nearest inch, called out a head–eye posture from a random sequence, unknown to me. Once I assumed the required head–eye posture, I closed my eyes while maintaining both postures and pointed at the just-seen marker tape (vision-based pointing).

Following each pointing with the right and dominant arm, which consisted of one smooth, ballistic movement, I maintained that arm position so that my companion could record the deviation between the intended (foveated) and obtained location. I then dropped the arm to its pretrial location—at the side of the body, out of the FV. I then returned my head and eyes to the primary position, opened my eyes, and waited for further instructions. To double check how well I had maintained the intended head–eye posture, I occasionally opened my eyes right after having pointed but after my arm was out of the FV and before returning the head and eyes to the primary position. I was quite successful, based on these spot-checks for accuracy. Prior to each pointing response and while my eyes were still open, I called out the seen pole position number to avoid error. I was given no knowledge of the results at any time.

A daily session consisted of 27 random trials or 3 pointing responses for each of the 9 head–eye combinations. The only limitation on randomness was that the same head–eye combination was not to occur more than twice in succession. The with-spectacle pointing sessions began on the ninth day of Stage 3 and continued daily through the fifteenth day in order to provide a process assessment of adaptation in this task. The aftereffect data were collected 15 minutes after I switched from the reversing prisms to the nonreversing glass. I continued daily aftereffect sessions for the entire 5 days of Stage 4. Two sessions were devoted to collecting "prespectacle" baseline data: the first one was on Day 5 of Stage 4; the second one, during the following winter at Cornell. Because both sets of baseline data are indistinguishable from one another, are very close to physically exact pointing, and display practically zero within-group variance, they were accepted as representative

[10]That I took Position 5 rather than 6 as my primary position for the eye–head system suggests that I judged my primary position to be 13–17 cm lower than I would have without prisms (see Figure 8.7 for my normal point of observation).

of the population pointing performance of Stage 2. No Stage 2 (prespectacle) baseline was taken because I had no inkling that different eye–head posture combinations could produce differential pointing behavior: Less precise observations on other pointing behavior during the first several days of Stage 3 led to the question of how the 9 different combinations of head–eye posture might influence ballistic pointing without optical knowledge of results, requiring a more rigorous test. Thus, the first with-spectacle data were not collected until Day 9 of Stage 3.

Results and Discussion

The results are shown in Table 8.1 and four representative head–eye postures are graphed in Figure 8.6. Two of these four conditions are also portrayed in Figure 8.5, which shows the mean deviation of the three daily trials from the foveated location, summed over the 7 days of testing. The bold-faced number indicates the pole position foveated by the observer. The results depicted in Table 8.1 show that as I raised my eyes, the initial pointing error increased linearly. This held for all head postures. The contribution of head postures to the initial pointing error decreased linearly as I raised my head, irrespective of the eye posture I assumed. The results show that there is something quite different about the "eyes up" posture when compared to the other eye postures, particularly when combined with the "head down" and the "head center"

TABLE 8.1
Pointing Error as a Function of Eye Posture and Head Posture While Wearing Up–Down Reversing Spectacles

Eye posture	Head posture	Target (pole) position	Mean deviation[a] from target (in inches)	No prism baseline	No prism aftereffect
Up	Down	1	42 (Figure 8.5a)	2	2
Up	Center	4	25	2	1
Up	Up	7	13	1	0
Center	Down	2	18	4	3
Center	Center	5	9	2	0
Center	Up	8	5	2	1
Down	Down	3	0	1	3
Down	Center	6	0 (Figure 8.5b)	2	0
Down	Up	9	−4	0	0

[a]A positive indicates observer pointed above the foveated location (pole position); a negative, below it. All deviations are positive unless otherwise indicated and are rounded to the nearest inch. Each mean is composed of three scores. The test results are from the first day on which the pointing test was conducted (the 9th day of Stage 3).

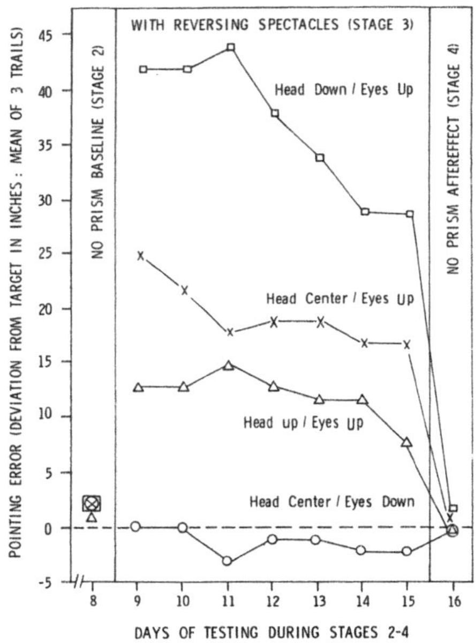

FIGURE 8.6. Pointing accuracy and its adaptation while I wore up–down reversing prisms during the Prism Study. I closed my eyes and attempted to point toward the place I had been foveating the moment before.

positions. The magnitude of error here is considerably greater, suggesting that the eyes were able to deviate more in an upward direction while the head was down or centered. If the degree of deviation directs the direction of the pointing arm, then errors of the greatest magnitude should occur where they did. Both Table 8.1 and Figure 8.6 reveal that pointing the eyes up in the head is followed by pointing more nearly in the direction of the line of fixation than foveation. This is depicted in Figure 8.7. In short, the observer points where his or her eyes are pointing, not where he or she is foveating, irrespective of head posture.

It is interesting to note that contrary to expectations, there was no aftereffect in the opposite direction once the spectacles were removed. This finding underscores my contention, further developed in Chapter 10, that the adapted observer has become *biperformatory:* He or she has learned to function competently, with or without spectacles. Operational definitions of adaptation, which depend upon an aftereffect criterion, may be sacrificing much information available in a process description of adaptation or may even arrive at the misleading conclusions that no adaptation occurred.

Overall, the data suggest that even as late as 9 days after donning

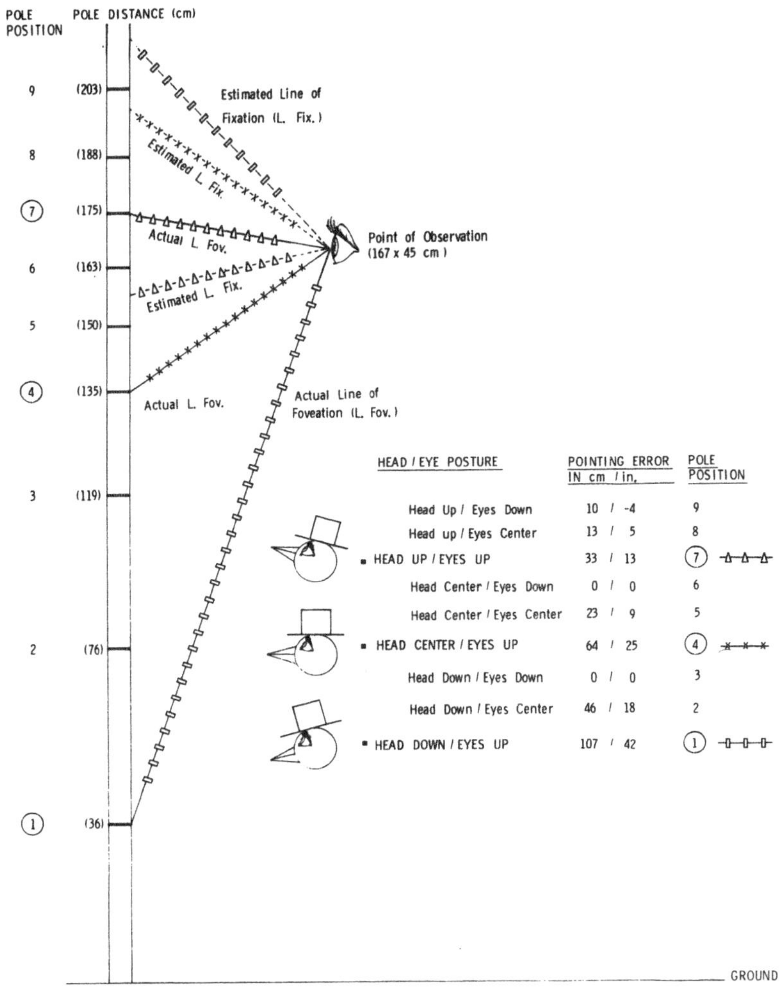

FIGURE 8.7. My estimated lines of fixation and foveation during pointing test. Data points are those shown in Figure 8.6; two are depicted in Figure 8.5 (also see Figure 3.4).

reversing spectacles, ballistic arm movements, which follow foveation of a marker and closing of the eyes, are vision-based in that they approximate more nearly the observer's line of fixation rather than his or her line of foveation. Furthermore, this vision-based action increases in accuracy, presumably benefiting from direct optical information for pointing and reaching errors witnessed by the observer before each new pointing test.

Visually Guided Reaching

New Invariants: Misleading Information during Arm Movement

Assume that it is an observer's task to reach for an object located at knee level and that his or her head remains stationary; the arms are at the sides, out of the FV. At first, the observer reaches skyward for the object, in the same direction as its virtual image and where the eyes are pointed. Moreover, the observer judges that the hand and arm entered the *top* of the FV, proceeding downward. Thus, he or she judges the direction of movement of the arm to be appropriate to the task: The reaching movement *looks like* a groundward reach. The observer makes this erroneous perceptual judgment because the direction of the optical shift during a skyward arm movement is indistinguishable from the optical shift that, in prespectacle days, specified a downward arm movement. Hence, the observer is surprised once the arm movement has ceased. The surprise is based on a visual–visual discrepancy over time: During the ballistic movement, he or she saw the arm move toward the bottom of the FV, yet, a moment later, it pointed in a direction other than the one he or she visually moved it in.

Old Invariants: Veridical Information During Arm Reaching

The observer comes to adapt in the face of such misleading optical information because he or she gets optical knowledge of results both during and after any reach. As the observer reaches skyward, while trying to reach toward the knee, the visual distance between the intended goal and the reaching hand is seen to progressively increase rather than decrease! Thus, instead of progressively concealing places closer and closer to the desired object until it is hidden by the observer's hand—the essence of grasping—the observer instead visually perceives that the hand reveals progressively more background close to the object. During the early stages of adaptation in the Prism Study, when I reached slowly for an object, I observed my hand as it alternately approached and veered away from the object—as if pulled by two equally strong magnets that ceased working intermittently, each allowing the other temporary control over the direction in which the arm proceeded. This is a vivid example of performing on the basis of two sets of concurrently available *optical* information—one confusing the observer by erroneously specifying the *direction* of arm movement and the other veridically specifying the *distance* of the hand from the object and thereby also the appropriate direction in which to move. (I have deferred until Chapter 11 a discussion of Harris' assumption that "adaptation results from a discrepancy between proprioceptive and visual information [Harris,

1965, p, 440].''). Thus, during adaptation, I attempted corrections of the trajectory of my arm, based on (*a*) veridical end-point information from the last reach and (*b*) veridical information about progressive distance from the goal during the reach.

More Veridical Information Available at the Conclusion of an Arm Movement

The visual contradiction during arm movement is optically reaffirmed after the arm comes to rest: The observer notices the discrepancy between the intended goal and the achieved result—he or she has reached toward the head for an object actually at knee level. This visual discrepancy became most informative during my study when (*a*) there was a maximum separation or visual ''gap'' between the final position of the hand and the reached-for object and (*b*) when both the hand and the object were simultaneously in the FV at the conclusion of an erroneous movement. Moreover, the longer I was able to view this discrepancy at the end of the reaching movement, the more aware I became that there was a discrepancy between the visually judged trajectory and the end-position of the arm. Finally, the slower the reach, the more obvious was the contradiction between the visually judged direction of arm movement and the progressively increasing distance between the hand and the object for which I reached.

Dynamic Adaptation: Eye–Head–Arm Pursuit and Errors in Head Movements

The data for visually guided actions like pointing and reaching for stationary objects and pursuit of moving objects suggest a distinction between static and dynamic adaptation. *Static adaptation* concerns tasks that require saccadic EMs for successful completion and are readily accomplished. *Dynamic adaptation* concerns tasks that require eye-head-arm pursuit, characteristically mixed with saccadic and compensatory EMs. Such tasks were exceedingly difficult to accomplish competently. Indeed, despite many hundreds of practice trials, I was unable to learn the eye-head-arm coordination required to catch a ball or return a tennis volley—to keep an oncoming object in the FV and to intercept it.

Static and Dynamic Adaptation: A Function of of Saccadic versus Pursuit Eye Movement Control Systems

How adaptation proceeds, how long it requires to be achieved, and what final level of accomplishment may be reached are cofunctions of two factors: (*a*) The type of EM demanded of the observer and (*b*) the unique adapting requirements that link those EMs to how the observer now must move the head and arms to act competently. A stationary observer with reversing spectacles must learn that when the eyes point *up* in the head by a given angle relative to the primary position while the head is in a known position, if he or she points *down* by the *equivalent* deviation from the primary position, he or she will point correctly (cf., Figures 3.4 and 8.7). In that sense, a perceived change in the meaning of directing one's gaze is a component of the adaptation process.

Clearly, such a change in the perceived *direction* of gaze is quite unsatisfactory as an account of adaptation when eye-head pursuit or eye-head-arm pursuit are required for action. Successful pursuit of an event requires that the observer move the head and arm in a direction opposite to the eyes (cf., Chapter 3). As in prespectacle days, I tended to move my head in the direction of the pursuit EM. With spectacles, such HMs produce an apparent shift of the border of the FV opposite to the direction of object motion, thereby defeating continued foveal pursuit. Meager veridical information for adaptation is available to the observer during pursuit tracking and at its conclusion. Provided the observer can already distinguish between his or her own HM and the swaying motions of the FV, the object's movement out of the FV when the observer makes an incorrect HM constitutes direct optical information for the error. Moreover, at the termination of the head or arm movement, the observer gains end-point information for having moved in the wrong direction: He or she sees sky at the end of the HM and sees himself-herself pointing skyward. Significantly, the observer is handicapped in two ways for detecting what the nature of the error was and how he or she can correct the situation (i.e., how to adapt). First, the faster the moving object to be pursued, the less time the observer has to visually perceive and act upon simultaneous optical information *during* the head and arm movement about the direction in which he or she is moving relative to the direction in which the object is moving. Second, the observer does not have the luxury of comparative discrepant optical information after this head and arm movement have been executed because the event is over: The ball is rolling on the ground before the observer has a chance to see how he or she misreached.

Dynamic Adaptation: Two Requirements

Two requirements must be met by the visuomotor system to bring about competent eye-head-arm tracking. First, decoupling of the head and arms from their evidently firm dependence upon eye pursuit: From the direction in which the eyes *are moving*. Second, the motor commands the observer must learn to issue have to be quite different for the head and arm than for the eyes: They must conflict in the direction in which they "aim" their respective body parts. The evidence cited from the Prism Study suggests that the decoupling may be accomplished for the head but is much more difficult for the arms because I ceased making errors in the direction of my HMs, provided I did not attempt to reach concurrently.[11] The evidence suggests that the ability to move the head or the arms in the direction opposite to the optical events that elicit a pursuit EM is critically dependent upon the rate of the optical shift. A slow event such as a large ant walking up a wall produced no problem: Even if a HM in the wrong direction was initiated, I had enough time to introduce a correction. However, a rapid event such as the flight of doves or a flying ball frequently resulted in an inappropriate HM and invariably elicited an incorrect reaching movement: Even after many hours and many hundreds of attempts at catching balls, spaced over the full 15 days (200 hours) of exposure to reversing spectacles, I was unable to succeed with any degree of consistency.

Introspectively, the head seemed to be used as just another visually guided appendage: The errors in the direction of HM seem induced by EMs that precede the HM in time and determine its direction. On a good number of occasions, I experienced surprise that my head looked and felt, not as if I had carried out an intended HM, but as if it had been ordered to move or as if it had *been* moved before I had a chance to do so intentionally. Moreover, the initiation of the HM appeared to precede the start of the arm movement. In the pursuit situation, the visual system appears to function as a hierarchical control system in which the optical information that is used to direct the eyes also directs the head, then the arms, then the legs, and finally the body as a whole. A direct relationship with the specific direction in which the eyes are moved is established and functions fairly rigidly, particularly *during* pursuit tracking of events.

Complex Dynamic Adaptation

The perceptual control of complex action (e.g., playing soccer, handball, Ping-Pong, or tennis) requires split-second reaction and coordinated precision. What really happens when the spectacle-wearer tries to catch a ball that is closing fast? Several EM control systems (cf., Carpenter, 1977; Sanderson & Whiting, 1978) participate in this form of

[11]Haptic information was of some limited use in inhibiting errors in the direction of HM, provided I made a special effort to consciously monitor its presence and to use it at that time.

visual guidance, and all are capable of directing a HM and reaching movements. The typical scenario, especially for events not anticipated by the observer, is this: As the ball enters the FV, the observer intercepts it with a quick saccadic EM, followed rapidly by a HM in the direction of the saccade. The HM almost instantaneously elicits a vestibular compensatory EM to keep the fovea "on target." This vestibular compensatory EM is then rivaled by a light-dependent compensatory EM (see Chapter 7), which attempts to move the eyes and the head in the opposite direction. Finally, a coordinated eye-head-arm pursuit sequence is initiated to track the moving object at its velocity, moving the head and arms in the same direction as the eyes and precisely opposite to the ball's actual direction of motion.

This much seems clear: The evidence of the Prism Study—underscored by the evident complexity of coordination among the saccadic, compensatory, and pursuit systems of controlling EMs, HMs, and limb movements—militates strongly against a simple interpretation that suggests that adaptation consists of proprioceptive changes—changes in the felt location of body parts (Harris, 1965; see Chapter 11 for an expanded discussion).

The information that is normally available to the nervous system or that is made available by moving any body part is critical for establishing and maintaining normal competent action. Reestablishing disrupted action, following exposure to optical transforming spectacles, is no less dependent on these sources of information. The information the observer uses in both situations is in three basic forms: (*a*) Current and past perceptions of himself-herself in the world; (*b*) current and past motor output (efferences) to the musculature, produced by the observer to initiate bodily movements; and (*c*) various forms of (perceptually) preparing for and predicting the motor output before it is executed, monitoring it while it is ongoing, and changing the motor output after its occurrence. Even though I have emphasized the role of afferent optical information in renewing competent action—and I am convinced of its preeminent importance—it is clear that the great variety and flexibility of performatory capabilities require postulating the following mechanisms. They can work sequentially, concurrently, cybernetically, synergistically, in consort, and in ways as yet dimly understood (cf., Stelmach, 1976, on motor control mechanisms).

1. *Current perceptions:* Normally the observer has available afferent optic, haptic-kinesthetic, acoustic, and other forms of information before, during, and after engaging in any bodily movement. These forms of information covary, redundantly specifying the facts as they are. The

information gained is relational and direct, informing the observer about the contingency relations between his or her actions and environmental events. Example: awareness or registration of how reaching for an apple fared.

2. *Past perceptions:* Current perceptions are supported by a progressively richer pool of stored past perceptual schemas and may be said to contain *predictions* as to the nature of forthcoming perceptual change once the observer initiates action, based on past actions and how they looked, felt, sounded, etc.

3. *Current and past efference:* To direct action, the observer has available a vast known repertoire of ready motor programs for appropriate, situationally contingent actions, based on past perceptual information that specified the task requirements in similar circumstances. Current efferences are thus also *predictive* since they are rooted in past efference. Yet current efference depends on current perceptions for competent action.

4. *Produced efference:* To affect action, motor commands are executed, based on current perceptions and current efferences. Produced efference produces feedback that is perceptually available. This reafferent information is used to modify and direct subsequent produced efference. Example: the power, direction, speed, and extent of the reach used to get the apple.

5. *Efferent monitoring of efference:* It is likely that the system is capable of monitoring and comparing predictive efference with produced efference and either or both of these with produced efference. The system may also be able to compare predictive efference with predictive perception. As indicated earlier in this chapter, I doubt the *necessity* of these steps.

6. *Perceptual monitoring of efference:* Similarly, it is likely that the system is capable of comparing, via afferent perception, predictive perception, and predictive efference with concurrent afferent information. Again, I question its necessity. What the system does undoubtedly do, and to good effect, is directly perceive its own performance, introduce midcourse corrections on the basis of that afferent information, and modify future action. This inevitable acitvity is best thought of as perceptual monitoring of action and leads to reestablishing competent action by optimizing predictive perception and predictive and produced efference.

7. *Modification of produced efference and of predictive perception:* The original motor program and predictive efference are "fine-tuned." Similarly, perceptual schemata are brought in line with the perceptions available during and following action (cf. Williams, 1978).

Competent action, disrupted by optical transformations, can be reestablished as long as some invariant relationship can be discerned among current perceptions, produced efferences, and perceptual monitoring of efference. I have argued that perceptual monitoring is the key to apprising the observer of the new requirements for competent coordinated movements: Most importantly, the observer *sees* the consequences of his or her movements during and after their execution.

Hybrid Actions

Visual and Haptic Perceptions during Incompetent and Competent Action

An action can appear visually to be performed competently or incompetently: Doing something can "look" "right" or "wrong" to the observer; concurrently, body movements, particularly arm–hand movements, can be haptically experienced as "feeling" "right" or "wrong";[12] and of course, actions are well or poorly coordinated and more or less competent, all relative to prespectacle days. During the adaptation of a wide variety of tasks in the Prism Study, I experienced every combination of right and wrong looks and feels while I found myself performing highly atypical actions that ranged from being highly incompetent to highly competent. I call these *hybrid* actions.

The hybrid actions described here are unique for two reasons. First, the actual movements I executed differed greatly with respect to the way in which I moved and twisted my whole body (e.g., the way I twisted my shoulder, elbow, and wrist joints in order to grasp and handle a fork). I even moved and positioned my head in novel ways to guide and inspect limb movements. The relationship among all these body parts was often entirely uncommon, much as it might be if a novice made a clumsy attempt to imitate some complex movement sequence demonstrated by an expert. Second, the visual and haptic-perceptual accompaniments to such actions were also unique, featuring all combinations of right and wrong looks and feels during and after a movement sequence. Moreover, the visual and haptic-kinesthetic perceptions at the termination of an action often did not concur with the look and feel during the action, either with respect to the perceived *location, orientation,* or *direction of movement* of the body part used.

The principles of the analysis offered for visually guided reaching

[12]For ease of expression, I will call these perceptions the "right" or "wrong" "look" or "feel" of (accompanying) action. Quotation marks will no longer be used.

can also be applied to hybrid actions. What looks wrong about a correctly executed action is (*a*) the point of entry of the hand into the FV and (*b*) the direction of the trajectory of the hand and arm. Optical end-point information appears more easily utilized when the reach is up or down than when either a near-far or clockwise-counterclockwise arm movement is executed. The near-far confusion (reversal) proved particularly resistant to adaptation. An added difficulty was the perception that my hand appeared to be pointing toward my midsection when the fingers were actually pointing away from the body. While the "static" distance-from-self to some stationary object was judged correctly, such that an already extended arm was visually perceived to be extended, the perception of the "dynamic" distance-from-self was another matter. With the initiation of an arm movement toward an object straight ahead of the body, moving away from self was at first judged visually as moving toward, even "into," myself. Consequently, I arrested and often drew back the extending arm. Once stopped, end-point information clarified that I had not moved far enough to make contact with the desired object, and the cycle began anew. The haptic-kinesthetic perceptions that accompanied such maneuvers were nothing short of physically uncomfortable, sometimes even painfully reminiscent of a cramp. In reaching for an object such as a glass, the orientation of the hand relative to the object was at first misjudged, resulting in bizarre contortions of the arm and hand so that it might "look right." At some extreme, haptic-kinesthetic information obtruded itself upon consciousness and signaled the onset of possible damage if the contortion should persist. For example, I twisted my right hand by approximately 200° counterclockwise in an effort to get it to look right as I reached for and began to grasp a glass.

Hybrid Actions Outside and Within the Field of View

In describing the process of adaptation, it is important to distinguish between the conscious visual and haptic-kinesthetic accompaniments of actions inside as opposed to outside the FV while an action is ongoing. As a rule, if the action occurred *outside* the FV (i.e., not under direct visual inspection), then adaptation proceeded thus: (*a*) At first, the feel of actions was stable, unhesitating, secure, and competent (e.g., observation 1/4–2/14, p. 165); (*b*) actions occasionally felt wrong, awkward, incompetent, insecure, and they were, in fact, incompetent (e.g., observation 2/20–12/200, p. 169). "Pure" examples are hard to find. Moreover, visual information was often available just before and may well have "carried over" to influence the haptic perception; (*c*) during the later stages, actions were accompanied by feeling right, though the actions in question were incompetently performed (e.g., observation 2/14–11/143, p. 166); (*d*) finally, performing both felt right and was competent (e.g., observation 10/138–10/138, p. 177).

If, on the other hand, the action was under direct visual inspection, then adaptation with its accompanying perceptions proceeded thus: (*a*) At first, actions felt wrong but looked right (haptic-visual conflict), even though they were hesitant, unsuccessful and frustrating (e.g., observation 1/2.5–2/20, p. 175); (*b*) not infrequently, actions both felt and looked right (haptic-visual agreements), though they were incompetent (e.g., observation 1/2.5–7/87, p. 165); (*c*) at a yet later stage, adaptation was occasionally accompanied by feeling right and looking wrong, though the action was competently performed[13] (e.g., observation 1/4–4/46.5, p. 176. Very few, if any, "pure" cases were noted.); (*d*) finally, actions both felt and looked right and were competent, (e.g., observation 6/73–6/73, pp. 176–177). When actions were competent they typically felt right before they looked right: Wrong looks persisted longer than wrong feels.

Perceptual End-Product: Visual Meaning Attained

The most salient accompaniment of an action coming to look right was a change in the *meaning* of that action. Indeed, one end-product of adaptation was that relationships between the performing self and objects and events began to make sense once more. These relationships took on an air of predictability and of a newly wrought familiarity that, though distinguishable from the old, prespectable familiarity, was coming to be just as sound functionally and beginning to provide usable information.

Performatory and Perceptual Adaptation: Metamorphosis and Meaning Change

Many visually guided actions went through a complex metamorphosis until a meaning change was achieved. The adaptation of action, with its conscious perceptual concomitants, did not proceed from simple errors attended by "misperceptions" to errorless action accompanied by veridical and unconfusing perceptions. Adaptation did not advance

[13]The apparent rule, "once an action is performed competently it will both look right and feel right," was not without exception. For example, on the second day, I attempted to write under visual guidance. Performatorily, this attempt was a conspicuous failure, and the visual and haptic accompaniments were that writing looked and felt inappropriate, awkward, and as if it were a uniquely difficult skill. Writing was surprisingly smooth and legible after 128 hours (75 waking hours), although I had not touched a pen in the interim. Yet, writing looked *and* felt wrong.

simply, efficiently, and smoothly. Rather, several forms of adaptation went through a complex perceptual and performatory metamorphosis that cannot be adequately characterized within a simple touch-vision dichotomy. Before perceptual consistency and performatory competence are achieved, this metamorphosis is typically composed of every possible combination of experiencing the action as visually and haptically correct and-or incorrect and of actually being incompetent or competent. At the conclusion of this variable process, the end-product of adaptation frequently includes a change in the felt position of body parts, as Harris (1963a,b, 1965) has emphasized (see Chapter 11 for a full discussion of this position).

The most conspicuous perceptual end-product of adaptation to visually guided action, however, is visual, almost cognitive. Both incompetent and competent actions were accompanied, more and more, by a new, visually gained understanding of what events signified and what my actions meant. These perceptual changes were exemplified by realizing and anticipating that flicking my eyes up in the head by means of a self-directed eye jerk would yield a view of the ground underfoot. At a more complex level, such meaning changes enabled me to predict accurately the trajectory of a moving object or they helped me to know, even before the conclusion of a reaching movement, whether the reaching hand would arrive at the desired place or that my hand was twisted in the wrong direction to succeed at grasping an object. I contend that these newly gained forms of predicting the consequences of simple events and actions and the newly achieved understanding of the meaning and affordances of more complex interactions with the environment are based on this: The observer once again notices optical invariants that veridically specify the true meaning of his or her actions and the true characteristics of environmental events. Moreover, I contend that the novel invariants that at first confuse and mislead the observer take on a new meaning, congruent with what the old invariants have specified all along. Thus, the observer's actual skyward reach at first confuses him or her because the arm looks as if it were moving groundward; however, many repetitions of this optical event produce a meaning change. These optical motions come to signify the observer's action in accordance with the true facts—as a skyward reach. Moreover, the true meaning of the optical event, provided by end-point information, becomes superfluous.

In summary, the rate and course of adaptation to visually guided action appears to be a function of the unique adapting requirements demanded of the observer during action (i.e., the kind of eye-head-arm-hand-foot-body combinations required by his or her task. The kind of EMs necessitated is particularly crucial in establishing whether an observer will adapt and in limiting how quickly and how well he or she will come to perform in a well-coordinated and competent manner. EMs and task requirements that maximize attending to veridical invariants will facilitate adaptation. Also, the frequency with which such movements are attempted and viewed undoubtedly figures in the rapidity of adaptation.

SUMMARY

The information in this chapter, more than in any other, helps answer some basic questions that constitute the epistemological context of this book: "How dependent is knowing and doing on perceiving?" and "How do humans perform successfully in the real world?" In this chapter I begin to answer these questions by offering a description of the interdependence of perceiving and acting. A discussion follows of the optical information that permits a spectacle-wearer to achieve three accomplishments upon which successful action depends. The first two constitute the phenomenon of *visual direction constancy* (VDC): First, VDC exists when objects in the field of view (FV) do not appear to move during eye movements (EMs). Second, VDC exists when objects appear to remain in the same direction relative to the observer even though he or she has moved the eyes to a new position. Third, competent action depends on having accurate information for the position of the eyes and other body parts.

Using Stage 3 of the Prism Study as a paradigm, I then describe the immediate effects of and adaptations to wearing up–down reversing prisms for a variety of visually guided actions. In the concluding section I discuss the information the observer has for the adaptation of three classes of visually guided action: vision-based pointing and visually guided reaching; dynamic adaptation represented by eye–head–arm pursuit; and hybrid actions.

I argue that objects in the FV do not appear to move during saccadic EMs because they do not and because the observer has direct optical information for that fact: Objects retain their relative position before and after an EM. Moreover, the observer can *see* that he or she has moved the eyes as soon as he or she has done so because the observer can see that he or she is now looking at a different place than before. Both discriminations may suffice to assure the observer's experience of a stable world during saccadic EMs. Three other accounts of the phenomenon are considered less plausible: (*a*) That vision is "suppressed" during saccades; (*b*) that the visual system continually accounts for the effort of will required to execute any saccade; and (*c*) that storing and "canceling" the motor commands issued to the eye muscles is required to differentiate environmental and retinal motion during a saccade.

Many visually guided actions (such as being oriented, successful locomotion, and reaching) also depend on stationary objects appearing to remain in the same direction relative to the observer's point of observation before, during, and after an EM. I contend that this second aspect of VDC is given by afferent optical information. First, the visual system can distinguish between a body movement that generates changes in the optic array that fills the observer's FV and those that do not because, if the observer moves his or her eyes back to their previous position, the object he or she fixated will still be *there* and will not appear displaced. Second, the observer *sees* that the relative positions of objects visible during the fixation have remained constant once the second fixation commences. Third, objects, places, and body parts visible during the first fixation go out of sight, and objects and body parts that were not visible come into view during the next fixation. These forms of optical information are available concurrently and they covary: The observer is thus directly apprised of where objects, places, and body parts are located relative to one another even though the light reflected from them falls on different places on the retina during and following changes in fixation.

I then show that effective visually guided actions are dependent on the accurate perception of the location and orientation of the observer's stationary and moving body parts relative to one another and relative to objects, places, and events in the environment. In particular, the observer cannot be expected to achieve VDC or to act competently unless he or she has accurate knowledge of the position of the eyes and the location of other body parts. I argue that by far the most precise and reliable information the observer has for the position of the eyes, as well as for having moved the eyes from one fixation to the next, is available in the optic array that fills his or her FV. The observer knows the position of the eyes in the head because assuming any eye posture yields an unique and invariant view to each eye of a particular portion of the eye's bony orbit, nose, head, and other body parts. Moreover, these unique sights are embedded in an *optical frame of reference,* a richly textured environmental context that allows the directing of EMs and the monitoring of each relative eye position by the visual system. The fine optical structure visible during the last fixation is uniquely different from the present fixation, and hence the observer knows that he or she is looking at a different place in the world. The extent and direction of the EM and the new eye position are specified by the *relational* optical information the observer picks up about the body parts relative to the portions of the environment visible because of changes in fixation. Thus, maintaining an eye posture, as well as any change in eye posture, yields a unique view of the observer's own body relative to unique portions of the environment. Eye position is then specified by the special *seen* relationship between particular parts of the visible body and the environment. Information about eye posture is also shown to be made available to the observer during compensatory EMs, in the dark, and whenever the observer "parks the eyes" in the primary position.

That this book is a treatise in defense of visual knowledge is best illustrated by the results and adaptations of acting in a world transformed. When an observer dons spectacles, his or her perceptions of the environment and himself–herself are reshaped. His or her actions, which are based on these perceptions, are changed accordingly. Only after visually guided actions in the transformed world are performed and perceived by the visual system and performed again will adaptation to the new world begin. Indeed, *perceptual adaptation* to watching myself act proceeded from an initial stage of confusion and surprise to a final stage of perceptual–performatory consistency, lack of surprises, and an understanding of the perceptual meaning of actions. *Performatory adaptation* proceeded from an initial stage of disorientation, incompetence, and variability to a final stage of performatory competence. In particular, gross motor actions were accomplished most readily. Visually guided reaching during fixation or directed by saccadic EMs took longer. Fine motor coordination was achieved but presented even greater difficulty. Some visually guided actions such as catching a ball, which require the rapid coordination of eye–head–arm pursuit, were never executed satisfactorily in spite of 15 days of practice. Thus, the course of adaptation seemed to be a function of the kind of visuomotor control system that directed a given coordinated sequence of movements. This is a highly significant fact for theories of adaptation.

The directional characteristics of vision-based pointing (i.e., pointing after closing one's eyes) appear to be governed by the judged direction of positioning the eyes and foveating a target prior to closing of the eyes. The prism-wearer's initial mispointing and eventual correct pointing suggest that such vision-based action is also partly contingent on the observer having stored in memory visual–cognitive representations of the layout of the body within a context of familiar environments. Adaptation of vision-based pointing is a change in perception in that the new and quickly dominant transformed visual memories direct the initial mispointing. Correct vision-based reaching is achieved when the observer undergoes a change in the meaning of the judged direction of foveation along with a change in the meaning of the judged direction of the eyes before pointing. In that sense, a perceived change in the meaning of directing one's gaze is a component of adaptation.

When vision is allowed to guide action directly, as in reaching, the observer's task is to reach toward the true location of the object, not in the direction in which he or she points the eyes—not toward the object's virtual image. Adaptation consists of a process during which the observer at first reaches in the direction of the virtual object and visually judges the direction of that reach to be accurate during the arm movement. However, at the end of the reaching movement, the observer has veridical end-point information for having misreached. He or she uses this old invariant to correct the reach, even though an accurate reach now looks to be moving away from the desired object. One important aspect of adaptation is a change in perception, such that the originally novel sight of the observer's correct reaching movement during and after the reach are accepted as commonplace and the observer no longer suffers confusion about the relative location and orientation of arm-hand movements with reference to the object and its environmental background. Reliable changes in action are based on these perceptual adaptations, I believe. The process of adaptation of such visually guided actions is a vivid example of acting on the basis of two sets of concurrently available optic information: one confusing the prism-wearer by erroneously specifying the direction of arm movement and the other veridically specifying the distance of the hand from the object during the reach and thereby also revealing the appropriate direction in which to move. At the conclusion of the movement, the optical confirmation for moving in the correct direction during the reach and for having moved accurately constitutes the sufficient information for performatory adaptation. Control of action is thus partly the result of noticing any discrepancy between required and achieved action. More precisely, competent action disrupted by an optical transformation can be reestablished, provided some invariant relationship can be discerned by the observer among current perceptions, motor output to the musculature, and the perceptual monitoring of the consequences of that output.

With reversing prisms, successful catching, which consists of coordinated eye-hand-arm pursuit entails a unique adapting requirement: The head and arms must move in a direction opposite to the eyes. I failed to achieve this adaptation, remaining incompetent throughout 15 days of intermittent practice. In order for such dynamic adaptation to come about, two adapting requirements must be met by the visuomotor system. First, a "decoupling" of the head and arms from their evidently firm dependence on the direction of eye pursuit movements must occur, and second, motor commands radically different from those that direct the eyes must be issued to direct the head and arms. The evidence shows that coordinated movements that make use of eye fixations, compensatory EM and saccadic EM control mechanisms adapt. Coordinated head–body movements that are directed by the pursuit system are, to say the least, considerably more refractory to adaptation. Consequently, the data make necessary different interpretations about the nature of adaptation depending on two factors: the type of EM demanded of the observer and the directional characteristics of eye and body movements that link those EMs to how the observer must move to act competently. It follows that we must abandon any simple interpretation of the nature of adaption as consisting of one kind of change rather than another. Indeed, achieving coordinated precision of split-second reactions should be described as *complex dynamic adaptation* because all forms of visuomotor control are recruited in such actions. The preeminent importance of afferent optical information in the process of restoring performatory competence for the prism-wearer is amply illustrated.

That the nature of adaptation to optical reversal is complex is underscored by the adaptation phenomena I call *hybrid actions:* As the observer, I moved in entirely uncommon ways, frequently combining components of actions that were incompetent and competent in brief succession. Moreover, I visually and haptically judged such actions to be correctly or incorrectly executed, irrespective of whether they actually were competent. Before adaptation was accomplished, many visually guided actions went through a perceptual–performatory metamorphosis rather than a linear-sequential correcting of "misperceptions" and "simple errors."

9

Perceiving in a World Transformed: The Self and Events

Changes in appearance noticed in everyday life are often difficult to pin down. When, precisely, did the city block to which I recently moved begin to look unmistakably different from the way it appeared when I first saw it? When did I cease caring that the toes of my feet, seen through up-down reversing prisms, appear to point toward myself rather than away from me? When did walking forward, which at first looked as if I were walking into myself, begin to mean (signify) that I was walking forward? Indeed, when did the many incongruous and aesthetically morbid sights, including print, facial expressions, and people's walking movements, assert their congruity and become aesthetically pleasing sights again?

This chapter is specifically about how the world and the self look when one gazes at them through reversing spectacles and how the world and the self change in what they mean and how they appear over the days. Because appearances and meaningfulness are closely tied to the perceived location and orientation of both the regarded objects and the seen body (Howard & Templeton, 1966; Rock, 1966, 1974), I treat the relationship between perceiving oneself and the environment. The spectacle-wearer's perception of the self is emphasized because usable data on the subject is sparse (Peterson & Peterson, 1938; Stratton,

1897b). The observer's perceived body–environment relationship is divided into two overlapping categories, primarily *world-relative observations* (event perception) and primarily *self-relative observations*. World-relative observations are those during which the observer primarily attends to the characteristics of the environment with rather less awareness of body parts and point of observation. Self-relative observations are those during which the observer is clearly aware of the location and orientation of seen body parts, including the point of observation.

RESULTS OF THE PRISM STUDY

Immediate Effects: Perceptual Disorientation and Confusion

1. I experienced what I call *initial massive meaninglessness*[1] (perceptual confusion) regarding the location relative to self of places, objects, and events.
2. Particularly when regarding once *familiar* places, objects, pictures, script, facial features, and events like smiles, I applied such labels as "uncanny," "weird," "novel," "surrealistic," "strange," "bizarre," "uncommon," and "surprising." Thus, I had the greatest difficulty in recognizing once familiar persons and reading normally oriented print.
3. I initially judged both the *orientation* and *location* of my head to be somehow different from what it had been preexperimentally and different from that of other persons.

I did not experience any initial uncertainty about the *visually* perceived orientation of my hands and feet: Fingers and toes were clearly perceived as pointing toward my midsection (see Figure 9.1). Moreover, the feet were now perceived to protrude into my field of view (FV) from its top border, extending toward the bottom edge. Mostly, the *haptically* perceived orientation and location of my head and other body parts were *indeterminate,* or I had difficulty attending to them or noticing them.

[1]The reader may attain some appreciation of this phenomenal experience for an observer with a stationary head by looking at Figure 7.1 through a rolled up paper tube and by inverting any other photograph depicting a natural scene, even those that include people. Some perceptual confusion may be experienced even though the reader does not have the optical information specifying reversal of the self vis-à-vis the optically projected environment and even though these are but static pictorial representations. A more strenuous method is to look at the world from between one's legs.

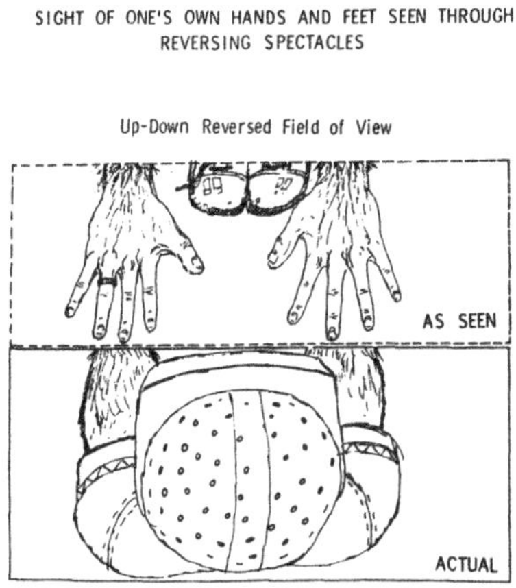

FIGURE 9.1. My visual perception of the orientation of my hands and feet (relative to the rest of my body) through the reversing prisms of Stage 3. These unique sights contributed significantly to my initial perceptual confusion and incompetent action.

Observer's Direct Report

Immediately after gazing through the reversing spectacles, I made the following world-relative observations (1/0–1/0)[2]:

> *Whatever I view has an aspect of entire irreality. . . . Somehow the mountain does not enter the calm sea. It simply sits upon it; it's placed there—cut out from cardboard and gently placed upon the water. I see some children batting about a tennis ball with a PingPong size racket; what is unreal is that the* shadow *they appear to be batting about can hardly stay in the air; it flops down all the time as if suddenly pulled down by hidden magnets; the motion of the ball is unlike anything I've ever seen.*

(1/0–1/4):

> *There is nothing odd about the movement of the branches or leaves of trees. Sitting here, gazing upon the sea and sky is really a dissociated and dissociating sort of experience.*

(1/2–1/2):

> *My son was standing, facing me, and moving his head repeatedly left and right. I was totally unable to judge which head-turn was to the right and which to the left,*

[2]See Footnote 1 in Chapter 7 for an interpretation of the time code. This particular observation was recorded for the first and last time on Day 1 of Stage 3 and within the first one-half hour of donning the spectacles.

that is to say, when *he was turning* which *way. I only know that he was turning his head.*

Immediately apparent self-relative observations (1/2.5–1/2.5) were:

I glanced at the portable tape recorder standing on the edge of the table. The remote on-off control, made of soft, plastic-covered wire, appeared to be standing *straight up into the air. (The ground was not in the FV.) This in spite of knowing that it had to be hanging toward the ground.*

(1/4–1/4):

Gravity defying waitress: The waitress at the restaurant just brought two plates of soup and two glasses of water. Somehow, by some magic of her own, none of the liquids poured out of their containers as they visually should have for they were pointing toward the ground.

With respect to the immediately perceived orientation and location of my head, I said (1/0–1/0):

Suddenly I visually perceived that I was geographically down there, below me, standing on my head, looking up *at the sky. It's when I sit here quietly, gazing upon the sea, the sky, that somehow my head is dissociated from my body or hanging upside down, or that I'm simply standing on my head gazing upon the entire scene. It's when I pat my helmet or move about that I come to realize that I'm really sitting, or if I pay attention to my arms on the chair, my seat on the chair, stamping my foot,* that *is definitely below so my head needs to be above; but something isn't right about that. On the other hand, I'm sitting quite normally and comfortably, but my head isn't oriented quite right, that is, it isn't sitting on my shoulders the way it should be, and that, despite moving it to the left or right, though when I moved my head up and down, oddly enough, it seems to be on my shoulders again.*

Gradual Modifications and Final Accomplishments: Perceptual Consistency, Meaningfulness, and Congruity

In the Prism Study perceptual adaptation to these effects proceeded from a stage of massive perceptual confusion, uncertainty, and unfamiliarity to a stage of what I call *perceptual consistency* and a lack of perceptual uncertainty and surprises. Thus, I came to describe with consistency the visually perceived location and orientation of places, objects, head, and body parts of other persons relative to the perceived location and orientation of my own head and body parts. The result of this adapta-

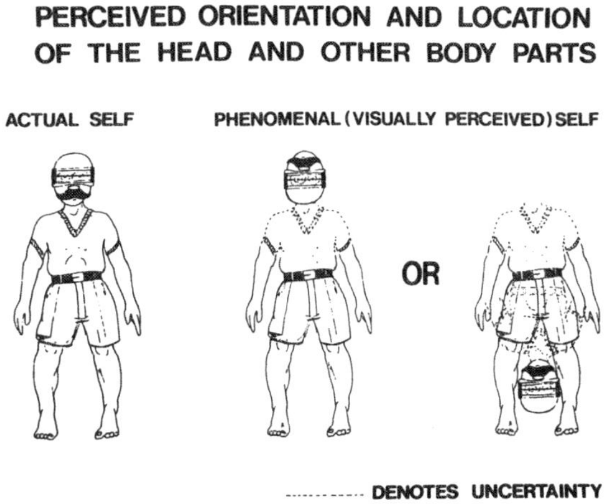

FIGURE 9.2. My visual perception of the location and orientation of my head and other body parts seen through the reversing prisms during Stage 3.

tion, I will claim, was that the orientation-*relationship* among visually perceived places and objects relative to me began to "make sense" once more. I achieved (visual) perceptual orientation thus facilitating oriented action. Further, the visually perceived *orientation* of my head was very quickly and consistently judged as up-down reversed: The top of the head was judged to be closer to the ground than any other part of the head. The visually perceived *location* of my head was variable, though my effective point of observation was mostly judged to be just inches above the ground (see Figure 9.2). I also found that I came to recognize again facial features and expressions, particularly of persons once visually familiar; I was eventually able to read and identify again once familiar print, writing, pictures, and photographs. I began to describe these sights as "normal," "common," "aesthetically pleasing," and "symmetrical." Thus, there *were* striking changes in the way things looked while I gazed through reversing spectacles.

Observer's Direct Report

Gradual modifications and final adaptations of appearances that may be characterized as primarily world-relative were (3/32–3/32):

> *Oddity of other persons' head movements (HMs): The HMs of others, as they walk along normally, is very like the up-down bobbing of an ostrich when it runs. This impression is most pronounced when I also am walking. The special rubberiness of others' walking movements themselves are remarkable.*

(9/118.5–13/170):

> *During inactivity, perceptual consistency [and "normalcy"] is the rule. However, during head or head and body movement, perceptually it's a long way from "normal," "common," "usual," "stable," "natural" or unsurprising. Particularly during actions like walking or bicycle-riding, which involve quick HMs, it becomes apparent that there is a huge difference between gazing upon the scene while stationary and while carrying out some action; that is, what one perceives (what information one is confronted with) and how one perceives that information (to what use one can put it) differ greatly in these situations.*

(11/148–11/148):

> *Foward pedaling of bicycles is visually judged to be pedaling in reverse. There were only two bicycles in the village. Neither had gears. Hence I knew that a counterclockwise movement of the pedals meant the rider was applying the brakes. To my utter amazement, I watched a boy ride the bike down the main street backpedaling all the way. Knowing that this was impossible had no influence on my judgment that his legs and the wheels of the bike were revolving counterclockwise while the bike was moving forward.*

(13/175–13/175):

> *The geographically* up *posture of the eyes is beginning to signal (mean) (seeing something) geographically down: This has been a subtle and gradual process which has by now gained a good measure of consistency. For example, I may be sitting and attending to writing, flick my eyes up in the head without thinking about it, and it's quite clear to me that I am (i.e., I* expect *to be) looking down, where the top of my head is phenomenally and where the ground is visually and geographically.*

Primarily self-relative adaptations were these (2/18–2/18):

> *I was just handed a glass filled with water to within one-half inch of the top (so I was told later). Visually, there was only one-half inch of water in the glass, but the odd thing is that this one-half inch of water appeared to be* from its brim down*—in the portion of the glass which was, in fact, empty. The rest of the glass appeared to be empty. Moreover, the brim of the glass was facing the same direction as my forehead—geographically down. These observations are not based on simultaneous or successive comparison with the ground, which was not in the FV.*

(2/18.5–2/18.5):

> *[I walked on the village road when] an open convertible with four people in it passed by. The instant I saw that, I experienced a pit-of-the-stomach apprehension for them, and exclaimed that I hoped they were strapped in with seatbelts for otherwise they would surely fall out.*

(2/22–2/22):

I have the definite impression that a stable "reorganization" of the self–world perception *relationship has taken place. I know that this "impression" is based on visual information, for when I close my eyes, it is no longer true. I'm sitting at the dinner table. Every moment I fear that in picking up a glass to drink, I will invert my hand and pour the contents of the glass on the table because the rim of the glass is no longer pointing in the same direction as the top of my head—the rim of the glass phenomenally faces skyward, the top of my head geographically down. My head is in the primary position. I am convinced that if I moved my head parallel to the ground and toward the table, the top of my head would touch the table-top. In spite of the fact that my chin is about 12 inches above the table edge, I'm convinced that the top of the helmet would come in contact with the tablecloth. In short, the table top is judged to be almost at eye level. When my head is in the chin-to-chest position, I am visually convinced that my head would disappear under the table if I moved forward toward the table top.*

(2/25–2/25):

I picked up the portable tape recorder and this time the remote control was hanging *down toward the ground from it rather than standing up into the air. The hanging remote control was pointing in the same direction as the phenomenal top of my head—geographically down.*

(6/77–6/77):

Disorientation as to how chess pieces move: In the end game of a game of chess, besides the two kings there were three pawns and two castles left. All of a sudden I simply didn't know which way my own or my opponent's pawns were supposed to march, even though I still knew I was playing white. I had to ask him repeatedly to slowly show me (by moving his fingers or one of the pawns) which pawns had to move toward or away from me. He had to demonstrate because I did not comprehend his verbal instructions. I simply did not know how to "translate" his verbal instructions into action.

(6/77–15/209):

Slanting of chessboard or table top: I'm sitting at a table playing chess. Visually, the top of my head is almost touching the tops of the chess pieces. In spite of the fact that I maintain a constant head posture, the chess board at times does not appear to lie parallel to the table top or ground; it is tilted away from me by about 45°. By "tilted away from me" is meant that the edge of the chess board or table farthest away from my midsection is closer to the ground than the edge closest to my midsection—as if the pieces would slide away from me. The same phenomenon is at times observed with the table top.

(12/164–12/164):

Perceptual contradiction tolerated: Smoke is seen to come down toward the top of my head yet is also seen to rise toward the sky. I was smoking for the first time. Visually, smoke very clearly went down toward the top of my head, which is pointing toward the ground . . . [moments later] the smoke was perceived to be rising upward toward the sky (geographically speaking) because [now] I had a portion of the floor in my FV. Logic will tolerate no contradictions but perception will! So the geographic judgment is that smoke is going up, and the ego judgment is that smoke is going down. With respect to one reference system, the smoke is perceived to be rising upward; with respect to the other, downward. There is no contradiction in this (i.e., I am certainly not bothered by such perceptions). [The two judgments were rendered successively, in very close temporal contiguity.]

The adaptations to the perceived orientation and location of my head (and other body parts) were (1/2.5–2/14):

Again, visually my head is strictly upside down. In spite of stamping my feet, I'm perceptually standing on my head or looking through my legs, again without the haptic information that my head is supporting my body weight. What has changed is that I'm quite convinced that my blood is flowing toward the ground and toward the top of my head rather than pumping, as I faintly know it to be.

(1/6–4/55):

The most consistent impression—the visual as well as haptic perception—is that I'm suspended with my head toward the visible ground. This is true even if I'm in a room with homogeneous white walls which fill my FV. Saying that I am convinced that my head is upside down means that I judge the top of my head (helmet) to be closer to the ground than my chin; it means that I judge my head to be located on my shoulders but after my neck comes the top of the head, my forehead, eyes, nose, mouth, and finally, my chin. My chin is phenomenally closer to the sky than is the top of my head.

(2/14–2/14):

The pain on top of my head due to blisters created by the chafing of the heavy helmet has now become perceptually comprehensible. The pressure on my head is perceptually the result of the weight of my head pressing geographically downward against the helmet—the result of gravity—rather than the result of the helmet resting on top of, and pressing against, my head.

(2/14–13/170):

Shift in the point of observation from shoulder or head level to a level just above the ground: What perhaps goes along with the above entry is the perception that, at times, *my head, though still up-down reversed, is located visually very low off the ground rather than above neck level. For example, what I perceived as I sat on the beach watching small waves come ashore was unequivocal. If I were sitting any closer, these waves would first wet my hair, then my forehead, and finally, reach my mouth and chin.*

(2/22–9/110):

The visually and haptically perceived orientation of all body parts other than my head is the same as it was before I put on the reversing prisms—the same as that of other persons. This is true while I'm upright. Moreover, excepted are my feet, which visually point toward my midsection though at the level of the ground [and my hands when they are in the FV.] The visual and haptic perception of the direction of the top of my head and of my forehead is geographically down. That of my eyes or other parts of the head is indeterminate.

(3/27–3/27):

Before putting on the prisms this morning (eyes closed), I judged my head to be oriented as it was preexperimentally. This judgment is based on passive haptic appreciation (no active touch involved). Moreover, for about 1 hour after putting on the prisms, I'm not at all sure that my head is up-down reversed on my shoulders. Sometimes I have the impression—based on visual information—that it is the environment and others in it who are up-down reversed relative to me.

(3/38–3/38):

The classic picture of the distorted man: I'm sitting on the veranda in a chair with the soles of my feet actually resting on the railing of the veranda, which is 3 feet high. I present a strange sight to myself. If I had to sketch myself in this posture, I could not do it. Visually, the top of my head is pointing toward the floor of the veranda. The tips of my shoes are, though actually pointing toward the sky, visually pointing down toward my mouth, and pointing in toward my chin are my legs and knees. If this is where my legs are, then where is my chest? Even with my head in the chin-to-chest position and eyes in the extreme up position, I cannot catch a glimpse of my belly or chest. This person I'm describing is extremely dependent upon head posture *for* how *he looks to himself. If I throw my head back, the tips of my shoes are far off there, pointing down at me. Now, when I move my head into the primary position, my feet appear to be only slightly above me—they're simply over there, and I can now point straight over there. My feet somehow don't seem to belong to me but it isn't nearly as bad as looking at them with my head thrown back: Then my feet appear to be way up there somewhere, floating and dissociated from me.*

(4/46.5–5/67):

The apparent location of my head is about 6 feet above the ground: When I'm sitting above someone on an incline or a stairway, head positioned slightly below the primary position, the other person seems to be very far below me, some distance certainly not reachable by arm movement it seems. In fact, if I did no more than move my elbow, I would touch the other person's midsection.

(14/191–16/210):

Information for head orientation *is visual and tells me my head is "down there": When I touch the top of the helmet or remove the helmet and touch my head in the dark, I'm often simply confused as to which way my head is oriented and whether I'm touching it from below or whether it's on my shoulders and I'm touching it from above. When I close my eyes in the daytime, I waver. I may fancy my head to be upright or reversed; in fact, the orientation of my head is indeterminate, but this is so without action. Indeed, when I knock on top of the helmet with my knuckles (eyes still closed), the top of that helmet is geographically up toward the sky and also up relative to me, the ego, sitting. The instant I open my eyes, that impression dissipates like a mist suddenly lifted—the visual information is compelling and unequivocal. There is someone knocking from* down there *on my head. At times there is a hint that the haptic ("felt") aspect of that action is geographically up, but the visual ("seen") aspect is still down toward the ground. Even dropping objects on the helmet doesn't contradict the visually gained conviction that the top of the helmet is just inches off the ground. That simply isn't a contradiction because it isn't a game of logic that's being played, but the game of perception. (Note that the portion of my FV which sweeps across the world is attached to the helmet on my head. Thus, I have uninterrupted information about head position and head orientation provided I keep my eyes open and provided there is sufficient light about.)*

Evidence, supportive of the conclusion that I perceived my head orientation as up–down reversed from the early hours onward, is as follows (1/4–12/160):

Eating with my forehead: My luncheon companion just spoonfed me. The spoon with food was seen to be coming directly toward my forehead, and I experienced great surprise when the spoon touched my closed *lips. While the spoon was on its way, I recall thinking angrily, "What's the idea of trying to stick food onto my forehead?" On Day 12, the same thing happened. This time her* hand *never entered the FV and haptically, the "feel" of the food on my lips was* wrong*—haptically, my mouth should have been somewhere else... up there somewhere... at the top of my head.*

(1/6–13/170):

While in the shower, my head still seemed suspended upside down on my shoulders; the water was seen to be running down toward the ground—first past my eyes and then *toward my forehead.*

(1/12–1/12):

On several occasions I made the observation that if I were to kiss someone (sitting across the luncheon table) on the mouth, my forehead would come to rest against her chin and my chin would touch her forehead.

(5/69–5/69):

Cartwheel communication: Two children just came by doing cartwheels on the concrete road. And just when they were at the 180° point of their 360° rotation, that is when their hair was touching the earth, I could commune with them—their heads were oriented exactly as mine was.

(7/87–7/87):

Pictorial perception and visually perceived orientation of my head: I'm looking at the cover of a magazine, which I'm holding as anyone else would. It is clear to me that the woman portrayed on the cover is facing in the direction opposite to the one I'm facing in. Now, if I turn the magazine 'round (180°), the woman's head is facing the same way I am. At this point, of course, I'm holding the magazine upside down for someone else. The top of the head of this represented woman is facing the ground, geographically speaking, and that is the way I'm facing too, regardless of head posture.

(2/18–2/18):

As I'm walking on the paved road, I'm not really walking on the road, I'm walking on the ceiling—the road is *that ceiling—and so are the people that are approaching me. They, too, are walking on this ceiling. But the odd thing is that whereas their* feet *are attached to the ceiling, my head is visually "attached" to (very close to) that ceiling. The fact that I am unaware of haptic* contact *of my head with the ground and the fact that I* am *aware of haptic contact of my feet with the ground does not alter this observation.* [*See Figure 5.2*].

(2/22–2/22):

My ear was hurting from being pinched by the side of the helmet. At no time was my hand or arm in the FV; although I reached up into the helmet to move my earlobe into a more comfortable position, the haptic perception was that my thumb was pointing toward the ground.

(3/37–3/37):

The helmet was getting quite uncomfortable again because phenomenally, my body weight is pressing against it and my head has to support it. As I lifted the helmet off

> *my head by one-quarter to one-half inch, it was visually distinctly like doing a* hand stand.

(13/170–13/170):

> *Perceptual contradictions are tolerated: In the shower with the (up-down reversing prism) backup system on my head, I patted my head. Visually, my head was down there, close to the floor. That didn't change. As I patted my head, the apparent direction in which my arm was moving alternated though. Sometimes, I visually judged my arm to be coming geographically* down *to pat the top of my head, and that wasn't strange; after all, that's where my head was visually located at all times. At other times, not 5 seconds later, the arm was perceived to be moving* up *toward the ceiling. (Head posture was constant in the primary position.) Yet, I failed to experience the surprise formerly attending such contradiction.*

Perceptual adaptations to recognizing facial features and expressions were as follows (1/8–5/69):

> *Facial expression recognition: It is just as easy as ever to judge the direction of gaze of another person (i.e., to know where, in the world, another person is looking). What is most prominent about another person's eyes are his sclera when the eyes are moved up in the head and the Chinese-appearing eyebrows (see Figure 5.4). Also, people's lips move in the most peculiar fashion while eating, smiling, or talking. (I'm reminded of the oddness of watching a film of someone walking presented in reverse.) Yet I do not find smiles difficult to recognize or distinguish from other facial expressions. These effects are particularly vivid for persons I have known for a long time. With strangers, these effects are quite apparent but not as striking.*

(2/20–15/200):

> *Getting to know someone for the first time with reversing prisms: I met the village baker today for the first time. I carefully looked at his face. I will visit him daily and then describe what happens after prism removal.*

DISCUSSION: THE INFORMATION FOR THE TRANSFORMED SELF, EVENTS, AND APPEARANCES

From these data three classes of results are analyzed in detail, following a brief historical survey: (*a*) The observer's orientation, that is, the reciprocal relationship between the perceived location and orientation of objects and events and parts of the self visible in the FV; (*b*) the perceived reversed orientation and shifted location of the observer's head; and (*c*) the recognition of facial features and expressions and perceptual familiarity. Other results from the protocol are presented in Tables A9.1–A9.2 of Appendix A. The effects of sleeping are discussed in Chapter 12.

Historical Precedents: Stratton's Observations

Stratton (1897b) was the first to describe observations that suggest that the visible self is changed in appearance when viewed through transforming spectacles: He perceived his head as inverted and located below its accustomed position with respect to his body (discussed in detail in Chapter 11). To date, no explicit observations or analysis of the shifted point of observation have been reported. Although J. Peterson did not explicitly describe experiencing his own head as inverted, he did report on the anomalous sight of seeing his feet pointed toward his body. His notes read: "I saw my feet approaching me on the rug which was seen somewhat ahead of me when I looked down. That was my first experience with such striking appearances as my walking toward myself [Peterson & Peterson, 1938, p. 21]." Unfortunately, Kohler's reports cannot be interpreted with respect to the issue at hand, as I will show in Chapter 11. Even if the reader is willing to assume a fixed frame of reference, his descriptions mix observations with explanatory inferences (e.g., Kohler, 1964, p. 33; Kottenhoff, 1957, p. 85). It is simply unclear what the facts are, given the reported descriptions. Descriptions in search of a meaningful interpretation should be presented within a consistent framework that relates the phenomenal self to phenomenal objects, and vice versa, as Rock has pointed out (1966, p. 16).

Again, it was Stratton (1897b) whose descriptions of the appearances of things seen through inverting lenses over time led the way. Both J. Peterson (Peterson & Peterson, 1938, p. 29) and Snyder (Snyder & Pronko, 1952, pp. 135–140) described the appearance of the inverted scene as well as attempts at reading. Kohler (1964, p. 160) also considered the phenomenal world of recognition. The more naturalistic spectacle-observations of the pioneers have their analogs in the laboratory (e.g., Goldstein's, 1975, or Yin's 1969, study of looking at pictures of upside down faces). The perception of facial feature recognition during different conditions of orientation is extensively surveyed by Howard and Templeton (1966, Chapters 12 and 13). A most lucid discussion of how things look while viewed through various spectacles is presented by Rock (1966), whose views are surveyed in Chapter 11. Rock's (1973) monograph constitutes a valuable addition to our study of form and orientation.

Orientation of the Self and of Things

One of the requirements for achieving functional adaptation in the real world is being perceptually oriented in one's immediate surround. That includes being able to describe as well as competently act upon where one is in relation to places, objects, events, and persons for which one has immediate visual, haptic, acoustic, or nosmic information. Importantly, the relative location and orientation of the observer's head, shoulders, hands, feet, and body are readily discoverable by appropriate eye-head movements.

The Observer's Perceptual Task: Discern Meanings in Confusion

With spectacles, both the phenomenal location and orientation of places, objects, events, and body parts within the FV are up-down reversed relative to their actual location and orientation. Consequently, the observer is confronted with a discrepancy between the direction of surfaces where they appear in the FV and where they are. This invariant fact is not only responsible for the observer's confusion about the location and orientation of visible parts of the body and things in the environment but also for the novel appearances of once familiar things and events. I contend that in perceptual adaptation, the task of the observer is to make perceptual sense again out of the disturbed relationships that now exist between the experienced self and the perceived environment: where visible surfaces are located; how they are oriented; and how they look.

World-Relative Observations: New Expectations Accompany Eye Movements

The initial perceptual confusion I experienced when I primarily attended to events in the world included the inability to attach the verbal labels "up" or "down" or "up relative to some visually perceived or out-of-sight body part or object"; my verbal descriptions were neither correct nor consistent. This observation is not surprising, given that the orientation of objects was phenomenally ambiguous, confused, or "reversed." For example, I was unable to tell immediately whether another person was ascending or descending a set of stairs; I only knew that someone was moving. Nor were places directly localizable as "up" or "down," for these terms have and had no perceptual meaning without a specific place of reference, either relative to me or relative to some locus external to me or relative to the sky-earth axis, which I in turn could refer to myself. I *was* aware of difference, chaos, flux, and perceptual instability. Indeed, the process of specifying the location or orientation of an object is best described as a laborious, error-ridden quasi-perceptual-reasoned judgment.

However, after 9 days and uncounted repetitions, I became aware of a new expectation: I anticipated seeing sky just before I moved my eyes *down* in the head and terrain just before I moved my eyes *up* in the head. The advent into awareness of this adaptational process was preceded, and possibly prompted, by consciously assuming extreme eye postures for the purpose of looking at the sky or the ground underfoot. This form of adaptation was characterized by a change in the experienced meaning relationship between repositioning my eyes and the information yielded thereby. Moving and positioning the eyes up in the head came to *mean* foveating a place down in the world, and vice versa.

Self-Relative Observations: Visual Contradictions Tolerated

Some of the confusing sights that I witnessed and was unable to describe clearly or act upon gave way to percepts that constituted blatant logical contradictions, yet were perceptually accepted by me as "natural" and "commonplace" and elicited no surprise or bafflement. I call such sights *hybrid perceptions.* They constitute another form of perceptual adaptation, a curious, developed capacity to tolerate visual–visual contradictions. For example, when, after only about 2 hours of wearing spectacles, I tried to make sense of what I perceived as I watched someone else smoke, I was quite unable to describe the direction of the moving cigarette smoke. I attempted to reason it out, based on the visual information available. This literally required minutes. My description was incomprehensible to anyone and quite contradictory from one instant to the next, reflecting the great difficulty of applying labels like "up" or "down": a testament to the difficulties of coordinating a factually accurate and linguistically and conceptually consistent world- and observer-relative description. However, after 12 days (164 hours) of wearing spectacles, a "consistent" description emerged that presented me with no difficulty, though someone else listening to that description would have been confused by it. I, a nonsmoker, lit a cigarette for the first time. Smoke phenomenally entered the top of my FV and was seen to proceed "downward" toward the bottom of the FV—in the direction in which I judged my forehead to be; yet, upon looking a moment later, smoke was perceived as proceeding geographically upward toward the sky. The environment-referenced description, on the other hand, is based on noticing that the smoke in fact traveled skyward: As I raised my head, my FV included part of the sky. Thus, I based my judgment on information gained by a simultaneous comparison of the direction of smoke and visible sky. Yet, neither description nor judgment *perceptually* contradicted or dislodged the other during such relatively passive viewing. Moreover, logical conclusions based on the abstract knowledge that the top of the head must in fact be pointing skyward had no force whatever in affecting either perceptual judgment. It is evident, however, that this form of perceptual coping (lack of perceptual surprise and tolerating such contradictions) cannot be the sufficient answer to the adaptation of action (e.g., to competent reaching in the direction of the moving smoke).

Anomalous Sights Lose Their Surprise Value and Look Natural. Seeing my own feet pointing toward my midsection at the level of the ground proved to be a particularly disconcerting sight and a stubborn obstacle to getting into a pair of slippers. Moreover, whenever I walked and my feet were in the FV, I saw myself walking toward myself—an anomalous sight, indeed. Yet, this constant condition came to be accepted as the natural state of affairs; after all, it now represented a new invariant that was neither challenged by haptic-kinesthetic perceptions nor contradicted by optical events nor, indeed, contested by visual or other memory images from prespectacle days.

Observer Accomplishment: Self-World Relationships Make Sense Again

In the broadest terms, the perceptual end-product of adaptation is this: The observer must achieve a new understanding and gain new perceptual meanings that functionally will serve the same purposes as those served prior to donning spectacles. I propose that active processes of perceptual learning are at the root of the goal of gaining new meanings. The observer must learn to differentiate and inspect the new and old optical invariants that specify a stable (i.e., a consistent) and predictable self and environment. I propose that what changes in adaptation is the *visual meaning* of the direction of the optical shifts (transformations over time) representing events, be they an object in motion or a moving body part.

The Observer's Visual Head: Reoriented and Relocated

The Observer's Perceptual Task: Know Where Your Head Is

The visually experienced up-down reversed orientation of the head was the most frequently noticed and most persistently confirmed self-experience during the entire Prism Study. Initially, I was only aware that somehow I was looking from somewhere else than before donning the spectacles or that my head had changed—that something was different or amiss. Within less than an hour, however, I judged the *orientation*, particularly of the *top* of my head, to be geographically up-down reversed and to be *located* very close to the ground relative to what it had been preexperimentally and also relative to the seen orientation and location of the head of other persons. This was so whether the ground was visible or not. Perceived head orientation was uninfluenced by anything I did to try to change it, be it stamping my feet, lifting heavy objects, dropping stones on the top of the helmet, or lifting the helmet ever so slightly; as long as I kept my eyes open, the head was perceived as upside down with respect to the rest of the seen or unseen body parts.

Pictorial Tests of Observer's Head Orientation

Within hours, I visually judged the orientation of my head to be the same as that of pictorial representations of heads or photographs of people that were presented up-down reversed or inverted, so that the tops of these heads were closer to the ground than the chins (see Figure 9.3).[3]

The problem was to ascertain my judged head orientation, using a repeatable method. The line drawings depicted in Figure 9.3 were presented individually to me several times daily. I saw them randomly in either of two orientations and either against a structured or homogeneous background while I kept my head in the primary position. In each case I responded to questions such as: "What do you see, a smile or a frown?" (Figure 9.3a). "How many hairs are on the head of the guy whose head is oriented the way you experience your head to be oriented?" (Figure 9.3b). Of Figure 9.3c, I said that the head of the king without the dot was oriented like mine and that if his crown were slid parallel to the ground toward me, it would come to be properly placed on my head. During these judgments, both my head and eyes were roughly in the primary position. For the drawing containing information for two different faces (Figure 9.3d), I was asked to describe what I saw, and once I did so, to "identify with" the sailor (or fellow with the striped cap, downturned nose, and beard). The results were, with but one exception, that over the 15 days, for a combined total of some 120 trials for all

[3]Figures 9.3a–c and f were used previously by Kottenhoff (1961, his Figure 6). Figure 8.3d is Thouless' "ambiguous" drawing, also displayed in Howard and Templeton (1966, p. 324). The reader should invert all relevant figures (or herself–himself) to get a fuller appreciation.

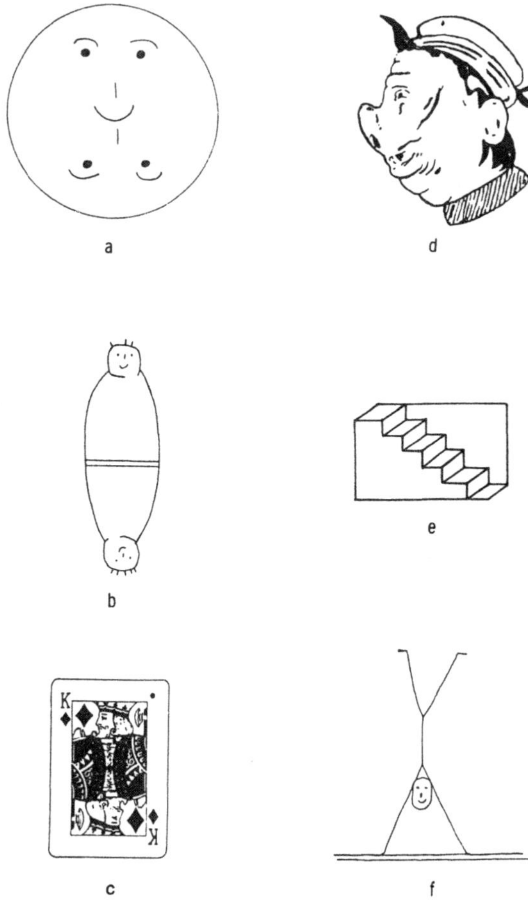

FIGURE 9.3. Pictorial tests of the visually perceived orientation of my head through the reversing prisms during Stage 3 (after Kottenhoff, 1961, Fig. 6).

pictorial representations, I identified the orientation of the heads in these drawings as would a person who looks at them from between the legs. For example, the moonface was perceived as frowning, and I perceived my own head as being oriented like the head with the five hairs on it, given the orientation depicted in Figure 9.3a and b. Head orientation, assessed by this method, was thus perfectly consistent beginning with the first presentation, after less than 8 waking hours of wearing the spectacles. Figure 9.3f is "ambiguous," as is the Schroeder staircase drawing (Figure 9.3e), which was also used. I reported "spontaneous reversals" throughout the 15 days of spectacle-wearing, much as I had preexperimentally during baseline observations, both when asked to just look at the stairs and report what I saw and when asked from which direction I would have to approach the stairs to ascend. Of Figure 9.3f, I said, without exceptions, that the depicted figure was doing a handstand rather than hanging. Preexperimentally, I had seen the drawing in either mode.

The Experienced Location of the Head Is Variable

For the most part, I judged my reversed head to be but inches above the surface on which I sat or walked; I also judged myself to be looking at the world from this novel place. This can only mean that *visually* I judged my eyes to be stationed, effectively, at that place. I was never aware of any haptic information that suggested that my *eyes* were located just inches above the ground. Generally, when my head was in a cocked-back position, and when I stood upright on a stairway or sat high above ground, I judged my head to be above its preexperimental shoulder level; when my head was in the primary position, its top was judged to be below shoulder level; when my head was below the primary position or in the chin-to-chest position while I walked or sat on a chair or on the ground, I judged the top of my head to be just above the ground, roughly between the groin and the ankles; the last of these was by far the most frequent estimate of head location (see Figure 9.2).

Visual Information for Head Orientation and Location

With a stationary head, the contents of the observer's rectangular FV and the physically lower border of his or her FV specify the direction of the top of the head, whereas the geographically upper margin of the FV specifies the direction of the observer's mouth and chin. During HMs, moreover, the perceived direction of optical shifts—the reversed occlusion-disocclusion relationship—now specifies an upside down head relative to the remembered location of the shoulders, which were not optically represented in the restricted FV.

What visual information does the observer have for judging the *location* of the head? I believe that *detecting* that the perceived point of observation has undergone a change leads to the observer's description that the head is located in a different position vis-à-vis the rest of the body and the ground. I propose that the observer's perceived point of observation is generally a function of the novel functional relationship between how the eyes must now be positioned in the head to continue foveation of a given place for any given HM and head posture; the perceived reversed orientation of the head is also a likely factor that biases the perceived location of the head; finally, the observer's near–far confusion may also constitute information for a shifted point of observation. The likelihood of this possibility is strengthened by observations that judged distance-from-self varies, as do judgments of head location and point of observation, as a joint function of head (eye) posture, the slope of the terrain within the FV, and the actual distance of the head from the ground.

Haptic–Kinesthetic Information for Head Orientation and Location

The spectacle-wearer's visual information potentially *contradicts* both the haptic information and the actual orientation and location of the head and other body parts; further, one might assume that the haptic information remains, initially at least, true to the facts. If that is so, then the agreement between visual and haptic information enjoyed during prespectacle days is destroyed. Before we can ask how any potential contradiction in visual–haptic information can be resolved, we must describe three types of haptic–kinesthetic information available to the observer that he or she might use to judge the head as being upright on the neck.

First, consider the passive haptic information from the muscles of the neck and the skeletal joints.[4] I did not notice any passive haptic information that told me that my head was still attached to my neck—either way. In fact, such information was conspicuously unnoticed. When I made passive haptic judgments with the eyes open, the orientation of my eyes, nose, neck, and shoulders—none of which were ever visible with spectacles—was judged to be *indeterminate* (see Figure 9.2). When I made such judgments shortly after a night's sleep with the eyes still closed, the orientation and location of my shoulders, neck, and head were judged to be as they had been preexperimentally. This did not work in the daytime with the eyes open. Accordingly, any contradiction between visual and haptic information was either not noticed or was "resolved" by the "supremacy" of visual information or by what Tastevin (1937) has called *visual capture,* a phenomenon further discussed in Chapter 11.

Second, consider the haptic information from my scalp, which itched due to the perspiration and chafing of the helmet, and from the pain on top of my head, due to blisters that had developed. Initially, I

[4]The following muscles are relevant: splenius of the neck; sternocleidomastoid; sternohyoid, trapezius; and the splenius of the head. Relevant skeletal joints are the first thoracic vertebra and the hyoid bone.

haptically localized the itching and pain to be in the same direction as the sky, though *visually* I judged the top of my head to be oriented toward the ground. By Day 2, after 14 waking hours of wearing spectacles, this contradiction was "resolved." The pain on top of the head had become *perceptually comprehensible:* I judged the pressure and pain on my head to be the result of my head pressing against the helmet, toward the ground, rather than the result of the helmet resting on top of, and pressing down on, my head. The visual information for the up-down reversed orientation of my head clearly influenced this haptic judgment and, indeed, seemingly overruled both haptic-gravitational information and my knowledge of how gravity would operate if one inverted one's head with a helmet on it.

Third, consider the haptic information gained from assuming extreme eye postures. Many researchers (e.g., Merton, 1964) are satisfied that an observer does not have any afferent haptic information for eye movements or for having moved the eyes by a moderate amount. Assuming and maintaining an extreme (up) eye posture was clearly noticed, felt like, and meant assuming and maintaining an extreme (up) eye posture—except that now it may simply have served as additional confirmation for the visually gained conviction that my head was up-down reversed. Yet, there was not a hint that the available haptic information from eye muscle tension and eyelid information ever changed. It seems to me that haptic information plays an insignificant role in providing the observer with information about the orientation or location of the head or eyes.

Finally, how was the only contiguously available visual-haptic discrepancy resolved? I first became aware of a discrepancy between the visually and haptically judged location of a specific part of my head upon seeing and then feeling someone else pointing at and then touching my forehead or mouth. For example, I was spoonfed. As the spoon with food, guided by the arm of another person sitting opposite me, dipped geographically *below* my primary eye position on its way to my mouth, I visually judged the spoon to be approaching my forehead. Note that the hand and arm with the spoon looked to me to be traveling toward the phenomenal top and hence, toward the geographically lower border of my FV. Since it is this physically lower margin of the FV that now specified the direction of the top of my head, the optical shift information available to me before the spoon made contact with my *closed* lips produced the visual expectation that the spoon would make contact with my forehead. The haptic information, however, served to quickly contradict the visual expectation that the spoon would touch my forehead "up there." To my surprise, "up there" was suddenly occupied by my mouth. Thus, the haptic information made me aware of the fact that there was a discrepancy between the expected and actual location, within the head, of my lips and forehead. Nevertheless, my (visually) perceived orientation of (the top of) my head remained up-down reversed.

In summary, it may be said that even though looking through reversing prisms provides the observer with optical misinformation about the actual orientation and location of the head and other body parts, haptic information either goes unnoticed or is not sufficiently specific or obtrusive to challenge the more precise and attention-demanding optical information.

Appearances and Events: Recognition of Faces, Expressions, Print

Recognizing Facial Features

If changes in meaning and appearance occur—and they do—they should, properly, be called *perceptual* adaptations. I am inclined to say, moreover, that such changes in appearance are changes "of" or "in" the visual *system*. However, understanding this interpretation first requires that one define some terms and thrash out the role played by stored meanings, memories, and aesthetic judgments.

Recognizing once familiar persons by their facial features (rather than by hair color, mode of dress, and time, place, or circumstance of meeting) proved to be virtually impossible at first. Even though I made use of all of this information and was thus doing more than facial *feature* recognition as such, I confused three adult women with whom I related most and who have similar facial features. At first I generally did not recognize the people I had known longest if I attended to their facial features and ignored other information.

It is hard to escape the conclusion that with reversing prisms the observer is forced to pay attention to novel optical information. Sometimes, that novel information visually "reminds" him or her of a fact long unnoticed. For example, when several years earlier I first met one of the three women, I was vividly aware of the fact that she had a permanently broken nose. Originally, this fact was apparent and attended to for perhaps a few weeks. For the following 5 years, I had been almost totally unaware of its presence until I put on spectacles. Then the broken nose once again became a vivid visual landmark—a very distinctive feature. By the end of the prism-wearing period, however, I once again stopped noticing it. An integral part of this novelty is the observer's phenomenal point of observation and how he or she has to cast the eyes to see. Moreover, the change in the light-intensity gradient contributes to the experience of novelty and strangeness in the scene viewed. What seemed most affected by the optical up-down reversal, however, was my visual standard of symmetry, good form, proportion and distribution of features, and congruity of arrangement. Hence, any arrangement (object, face) that conformed to this long-confirmed and laboriously acquired standard of visual symmetry was judged to be violated once I gazed through spectacles. In sum, during the course of adaptation, the novel optical arrangements became the critera and the new standard of symmetry, proportion, and congruity.

Recognizing facial features of familiar persons should be contrasted with describing facial features of total strangers. Here the distinctive identity of a person was readily established, presumably because visual memories of distinctive facial characteristics could not interfere in this process. Nevertheless, my standard of symmetry and composition of features contributed slightly to the "strange" character of the observed person's face, particularly of the eyes and eyebrows (see Figure 5.4). These considerations lead to the prediction, which was borne out, that I should not be able to recognize a person once I removed the spectacles after a prolonged period of wearing, provided I saw this person frequently but *only* while looking through reversing prisms.

Understanding Facial Expressions

Immediately after putting on the spectacles, I realized that I was responding to different levels of optical information; I was accurate and unfailing in noticing *that* someone's facial muscles were moving, but I was not always clear about the meaning of these facial expressions. Relatively gross changes, such as a broad smile, presented no problem, though the novelty of the optical transformation "carrying" that smile elicited everything from surprise to disbelief on my part. Nevertheless, the optical shifts reflecting such gross movements must have contained some invariant features, on the basis of which I made my differentiation and identification. More subtle facial expressions, especially those peculiar to a particular person (e.g., those conveying consternation or mild disapproval) were either missed or not understood at all. Such facial expressions are subtle in the sense that the magnitude of movement is slight and often of short duration; the situations in which they are used are also fewer and less predictable than for smiles.

From the first moment of gazing through spectacles, I became aware that I was forced to pay attention to a great many novel optical transformations that were unlike anything I had ever seen, including emotion-disturbing sights. By and by, the special combinations of symmetry of movements became the new standard, that is, special combinations and sequences of optical shifts came to signify or mean particular events. Presumably, this process is a form of perceptual learning that also relies heavily on old invariants in optical events as well as upon new consistencies that repeat themselves in each appropriate situation. For example, people seldom shout, get red in the face, hammer on tables, and smile at the same time.

In summary, through processes of perceptual learning, visually perceived and judged asymmetry of form, imbalance of composition, disproportionate distribution of features, irregularity of grouping, incongruity of arrangement, and even disharmony of aesthetic judgment eventually came to be perceived and judged as symmetry of form, balanced composition, pleasingly proportioned distribution of features, regularity of grouping, congruity of arrangement, and harmony of aesthetic judgments.[5] Such changes are the very stuff of which perceptual adaptation is made.

Reading and Picture Perception

Recognizing what is represented by line drawings, pictorial displays, and photographs and recognizing individual symbols, letters, words, and groups of words in handwriting or print was at best difficult and time consuming once I began to wear spectacles. With respect to line drawings and pictorial displays, my perceived orientation of my head seemed to play a role in my inability to recognize what was represented, and in my describing what was represented as "strange," "surrealistic," etc. With respect to symbols, letters, and words, on the other hand, the perceived orientation of my head seemed relatively unimportant. Initially, I was totally unable to read. I had to go through a laborious process of identifying each individual letter before I could read short words. Identification of the most confusable letters (e.g., p, d, n, and u) was clearly aided by the context of less confusable ones (e.g., c, s, l, and i). Confusability is related to the interchangeability of distinctive features in the two main orientations: the normal and up–down reversed orientation. Gradually, the character of "weirdness" and "strangeness" of printed materials disappeared. My ability to read improved and as it did, I began to judge the reading material as looking "normal," and "usual." Nevertheless, I continued to judge reading material as "different" than it had been preexperimentally, although I could not be more specific

[5]The relationship between orientation and aesthetic judgment has been considered by Braine (1978).

than that. On Day 12, I reported (12/155–12/155):

> *Reading becomes progressively more proficient:* [The] *"weirdness" character of written and printed materials has disappeared. Since Day 1, I have devoted 5–15 minutes to reading my own handwritten instruction sheet for observations to be carried out. This was prepared before the experiment. At first I was totally unable to read my own handwriting, but by now I'm beginning to be "at home" with it to the point where the "strangeness" of it has ceased.*

And two days later (14/191–14/191):

> *Reading of materials written and presented in four major orientations readily accomplished: I can read my own handwriting adequately, regardless of which way I turn the paper (except in-between orientations, which I have not tested) and whether I'm looking at the mirror-reversed writing, which I produced prior to Stage 3 by putting a sheet of carbon paper wrong way 'round behind the sheet on which I was typing. I can read it whether I look at it geographically right side up or upside down, or whether I look at what I have normally written upside down or right side up. Whichever way I look at these various productions makes relatively little difference as concerns ability to read what has been typed. The order of difficulty in reading from easiest to most difficult, is: carbon copy held geographically right side up; carbon copy held upside down; natural (pre-Stage 3) writing held right side up and read from left to right; and most difficult: natural writing held upside down and read from right to left (see Figure 9.4a–d, respectively, for an example).*

Perceptual Learning and New Visual Memories

The perceptual learning just described may be thought of as adaptations to the discrepancies between the perceived symmetry relations, rich in new perceptual invariants, and the visualized and remembered

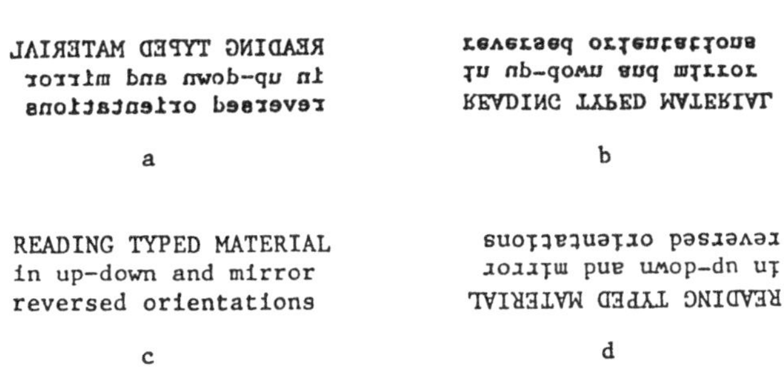

FIGURE 9.4. Typed material in various orientations. Before donning reversing prisms, ease of reading from easiest to most difficult was: c, d, a, b; immediately after, the order was a, b, c, d. When prisms were removed and aftereffects recorded, the order of ease of reading was: c, d, a, b.

ones. Progressively, the observer comes to recognize the now distinctive characteristics of a human face, in a landscape, in pictorial representations, and in written and printed materials. Moreover, this form of perceptual adaptation causes the observer to modify his or her initial comments regarding the strangeness, unfamiliarity, uncanniness, unrecognizability, novelty, bizarreness, and queerness of once familiar landscapes, objects, persons' faces, printed materials, and pictorial representations of all kinds. Such verbal descriptions and judgments are gradually modified until the observer can no longer visualize, image, imagine, or remember in any form what he or she may have meant by saying, for example, that the whole scene had an aspect of unreality about it when first glimpsed through spectacles; all is again familiar, common, usual, and instantly recognizable, yet different from the remembered or visualized past. The experience of "familiar, yet different" and all like descriptions and judgments seem to be the result of comparing visual memories from prespectacle days with more recently established visual memories and with on-the-spot perceptions. In turn, these immediate perceptions and recent visual memories depend upon the perceptual learning of new distinctive features.

Perceptual End-Product: Meaning Interchangeability

How does the adapted observer differ from the unadapted one? I am struck by the similarity between the way in which linguistic meanings for the bilingual reader and speaker[6] and perceptual meanings for the adapted spectacle-wearer appear to be interchangeable. Frequently, while reading a book in English with German passages in it (or vice versa), I have noticed suddenly that I had been reading German (or English) for an entire paragraph without awareness of having "switched." It usually takes a "10-dollar" word in either language to produce a break in the meaning continuity. Similarly, upon adaptation to a new perceptual "language," the observer is able to switch back and forth between spectacles and no spectacles (cf. Taylor, 1962, p. 204) and may not be clear at all times which condition he or she has just experienced. Such observations point to a very general capacity for developing meaning invariances that may operate on a set of basic principles that

[6]Professor Fabio Metelli of the University of Padova tells the story of Wolfgang Koehler lecturing in German to an English-speaking audience and therefore switching to English every so often to summarize what he had said in German. Koehler is said to have given the last part of his lecture in English rather than German. He then noticed he was running out of time and said, in German, in effect: "I'm sorry I won't be able to give you an English summary of what I've just said, please excuse me."

can subsume perceptual, linguistic, and other forms of meaning and the way in which one order of meaning may be substituted for another.

"Does the Upside Down World Come to Look Right Side Up?": A False Puzzle

This question, which predates even Molyneux and Berkeley in various guises, is based on an expectation without sound factual or theoretical foundation: Its very linguistic meaning must be questioned. Stratton was the first to formulate the question explicitly, as the titles of his 1896 and 1897 publications demonstrate. All three contain the inviting phrase, "vision without inversion of the retinal image," and the first in the series hopes, if not promises, to solve the riddle of "upright vision." Stratton's 1896 report was followed by swift criticism, in two parts, by James Hyslop of Columbia University (Hyslop, 1897a,b). He argued that to ask, "Why are all things seen upright when the image on the retina is inverted?" is to arrive at a misleading statement of the real problem because it contains a set of assumptions and ambiguites that render the problem, as initially stated, illusory. The real problem, according to Hyslop, is strictly visual and concerns "nothing but the real or apparent anomaly of opposition between the position of real objects and that of retinal images [Hyslop, 1897b, p. 147]."

Both the evidence and the analysis of the Prism Study make it clear that the original question with its built-in assumption, that somehow the perceived environment will "flip right side up again" given long enough to "adapt," is misguided, misleading, and linguistically ambiguous. The facts of *any* spectacle study are critically misrepresented by the assumption that only the places and objects of the external world are optically displaced, reversed, or inverted relative to an observer to whom we attach the device, whereas the observer perceives himself-herself as remaining unchanged in relation to this transformed environment. Studies of perceptual and performatory adaptation typically underemphasize or ignore the fact that an observer also has transformed visual information *about himself-herself relative to* the phenomenally transformed and visible environment. The facts are that at first the observer suffers massive perceptual confusion regarding the direction of the location—relative to the self—of places, objects, events, and even of the orientation relationship of body parts to one another within the FV. The observer shows this confusion by the ambiguous, confused, and downright contradictory verbal descriptions he or she offers when asked to talk about where places are, how objects are oriented, and in what direction an event is proceeding. To "adapt" means to achieve perceptual consistency in the sense that (*a*) the disturbed self–environment relationships make sense once again; (*b*) the observer experiences the body parts as being located and oriented in a clearly specifiable direction; (*c*) the observer's verbal descriptions of the location—relative to self—of places, objects, and of the direction of ongoing events no longer contain contradictions; and (*d*) the observer's verbal descriptions of the location and orientation of body parts to one another are congruent with the optical information that specifies them.

If the question, "Does anything re-reverse?" means "Are the new appearances *indistinguishable* by any criterion from the remembered appearances of pre-spectacle days?" then the answer is an unequivocal "no." The observer continues to be aware *that* whatever he or she perceives is somehow different from what he or she perceived without spectacles. The observer is often unable to specify, though, *how* what he or she sees through spectacles is different (with the exception of how the head is oriented relative to other body parts and relative to all that is visible in the FV). What is more, whatever the experienced differences, they no longer confuse, perplex, disturb, or bother the observer—even to the point of being differences quite unworthy of notice. In short, the observer accepts perceptually, cognitively, in action, and emotionally this new condition as the new standard of consistency and stability, as the model for aesthetic acceptability and familiarity, as the test of meaning, yea, as the gauge of everyday existence.

SUMMARY

Like the discussion in Chapter 8, that of Chapter 9 also helps answer some of the basic epistemological questions I asked at the outset. However, the questions are different: "How accurately is reality preserved in perception; how stable an index of reality is perception; and how do we perceive and represent mentally what there is to know about outselves in relation to the world?"

Again I use Stage 3 of the Prism Study as a paradigm and answer these questions by detailing three immediate effects of, and their perceptual adaptations to, wearing up–down reversing prisms: (*a*) Disturbed self–environment relationships; (*b*) the perceived reorientation and relocation of the observer's head; and (*c*) the difficulty I had as the observer in recognizing faces, expressions, and print as well as in understanding events. The apparent location and orientation of places, objects, events, and body parts within the observer's FV are up–down reversed relative to their actual location and orientation. This invariant fact accounts for the observer's initial perceptual disorientation and confusion about the true location and orientation of visible parts of the body and environment as well as for performatory incapacity. The optical reversal is also responsible for what I experienced as the bizarre and disturbing appearance of once familiar faces, of facial expressions and other bodily movements, and of print.

Perceptual adaptation consisted of gradually understanding the now disturbed *relationship* between the seen self and the seen environment: first, where visible surfaces were located; second, how they were oriented; and third, how they looked. During adaptation, I achieved a new perceptual consistency, congruity, and meaningfulness. Initial surrealistic, surprising, and aesthetically uncanny sights became identifiable print, recognizable smiles, and symmetrical and pleasing faces.

I was able to tell where visible surfaces were *located* by anticipating, after 9 days of prism-wearing, that whenever I moved my eyes up in the head, ground would become visible and whenever I cast my gaze in the direction of my feet, sky would become visible. Thus, the *perceptual meaning* of assuming extreme up–down eye postures changed.

Gaining consistency in verbally describing or recognizing how places and faces were *oriented* was preceded by the curious phenomenon of accepting visual contradictions as "natural." I call these sights *hybrid perceptions:* The same event (e.g., shower water) would appear to move geographically downward or "flow upward" in quick succession, depending on the nature of the background visible to me and depending on the direction of eye–head movements during the "switchover." The fact that the observer has a limited context of body parts and environmental places, due to the restricted FV, is probably a major factor in this phenomenon.

Perceptual adaptation to how the self and the world looked through reversing prisms was characterized by my awareness of unique and distinctive features from my novel, optically reversed, point of observation. Within less than 1 hour of donning the prisms, I consistently judged the orientation of my head to be up–down reversed: The top appeared closer to the ground than my chin. The visually perceived location of my head was variable, though I mostly judged my effective point of observation to be just inches off the ground. Perceived head location varied as a function of head posture, the slope of the terrain in my FV, and the actual distance of the head from the ground. I argue that direct visual information is responsible for the apparent orientation and location of the observer's head. Thus, even though looking through reversing prisms provided me with consistent misinformation about the actual orientation and location of the head and other body parts, haptic–kinesthetic information either went unnoticed or was not sufficiently specific to challange the more definite and attention-demanding optic information.

What seemed most directly violated by the optical reversal was my visually acquired standard of symmetry, good form, proportion and distribution of features, and congruity of arrangement for objects, faces, expressions, print, and pictorial displays. The fact that facial features of once familiar persons were difficult to recognize, whereas total strangers looked "queer" but identifiable, supports this inference: Old visual memories of distinctive facial characteristics could not interfere in recognizing the stranger upon a second meeting. Moreover, the one person whom I purposely saw only while I was wearing reversing prisms was not recognized when I saw him the first time without the spectacles. The fact that the initially anomalous sights become familiar and pleasing again suggests that novel optical transformation and arrangements became the standard of perceptual symmetry and aesthetic acceptability through perceptual learning. Such changes, which surely entail the establishment of new visual memories based on the new optical standard of reference, are the very stuff of perceptual adaptation.

The old question, "Does the optically reversed world come to look 'right side up' again," contains linguistic confusions and hence is a false puzzle. Because the seen self is transformed no less than the seen environment, the implication that the environment somehow "flips right side up again" makes no sense. If the question is rephrased to, "Can an observer continue to tell the difference between the appearances seen through prisms and those he or she remembers from prespectacle days," then the answer is a resounding "yes." In adaptation the observer comes to accept perceptually, cognitively, in action, and emotionally the initially disorienting, confusing, and disturbing sights. Perceptual and linguistic consistency and competent action become the rule. That the prism-wearer continues to judge the top of the head as being closer to the ground than the chin when reminded to do so is a guarantee rather than an obstacle to the validity of these contentions.

10

Returning from a World Transformed: Aftereffects of Adaptation[1]

As the adapted spectacle-wearer, I removed the reversing prisms from the helmet and inserted nonreversing glass, keeping the size of the field of view (FV) identical. Unfortunately, this control was not customary in the past (e.g., Stratton, 1896, 1897b; Snyder & Pronko, 1952). The observed aftereffects of adaptation to having up–down reversed the FV distributed themselves into two dichotomous experiential worlds: one of action, the other of appearances. Performatorily, I remained within or returned to a well-known and comfortable world. Basically, I experienced no surprises and was immediately competent, as if I had been practicing all tasks and had polished them to a high level of competence. Perceptually, however, I suddenly found myself thrust into a foreign world of uncanny appearances. I experienced amazement and required at least 5 hours of visual inspection before I began to feel (really *see*) perceptually, aesthetically, and emotionally comfortable in my new phenomenal environment. Also, I required at least 2 days (30 waking hours) of visual inspection and locomotion before I noticed a return to

[1]Aftereffect measures have become the most frequently used means of evaluating adaptation to optical transformation. However, as pointed out in Chapter 2, aftereffect measures, though informative in their own right, are an inadequate substitute for looking at the *process* of adaptation as it occurs.

the remembered spectacle and prespectacle magnitudes in the experienced minification of objects and in the apparent compression of distances along the ground to any visible place.

I have shown that living with a restricted FV produces several effects rather similar to optically inverting or reversing the FV (Chapter 4). It is therefore of considerable interest to discover what the aftereffects of having lived with a restricted FV are. Finally, the aftereffects of having increased the weight and size of the observer's functional head should be described before the observer can truly return to his or her former natural ecology.

Consequently, using the results of Stages 4, 5, and 6, respectively, of the Prism Study, I will discuss the aftereffects for perception and action of having (*a*) up–down reversed my FV; (*b*) restricted my FV; and (*c*) increased the weight and size of my functional head.

AFTEREFFECTS OF UP–DOWN REVERSING THE FIELD OF VIEW

From the results I have chosen three examples for discussion: (*a*) The seesaw effect observed during head and body movements (the original effects were discussed in Chapter 7); (*b*) visually guided actions (Chapter 8); (*c*) apparent object minification and distance compression (Chapter 9). The principles proposed in the analysis may be fruitfully extended to other results found in the protocol and described in Tables A10.1–A10.6 in Appendix A.

Aftereffects of Head and Body Movements

Results

1. Perceived global world motion during up–down head movements (HMs) was slight at first. Objects, people, and places were perceived to go out of the FV *downward* with *up* HMs and *upward* with *down* HMs, much as was phenomenally customary without spectacles but with a restricted FV. That is, the leading edge of the sweeping FV was again judged to reveal portions of the visible environment, whereas the trailing border concealed them.
2. After 50 minutes of wearing nonreversing prisms, the judged magnitude of apparent world motion with up–down HM was greater than immediately after removing the reversing spectacles.

3. During brisk up-down HMs while walking, I also experienced visually induced bodily instability: a milder form of the seesaw effect. These effects disappeared after 2.5 to 4 hours.
4. No aftereffect—no perceived world motion—was noticed by me even during rapid onto-the-shoulder tilt HMs.

Observer's Direct Report

During *Stage 3*, after 193 hours, I observed the following aftereffect:

> *On removing the reversing prisms in my room in almost total darkness [before going to sleep], I experienced global world motion in the direction* opposite *to my HMs; that is, the window, which was barely visible, went out of sight downward with up HMs and up with downward HMs.*

Immediately upon entering Stage 4 and gazing through nonreversing prisms once again (1/0–1/0.5)[2] after having seen through reversing spectacles for 211 hours, I reported:

> *Perceived global world motion with up-down HMs is slight, at best. Objects, people, and places go out of the FV* downward *with* up *HMs and* upward *with* down *HMs. Focal joggling is superposed on the global world motion, but the joggling is more obtrusive.*

After one hour, I reported (1/1–1/2.5):

> *After 50 minutes of wearing nonreversing prisms, the judged magnitude of global world motion with up-down HMs is much greater than it was at the beginning of Stage 4. Moreover, during brisk up-down HMs while walking, I also experience visually induced bodily instability.*

I then observed (1/2.5–1/4):

> *During slow to moderate up-down HMs, there is no perceived global world motion; it is very mild during rapid up-down HMs.*

Finally, I reported (1/4–4/59):

> *The perceived stability of the world is indistinguishable from what it was during Stage 2.*

[2]See Footnote 1 in Chapter 7 for an interpretation of the time code. This particular observation was recorded for the first and last time on Day 1 of Stage 4 and within the first one-half hour of removing the reversing spectacles and exchanging plain glass for them.

With respect to onto-the-shoulder tilt HMs, I reported (1/0–1/0):

> *Absolutely* no *perceived world motion with even rapid onto-the-shoulder tilt HMs (i.e.,* no *aftereffect is observed). I am aware only of my own HMs.*

Normal eye–head–body movements yielded the following aftereffects (1/0–1/4):

> *The focal joggling about the people, places, objects, and events which I foveate, particularly while walking, is quite considerable; the joggling, again, is very like the motions resulting from gazing at the world while pushing repeatedly against one's own eyeball. Focal joggling ceased after 4 hours.*

Discussion

Historical Precedents

The pioneers reported world motion and vertigo during HMs and walking. Stratton was again the first to describe the aftereffects of having worn spectacles and the *consequences* of HMs. Upon removing the inverting lenses from their narrow tube after 87 hours, he observed:

> When I turned my body or my head, objects seemed to sweep before me as if they themselves were suddenly in motion. The "swinging of the scene," observed so continuously during the first days of the experiment, had thus returned with great vividness. It rapidly lost its force so that at the end of an hour the motion was decidedly less marked. But it was noticeable the rest of the day, and in a slight degree even the next morning [1897b, p. 470].

The disturbance was more serious when Stratton began to walk. "While walking, there were distinct signs of vertigo and also the depression in the upper abdominal region, noticed during the earlier days of the experiment. The feeling that the floor and other visual objects were swaying, in addition to the symptoms just mentioned, made my walking seem giddy and uncontrollable [1897b, p. 471]." Ewert too, reported: "When I walked, the whole field of view was seen to be in motion. In order to recognize otherwise familiar objects, I had to cease moving about. When I got outside the building I was almost overcome with the vastness of the universe. The light also seemed unusually bright. When I walked, I became dizzy [1930, p. 348]."[3] The giddiness experienced by

[3]It is clear from this description that for this purpose, Ewert had already removed the tubes that restricted his FV, returning to a full FV. Although Ewert believed he was reporting on the aftereffects of inversion, he is evidently describing an aftereffect of restricting the FV. These observations underscore the importance of the role of restricting the FV in these experiments and are confirmed by the Cyclops Tube Study presented in Chapter 4.

Ewert lasted until the third day. Snyder also reported dizziness, nausea, and "swinging movements" into the second day after removing his inverting lenses and returning immediately to the full FV (Snyder & Pronko, 1952, pp. 142–143). J. Peterson suffered "immediate and severe nausea, with vertigo and vomiting [Peterson & Peterson, 1938, p. 30]." Finally, Kohler did not offer a description of aftereffects following the wearing of up-down reversing spectacels. Relative to right-left reversal, he wrote: "The immediate aftereffects lasted several hours; some, however, remained for much longer (up to two weeks; for example, apparent movement upon changes of position of the head and body) [1964, p. 159]." (Kohler's descriptions of aftereffects to the wearing of displacing prisms, on the other hand, are exhaustive [cf. 1964, pp. 64–67].) Unfortunately, none of these passages include a description by the above investigators specifying the *direction* of the world motion that was experienced upon removing their inverting or reversing spectacles.

Head Movements and the Seesaw Effect

Aftereffects are generally compared to the effects observed immediately after donning reversing spectacles. They are often comparable in magnitude but opposite in the direction of the pointing error, for example. The aftereffects of the Prism Study, however, were different from the immediate effects of reversal with respect to the apparent rate, direction, onset, and duration of the seen motions of the FV during HMs. First, the apparent rate of world motion for comparable rates of HM was so slight that it was hardly noticeable at first; not until 50 minutes after switching to the nonreversing spectacles was the world motion clearly noticeable and thus of much greater magnitude than at first. Moreover, its magnitude was such that the phenomenon should be called apparent *field motion* rather than *world motion*. Second, by far the largest component of field motion is attributable to self-produced HMs rather than to apparent self-instability or to being moved unpredictably. Third, no inclination to vomit was observed, suggesting that the prespectacle relationship between eye-head compensation was preserved and evidently remained in readiness. If this hypothesis is correct, support is given to the general rule that the adapted observer differs from the unadapted observer also in that he or she has accomplished a second viable system of functioning without relinquishing a former system of competencies. Fourth, apparent direction of field motion is congruent with prespectacle phenomenology and the reverse of the spectacle condition. Finally, the total duration of the field motion aftereffect was only one-twentieth (4 hours) of the length of time world motion persisted during adaptation.

These observations allow this conclusion: In addition to learning a new set of perceptual rules for distinguishing self-produced movements and object motion during adaptation, the observer perceptually recognizes and relearns the old HM-coupled invariants very quickly. Indeed, the observer seemingly preserves his or her prespectacle standard for doing so. Consequently, the adapted observer is *biperceptual.* Since the original standard is preserved, he or she experiences a contrast effect until the invariants that govern the new postprism HM-world-motion relationship are perceptually confirmed. The contrast derives from an attempt to continue to apply (in test–operate–test style) the spectacle standard—the newly learned rules about what optical shifts to expect, following any head or body movement. Further evidence, presented in Chapter 11, clearly shows that once adapted, the observer continues to be biperceptual, ready to apply the fruits of former perceptual learning almost immediately and with great skill.

Aftereffects of Visually Guided Actions

Results

1. There were no significant aftereffects of actions for the fully mobile observer. I was generally competent in carrying out all of the activities that I had engaged in while wearing spectacles. I did lift my head erroneously several times in response to a downward intentional eye movement that preceded the HM.
2. There was initial dizziness and unsteadiness during walking, but after 3 hours, I was more confident and generally more competent than I had been even after 15 days of wearing the spectacles.

Observer's Direct Report

Immediately after switching to the nonreversing prisms, I reported (1/0–1/0):

> *Errors in the direction of HM: On several occasions now I* raised *my head after deciding (intending) to look at a place geographically down in the world (i.e., following an intentional eye jerk downward).*

(1/0.5–1/0.5):

> *Writing: visually, writing appears quite normal, but haptically, it feels strange and unfamiliar. The result is quite legible.*

After going through many routines in fine motor coordination, practiced while wearing reversing prisms, I recorded (1/2–1/8):

> *There is no evidence of performatory difficulty in fine or precise, coordinated, visually guided arm-hand-finger movements during such tasks as clothing self, putting on shoes, reaching, grasping, twisting, etc. during pouring, drinking or eating, operating the tape recorder, handling tools and so on.*

I also noticed (1/1–1/1) that the overestimation of distance between self and objects ceased:

> *I can now correctly judge when I will make contact with an object, say a parked car along which I must walk. I no longer crash into such objects, convinced I'm 1–1½ feet away, as I did even until the last minutes of wearing reversing prisms. Similarly, the overestimation of the depth of stairs (enhancing of the visual cliff) has ceased.*

With respect to gross bodily action, I observed (1/1–1/3):

> *Walking, though fairly steady on a paved straightaway, causes dizziness. Moreover, I tend to bump into tables, chairs, and so on. I tend to stumble on rough terrain. Curious though it may sound, I do better and walk a little more carefully down stairs and steep mountain paths than I did even yesterday, after 15 days of walking down these stairs with reversing prisms. It's more uncomfortable today, but I am more efficient at it; that is to say, even though I feel dizzy and a touch nauseous, I feel more secure from falling—less danger-prone. Walking up these stairs produces a strange mixture of haptic ("motoric") familiarity and unfamiliarity—as if one mixed two familiar flavors and then had trouble distinguishing them. Walking downward still appears more dangerous and is considerably more trying, slow, and strenuous than walking upward—and this is how it was during Stage 3. One seems to be—and in fact is—much further from the surface of support in the event of falling when walking downhill.*

And thereafter (1/3–2/26):

> *After but 3 short hours I'm already more capable, confident, smooth, steady, and generally competent than I ever was, even after 15 days of wearing reversing prisms. This is true for general perceptual and performatory orientation exemplified by walking; climbing; sitting down on a chair; bicycle-riding; swimming; clothing self; rowing a boat; pointing; reaching; grasping; pulling; pushing; twisting; ball-heading, -throwing, -kicking, and -catching; and so on. Unless specifically noted, none of these activities posed any difficulty or entailed any visual system–haptic system discrepancies or surprises at any time during Stage 4.*

The next morning (2/12.5–2/12.5), I experienced a great deal of unsteadiness while walking. During the first hour of Stage 4, I also noted (1/0.5–1/1):

Ball-catching: Even though I caught the ball accurately, I clutched it in a spastic sort of way—as if afraid I wouldn't catch it and-or [would] drop it after having done so. The haptic perception of that action was quite novel and was enhanced by the fact that I assumed a rigid position and that all the muscles of my body were greatly tensed. Reaching out toward the ball as it approaches was done jerkily rather than in one smooth, flowing movement. After about 10 trials of catching this way, I relaxed my generally heightened tonus and the haptic perception of catching was now smoother and more "familiar" involving a small "clutching" component.

Discussion

Historical Precedents

Stratton reported that visually guided action was error-ridden following inversion; Ewert claimed it was not. Helmholtz was the first researcher to describe aftereffect errors in visually guided reaching in the direction opposite to the optical displacement produced by his wedge prisms (1962, Vol. III, p. 246). The first sentence of Stratton's brief description, following 8 days of living with inverted light, summarized his observations: "Movements which would have been appropriate to the visual arrangement during the experiment, were now repeatedly performed after this arrangement had been reversed [1897b, p. 470]." Moreover, Stratton now noticed errors in the direction in which he turned his head. Although Stratton did not report committing errors in the direction in which he moved his head while he wore the inverting lenses, once he removed them from their tube, he noted: "And in writing my notes at this time, I continually made the wrong movement of my head in attempting to keep the center of my visual field somewhere near the point where I was writing. I moved my head upward when it should have gone downward; I moved it to the left when it should have gone to the right [1897b, pp. 470–471]." Ewert's observations on visually guided action were opposed to Stratton's. Following 14 days of practice in card-sorting, which required eye, head, and arm movements to place the cards in their proper compartments, Ewert found that "Continued practice in card-sorting under retinal inversion does not cause interference in the ability to sort cards under normal vision. There is thus no noticeable persistence of the newly acquired habits upon a return to normal vision [1930, p. 320]."

Competent Action

The observations during the Prism Study suggest that performatory aftereffects to long-term reversal of the FV fall into two classes. First, I now committed errors of uncertainty and confusion because I continued to execute eye–head movement combinations that were functionally required of an observer wearing spectacles. I call these *carry-over aftereffects,* exemplified by the directional errors I made as I moved my head. Immediatedly upon removal of the spectacles, prespectacle invariants that govern the activity of the visual system become available to the observer. Moreover, since the adapted observer is biperceptual, as I have argued, *recognition* of these invariants is a truer description than relearning of them or relearning of their meaning. The finding that such carry-over aftereffects are transient supports the argument.

Second, I performed competently those activities that are not vitally dependent upon eye-head exploration because I continued to rely upon actions that I had learned to perform competently while I wore spectacles. These I call *persistence aftereffects.* We should not be surprised to find that the adapted observer, upon removing the reversing spectacles, performs with confidence and immediate competence. Then, as before, I had to accommodate myself to the invariant conditions of survival. A prism-wearer trapped in an empty room with a closed door and without sustenance must escape if he or she is to continue. A prism-wearer must walk toward the door, even though he sees himself walking toward himself; he must make contact with the doorhandle, even though he sees himself reaching toward it as he reaches away from it and even though he feels his arm where he sees it. It doesn't matter where the prism-wearer feels his arm to be. No change of any kind in the felt position of any body part can be equated with competent action, which is the only ecologically sensible definition of performatory adaptation. The prism-wearer must grasp the door handle, hide it from sight with his hand, and turn the door handle in the correct direction, even though he sees a clockwise arm-hand twist as a counterclockwise twist and even though he feels that twist either the way it used to or the way it looks now. Were it not for the novel adapting requirements for head-eye movements of which the casual onlooker knows nothing, or for the curious appearance of the observer's eyes, a naive onlooker should not be able to tell the adapted and acting spectacle-wearer from the wearer of plain glasses.

For the most part, I, the observer, acted competently after having worn reversing prisms. In fact, the more complete my adaptation to reversal, the more competent were these actions once the spectacles were exchanged for nonreversing glass. Because the spectacle-wearer who has adapted has, in effect, been *practicing* the same head, body, and limb movements he or she practiced prior to using spectacles, because he or she has come to open doors by reaching and twisting just so, and because he or she has come to reach for, lift, and bring to the lips a cup in a particular manner, we expect and observe basically competent action once the observer removes the spectacles. He or she can simply continue to do what was done in prespectacle days provided he or she pays attention to the old, prespectacle invariants such as optical end-point information. For an aftereffect encore, the observer simply needs to continue to perform on the basis of these old and tried invariants. The interpretation is underscored, moreover, by the following finding: Aftereffects of tasks that I had not managed to perform with adeptness during the study (e.g., catching a ball), were performed with uncertainty and hesitation.

Aftereffects of Having Seen the Self and Events through Reversing Prisms

Results

1. Immediately after I looked through the nonreversing glass, whatever I gazed at I described as "uncanny" and "unearthly."
2. After 5 hours, I was more and more impressed by a sense of familiarity and "belongingness" while looking about. There was a progressive decrease in strangeness, unreality, bizarreness, and asymmetry.
3. All of the distances along the ground from me to any visible place were judged to be much shorter than they were perceived to be when I gazed through reversing prisms or than I remembered them to be from prespectacle days. Moreover, I judged all people and objects to be greatly minified. That is, the difference between the judged and the actual (and remembered) distance along the ground from self, and the size of familiar objects, was enormous. This minification of object-size and underestimation of distance along the ground persisted for more than 2 days, or 30 waking hours, and then gradually diminished.
4. People I had known for years had only a foggy-vague familiarity.
5. I was unable to recognize a person I had met *only* while wearing reversing spectacles and whom I had visited for 1–3 minutes on each of the 15 days of wearing prisms.
6. The perceived orientation and location of the head was judged to be the same as that of other persons and as it had been preexperimentally (during Stage 2 and earlier).

Observer's Direct Report

The first aftereffect observation came unexpectedly. I had swum out several hundred meters about 7 PM on Day 15 of *Stage 3*. A strong wind blew up rather quickly, and the ocean became very choppy. My return swim against whitecaps and a current proved exhausting, and I swallowed some water. About 20 yards from shore, I came close to drowning and had to take off and drop my helmet. Relieved of this weight, I made it into shore. (One-half hour later, with my backup system on my head, I dove and recovered the helmet and began to wear it again.) I recorded the following world-relative observations while a companion went to fetch my backup system from the house (15/203–15/203.5):

> *Immediately after removing the helmet during Stage 3 (during an emergency), everything had the appearance of utter strangeness. It was a world I did not want to be in and did not belong in. An aspect of irreality pervaded whatever I gazed at. Despite persisting performatory problems, I prefer my "reversed world," my own world now, to the unknown and frightening world I now regard; I am glad to come back to my (reversal-prism) world as I now know it. My prism world is not bizarre as the so-called real world which today I experienced for just a few minutes. On the whole, I feel much more* secure and comfortable *with, than without, the helmet on even though* [*or* because?] *my FV is much restricted with the helmet system. This world I have known for 15 days is much more my world than the world I have just experienced on removing my prisms. This up–down reversed world is much more real and realistic and comfortable than the ugly, distorted, and horrible world which I can hardly believe used to be my comfortable and comforting world. I willingly reject this world of which I am supposed to have been part. I want nothing more than to remain in the up–down reversing-prism-world in which I am again, safe from the horrors of distortion and unrecognizability of persons. Were I not convinced of the relativity of this state of perception and perceiving, it would be difficult to convince me to remove my shell of security [FV-restriction effect also?].*

Moreover, I noted the following self-relative observations (15/203–15/203.5):

> *The most striking effects, after having to remove the reversing prisms, were the shrinking, in accordion-bellows fashion, of the world; that is, all of the distances along the ground from myself to any visible place, object, person, or event were unbelievably shorter than just an instant before. Thus, people appeared to be standing just 2 yards from me, though I had to take 25 steps to reach them. Moreover, there was an incredible minification effect.*

Concerning facial features and expressions, I reported (15/203–15/203.5):

> *People that I have known for years or months had but a foggy-vague familiarity. Several persons I had seen on several occasions prior to putting on reversing prisms and then daily for 15 days while wearing the prisms: I did not recognize them at all; that is, I knew it had to be them for they were with people I had known very well before Stage 3 and I knew that they almost invariably were to be found in the company of these others.*

Once the *planned* aftereffect stage was initiated, I reported these world-relative observations (1/0–1/5):

> *Upon initially gazing through nonreversing prisms, the whole scene looks uncanny and unearthly. There isn't anything that I recall being familiar with. It's as if I'm watching a very badly made movie or a cubist painting in which all sort of things are out of joint. Perhaps the most striking fact about "going back" to a world I had known for 30 years, is that after this 16-day "interruption,"* I simply cannot say things like: *"Ah, yes, I remember; that's just how this or that scene, person, object, or place looked." The "sense of familiarity" which Bertrand Russell talks about is nowhere to be found within me. The places I visit are strange to me—as strange as places I've never seen, or rather as odd as one seen through the half-occluding emotion-haze of a bad dream.*

At no time (1/0–4/59) did I experience any problem of perceptual orientation. Also, the rubberiness and springiness, so obvious and obtrusive a part and parcel of people's walking and running, has disappeared. After 5 short hours, I reported (1/5–1/5):

> *I am more and more impressed by a sense of familiarity and belongingness while gazing at the scene. There has been, and continues to be, a gradual decrease in strangeness, irreality, bizarreness, and asymmetry. This is so in spite of the fact that I am still aware of a huge discrepancy between the judged and actual (i.e., remembered from reversal days) size of objects and people as well as of the distances along the ground. Yet the magnitude of these discrepancies is slightly less than it was just 2 hours ago.*

Self-relative observations, concerned mostly with apparent object minification and distance compression, were as follows (1/0–1/4.5):

> *I'm standing on the balcony, overlooking the beach. People on the beach down there appear incredibly close to me; so close, that all I need to do, seemingly, is reach out to touch the people (never mind that I know it's well over 100 yards air distance to the beach). The people themselves are minified, and everything is shrunken relative to the last time I looked through reversing prisms. From the nearest house to the seashore (actually about 100 yards), it's 6 giant steps. I'm in the house now and minification of all* familiar *objects is also very obvious. Everything I look at looks tiny and dwarfed.*

And a bit later, down on the beach (1/1.5–1/4.5):

> *The discrepancy between the judged and actual (and remembered) distance along the ground between self and objects, persons and places is enormous. Thus, it appears to me that a very few steps, 10, 20 at most, would bring me to the edge of the ocean, yet*

> *the actual distance is between 60–70 yards. People, not quite half-way between where I stand and the water appear to be in reaching distance, and they are dwarfs—again, I am in the land of Swift's* Lilliput. *I also noticed a striking similarity between childhood estimates of distance and present distance judgments (see Appendix A, Table A10.3).*

In order to compare this aftereffect against my judgments of distance-from-self while wearing reversing spectacles, I physically inverted my head (1/1.5–1/5.5) and noted:

> *Looking at myself and the world through my legs: When I now put my head between my legs and look at the busy, heterogeneous scene, the perceived "rubber band of distance" has stretched itself out—houses and other fixed objects which I'm familiar with have assumed their former (Stage 3) size and distance along the ground from me and from one another. The instant I return my head to its former (upright) posture, the persons and places, which just a moment ago appeared normal in size and far off, "shrink back" to their minified size and into reaching distance.*

The relationship between perceptual and action ("looking versus doing") distance was assessed as follows (1/1.5–1/6):

> *Perceived distance along the ground, or the water surface, to a given place is quite small, but once I begin to walk or swim such a* visually *short distance, it begins to "stretch" perceptually and motorically (performatorily) and temporally speaking; it becomes visually perceived and haptically perceived distance* over time. *The only road in the village appears much narrower than it did only yesterday. I ask myself: "Will the perform*ing *or performed 'walking distance' be judged equal to the visually perceived distance along the ground?" Upon putting this question to the test from the width of the road to a distance of about 50 yards, I judged the "motoric"* (walking*) distance to exceed the passively perceived distance by 10–15%. Moreover, if I judged a given distance along the ground, then walked it, and then turned around and compared the* judged *distance before and after the walk, the "after walk" distance was decidedly greater. Yet, when I put my head between my knees immediately after such a judgement, the distance I've just walked appears 30–40% further off than I judged it to be just a moment ago with an upright head.*

The distance-compression effects prove robust (2/12.5–2/28):

> *Minification of object-size and shrinkage of distance along the ground persists.*

However, beginning with the third aftereffect day, I noted (3/32–4/44):

> *The underestimation of object-size and distance on the ground is becoming progressively less noticeable.*

Nevertheless, the process is not complete (3/35–3/35):

> *Upon exchanging the nonreversing prisms for reversing prisms for a moment, everything appeared to be a tremendous distance away from me. Moreover, on switching back to the nonreversing prisms again, the scene shrank as if by magic.*

On Day 4, an asymptote was reached (4/44–4/59):

> *I can no longer claim that I perceive any discrepancy or anything amiss as concerns object-size or distance-along-the-ground judgments.*

Other perceptual aftereffects, especially the recognition of persons' faces and facial expressions and their aesthetic quality were as follows (1/0–1/2.5):

> *The facial features and expressions of persons that should be familiar, like my son, . . . look totally "different"—not at all the way I remember them from Stage 3. For example, a person I had known for 6 years had a broken nose and even though I know this, before the experiment I neither noticed it when we were face to face nor when she offered me her profile. I had to be in a very peculiar or novel position relative to her (novel point of observation) to ever notice her broken nose. During the first few days of wearing reversing prisms, I couldn't help but attend to this long unnoticed fact and now, on the first day of donning nonreversal prisms, again I am forced to be aware of this fact. If it were not for dress, place, time, and circumstances of meeting, persons of association, hair color, and presences or absences of glasses, I would not give a nickel to back up my confidence in identifying* anyone. *People that I had* only *met while wearing reversing prisms and had come to regard as quite handsome or pleasing, today appear anything but handsome, perhaps even homely. Conversely, someone whom I had regarded as rather plain now appear as positively pleasing. The rough criteria of judgment of "beauty," which I seem to apply more or less consciously, have to do with symmetry, regularity, and composition of such features as shape of mouth relative to shape and size of nose, relative to shape of eyes, distance between eyes and origin of nose, shape of chin, texture of skin, location of ears, scars and wrinkles while smiling, and so on. When the complex aggregate of these characteristics seemed well harmonized and had symmetry, I would regard a person as pleasing or handsome. On removing the reversing prism this harmonious balance seemed suddenly upset—the symmetry disastrously altered. On the other hand, when I regarded a person as plain or not pleasing to look upon during Stage 3, on removal of the reversing prisms that person seemed to have acquired the evenness of structural composition, the symmetry and harmony of features which causes me to regard that person as beautiful or handsome.*

After 4 hours I noted (1/4–1/4):

> *Even though I now recognize people I had known for a long time, there was just something stubbornly new about them—as if they had just come out of the bath or*

beauty parlor, or had rearranged their face rather than their hair or clothing; as if they had had plastic surgery.

Looking at someone whom I had only seen through reversing spectacles for the first time through nonreversing prisms (plain glass) yielded this report (1/4–1/4):

Visiting the village baker for the sixteenth time: Every day during Stage 3, I had visited the baker. I had known the man only *while wearing reversing prisms, visiting him 15 times. To me, he was a rather handsome man with a most warm and winning smile. (When I came to see him the* sixteenth *time, I could not have looked any different to him. Only three people knew about the change of prisms, and unless one carefully looks at the* eyes *of the person wearing the helmet, one could not know that some change had taken place.)* I simply did not know that man. *Had it not been for the fact that he wore his invariant uniform, was in his shop, and was pulling steaming loafs of rye bread out of the oven, I should not have recognized him. That man before me was a totally different man—a stranger. In fact, this man was harsh and rather frightful to gaze upon. The scar on his right temple, which had "receded" over the days I had come to see him, bulged out in scarlet protest. Then the extraordinary par excellence happened: He smiled kindly, as he always had; I was incredulous for I did not expect* that *face to smile; I expected that face to break out in a red cloud of anger, matching the crimson scar; I expected that face to bellow or at least to frown, to do anything negative at all.*

Concerning the visually and haptically perceived orientation and location of my head and other body parts, I reported (1/1–1/1):

It is of note that it did not occur to me to be concerned about that until a companion administered some of the pictorial representation tasks (which I've been doing daily), at which time the question was directly asked and answered without hesitation. That change seemed to be instantaneous. I'm knocking on my helmet (as I used to during Stage 3), and it's definitely someone knocking from above down, geographically speaking. The perceived orientation and location of my body parts relative to places in the world and of places in the world relative to one another is as they were during Stage 2.

The following morning (2/13–2/13) I noted:

Today is one of those rare mornings on which the helmet does not feel to be part of (the weight of) my head. It is haptically perceived as independently heavy.

Finally, (3/35–3/35) I reported:

Upon exchanging the nonreversing prisms for reversing prisms for a moment, the visually perceived orientation of my head was instantaneously as it had been throughout Stage 3—the top of my head (helmet) was phenomenally closer to the ground than any other part of my head. Moreover, on switching back to the non-reversing prisms, the orientation of my head returned immediately to its normal (Stage 4 or preexperimental) orientation.

Discussion

Historical Precedent

Stratton was also the first to report the phenomenon of distance inversion and a shift in the apparent location of stationary objects: "On approaching the stairs, I stepped up when I was nearly a foot too far away [Stratton, 1897b, p. 470]." Although this is the only bit of evidence, and even though Stratton included this observation in his description of motoric aftereffect mistakes, it may be evidence for perceived distance compression. Indirect support for this contention comes from the following description, which suggests a shift in Stratton's perceived point of observation: "Objects in the room at a distance of ten or twelve feet from me, seemed to have lost their old levels and to be much higher than they were either during the experiment or before the experiment. The floor no longer seemed level, but appeared to slope up and away from me, at an angle of perhaps five degrees. The windows and other prominent objects seemed also too high [1897b, p. 471]." The hypothesized relationship between the perceived shift in the observer's effective point of observation and the phenomenal compression of distance is discussed below.

The Lilliput Aftereffect: Object Minification and Distance Compression

By far the most spectacular and obtrusive aftereffect was the disparity in appearance between Stages 3 and 4 with respect to (*a*) what size people and objects seemed to be; (*b*) how far apart objects and places looked to be; (*c*) from where in the world I appeared to be regarding the environment; and (*d*) how many steps I perceived it would take me to get to any visible place. I speculate that the aftereffect of apparent compression of distance along the ground and secondarily, object minification are the complex result of one or more of four phenomena.

First, consider the effect of the optical near–far reversal created by the reversing prisms. Without spectacles, near places are imaged large and high up on the retina, whereas far surfaces are imaged small and lower down (Gibson, 1950, p. 77). This relationship was reversed while I wore reversing prisms. Consequently, what was reversed was *where in the FV* near and far surfaces appeared to be. Specifically, with spectacles, physically distant places appeared at the bottom of my FV, whereas places closer to me appeared closer to the top of the FV. Although I did *not* notice that environmental surfaces near my body looked to be much more distant or that distant ones seemed near to me during passive inspection, the optical shifts produced by reaching away from my body, for example, did help me to confuse near and far. I also had to reckon with the reversal of retinal gradients while wearing spectacles: A ground scene inspected from above became, phenomenally, a ceiling scene seen from below (cf., Gibson, 1950, p. 85). I was faced with a novel correspondence, in effect.

Second, consider the effect of positioning the eyes up or down in the head on the apparent compression of distance. Casting the eyes up in the head without spectacles yields a view of the visible horizon and has generally been accompanied by seeing places that are off a greater distance from the observer than what is optically represented upon casting the eyes down in the head. Under these circumstances the observer certainly develops an expectation to see far-off places upon looking up and nearby places upon looking down. During reversal, on the other hand, positioning the eyes up in the head now yields a view of the ground close to the body. In fact, by Day 9 of reversal, I had become consciously aware of expecting to see earth and not sky and consequently, to see a place near myself and not far off when I cast my eyes toward my forehead. Alternately, I began to expect to see relatively distant places, objects, and often the horizon when I pointed my eyes past my nose toward my chin. Pointing the eyes down in the head came to *mean* seeing distant places—those above me, above my point of observation, and above the horizon line, including sky as background. Positioning the eyes up, on the other hand, came to mean seeing *relatively* nearer places—those close to the ground, those below my point of observation, and those below the horizon (cf. Sedgwick's challenging analysis of the visual horizon [1973]). Note that this rule held, irrespective of the head posture I assumed.

During reversal, I thus experienced a radical change first, in what parts of the environment and of myself became optically available as a consequence of positioning the eyes and secondly, in what I came to expect and what it meant to cast my gaze with respect to *what* I saw, *where* I saw it relative to my body, and approximately *how far* I judged what I saw to be from me. As soon as the reversing spectacles were exchanged for plain glass, these relationships were reversed again. I postulate that what positioning the eyes up or down in the head came to specify optically and came to mean during reversal of the FV contributed to the aftereffect of apparent compression of distance along the ground and to the phenomenal minification of objects and people. Finally, even though I did experience an enhancement of judged distances from self during reversal (e.g., of the visual cliff), its magnitude cannot account for the magnitude of the aftereffect. Curiously, during the entire period of wearing reversing spectacles, I continued to collide with objects because I was visually convinced that I was 45–60 cm (1.5–2 ft.) away. This "lateral estimation error" was no longer noticed during Stage 4.

Third, consider the possible effect of practicing inappropriate accommodation during reversal on the apparent compression of distance. As a likely accompaniment to the optical near-far reversal, I may well have engaged in a good deal of faulty accommodation in order to "hunt" for the appropriate accommodation-solution. Particularly, underaccommodating for optically near objects is known to decrease the perceived size of an object further away (Koffka, 1935, p. 237). The reversing prisms may also have produced a slight magnification, which would also necessitate novel accommodation practices and would tend to reduce the perceived size of objects as an aftereffect. The idea that a good deal of novel accommodation may have been at work while I scanned postprism light came from the observation that, during Stages 4 and 5 and for days following the study, I could read signs and posters and make out details on a movie screen from the same row with my 20/80 myopic right eye (monocularly) at distances over which I had been quite unable to do so preexperimentally. The suggestion is that "accommodation practice" with reversing prisms may be of (temporary) benefit to the myopic eye. These observations are in need of rigorous confirmation because I did not have the proper measuring instruments such as the Snellen chart used preexperimentally to check on my monocular and binocular acuity.[4]

Finally, consider the role of the apparent shift in my point of observation during the reversal stage and its influence on the distance compression aftereffect. During reversal, the top of the refrigerator in the house appeared to tower above me when I maintained my head in the primary position. Upon switching to nonreversing glass, it appeared below me, barely reaching my chest, which is its actual height. Similarly, the kitchen shelves, which seemed high up during reversal when my head was in the primary position, now appeared below eye level. The tops of things in general, such as the top beam of a door frame or a hanging clothesline, when at an actual distance of about 3 m (10 ft.), appeared now just at the level of the top of my head when it was in the primary position. At the same distance, I would have had to throw my

[4]The role of sustained near-far convergence in prism adaptation has been investigated by Paap and Ebenholtz (1977).

head back to pick up light from the same place during reversal. With nonreversing glass (Stage 4) and with the head and eyes in the primary position, I saw the top of the head of a woman who is 5 ft., 4 in. tall (I am almost 5 ft., 10 in. tall) when she was standing just a few feet away, and she appeared positively tiny. During reversal, I could not see the top of her head, given the same distance and position of the head and eyes. On the whole, stationary objects that seemed to be at eye level or appeared to be high off the ground during reversal appeared much lower and closer to the ground and phenomenally below me once I removed the reversing spectacles. As I walked toward the kitchen door during Stage 4 (for which I had to duck by about 2 inches in order not to hit the top of the helmet) and while keeping the head and eyes in the primary position, I veridically perceived that the top of the helmet would strike the crossbeam. However, while wearing reversing spectacles, I did not even notice the top of the door, unless I threw my head back and pointed my eyes groundward: Then the optical information specified collision with my throat—decapitation of an up-down reversed head.

It is interesting to note that in the Tube Study, upon removal of the tubes that restricted my FV (discussed in Chapter 4), I also experienced an upward shift in the effective point of observation, judging myself to be taller and to be looking down on objects that had previously appeared at or above eye level. This curious parallelism in the results of the two studies has other points of correspondence. When I first put on tubes I judged the distance from the head to the ground to be smaller than it had been, much as was true for the reversing spectacle case. In both instances, I had visual information for looking at the world from closer to the ground; moreover, in both situations I underestimated distance from self.

I postulate that the shift in the place from where I perceived myself to be regarding my environment—from close to the ground with reversing spectacles, to considerably higher above the earth upon their removal—also contributed to the compression of distance along the ground and minification of objects and people that I experienced as an aftereffect to reversal of the FV. When one's head is visually judged to be just inches off the ground or below shoulder level, as my head was most of the time during reversal, then objects will appear large and above one's head; on the other hand, when one's point of observation then suddenly shifts above shoulder level, as happened upon removal of the reversing spectacles, then objects should appear below one's head and relatively small. One additional influence that I had to contend with was the fact that the reversing prisms could not be fitted onto the helmet bars at the same angle as the nonreversing glass. Thus, given a constant head posture, 20° more of the geographically upper portion of any object in the FV was optically represented with reversing than with nonreversing prisms. It may well be that this fact biased how far I judged that the position of my head—my point of observation—had shifted once I exchanged the nonreversing glass for the reversing prisms.

Distance compression and object minification are contrast effects. I believe that during optical reversal, a new standard of judgment of distance along the ground from oneself and of the relative and absolute size of objects and people is achieved. It is this standard against which aftereffects are experienced and perceptually measured. Thus, what I experienced when I inverted the optical reversal by putting my head between my legs, even after 11 days of wearing spectacles, was indistinguishable from what I witnessed as an aftereffect: I was suddenly thrust into Swift's *Lilliput*. Thus, the aftereffect phenomena of compression of distance and minification of objects and people are hypothesized to be a contrast effect.

I experienced both a passive "gaze distance" and an active "locomotor distance." I was aware of a dual reality. First, objects appeared minified and distances along the ground seemed compressed, even if I attended primarily to external appearances. On the other hand, when I shifted my attention to what I could *do* in this minified and shrunken world, thus including myself in the observation, I had the distinct impression that compression of distance along the ground and, to a lesser extent, object minification were intimately a function of my point of observation and my own bodily size and how I could "use" my perceived self by walking or reaching, to pass over these distances. I was *perceptually convinced*, and I use the term advisedly, that if I took about 10 giant steps, of which I somehow perceived-thought myself capable, I could thereby reach the water's edge as I stood on the beach—an actual distance of some 55–65 m (60–70 yd.) away. That perceptual conviction reluctantly gave way, provided I actually began walking toward the water. The perceptual conviction yielded only by degrees when measured against the locomotor effort I perceived that I had exerted. As soon as I again regarded the visual environment passively, however, the perceptual conviction of how far I was from a given place returned with full emphasis. Distances from the self to the beach or mountain appeared small compared to how I remembered them from Stage 2 or 3. Only when I began to walk such a distance, did it begin to "stretch," motorically speaking. Gazing at this shrunken and minified world did not teach me anything, it seemed; behaving within it, on the other hand, brought the discrepancies in information from various bodily systems into contact. By and by, the stable facts of the environment asserted themselves, overruling, readjusting, or recalibrating the results of peculiar or transient perceptual modes of operation that were at first unconfirmed and untested by information gained from performing. Less than 4 hours after reversal, I swam in a rough ocean and had to exert tremendous effort to make it back to shore: actual distance, 6–7.5 m (20–25 ft.) or 3 waves to go. The shore appeared to be very far off, yet upon arrival, that distance appeared considerably shorter when passively inspected. "Walking distance" or "motoric distance" or "exertion distance," undoubtedly a messy time-tied set of variables, may well have increased experientially during reversal because the exertion needed to traverse a given distance was noticeably greater throughout the reversal period than before switching to reversing spectacles and was greater than after removing them.

In order to compare "motor" and "gaze" distance, I marked a conspicuous spot, regarded a clearly visible place at the other end of the long beach, and tried to fix that perceived distance for a visual memory comparison upon my arrival there. I estimated that I would get there in 3–5 minutes at my normal walking pace. I arrived *15* minutes later, wet with perspiration. I turned and looked back toward my starting location. The distance I had walked along the coastline now *looked* distinctly farther than it had before I started out. I then put my head between my legs and looked toward the place from where I had come. Even then, the distance looked to be greater by 30–40% than when I was standing upright and perhaps double what it had before I had begun to walk. These observations came 5.5 hours after exchanging the reversing spectacles. I repeated this procedure several times. Thus, "gaze distance" appears to be recalibrated to match "effort distance." The observed phenomenon can be described best as a gradual process of veridicalization (J. J. Gibson in Kohler, 1964, p. 11). "Event" distance or "motor" distance or "active" distance—all requiring the effort exerted in walking, swimming, cycling, or crawling—appeared to exert a "correcting" influence upon the phenomenally compressed distance from the self, registered during passive viewing of the visible environment. In this instance, at least, distance-from-self, perceived passively, seems to profit from visually perceiving one's performance, with motoric exertion as a likely guide to accuracy.

Event Perception and Visual Memories

During the aftereffect stage, I no longer needed to make the distinction between a geographic and ego frame of reference because they were one and the same: They yielded the same phenomenal experiences, verbal descriptions, and actions. For example, I once again visually perceived the top of my own head as pointing toward the sky.

A short 5 hours after removing the reversing prisms, but after more than 200 hours of viewing through them, I was already unable to remember or visualize or conceive of what the contents of the reversed FV had been like with respect to the relative orientation of objects. This observation was certainly true as long as I regarded my visual surrounding. I had to put my head between my knees to approximately recreate a rather recent and compelling reality. The implicit suggestion is that we may need to reevaluate how influential (visual) memory is in the process of adaptation and readaptation.

AFTEREFFECTS OF RESTRICTING THE FIELD OF VIEW

Method and Results

To initiate Stage 5, I removed the nonreversing prism unit from the helmet and put the front counterweight and skiing goggles in place, returning the FV to nearly normal size.

There were three main aftereffects of restricting my FV to 46 × 115° for 25 days (344 waking hours):

1. I continued to engage in small up–down HMs as though the FV were still restricted.
2. General geographic orientation and a wide range of performatory skills, particularly those requiring much head-scanning, were facilitated.
3. I was frequently unaware of objects, body parts, and events that were actually present in my peripheral FV; noticing an object in the periphery often required that I first attend to the object by foveating it.

Observer's Direct Report

The first aftereffects were recorded unexpectedly during Stage 3 (15/203–15/203.5):

> *When I removed the helmet with reversing prisms during an emergency, yielding a full FV, head-scanning persisted as if my FV were still restricted. My HMs, particularly in the vertical plane, were small, exploratory scanning movements which were now both unnecessary and inappropriate to the intended task. Thus, I applied HM*

scanning to all (visually guided) activities: to look at people, to put on my fins to dive for the lost helmet, and to directly guide my walking; I do not commonly walk with my head in the chin-to-chest position in order not to fall when I have a full FV but had perforce learned to do so while my FV was restricted. Virtually all of the HMs I executed were unnecessary. Ocular exploration would have sufficed to reveal details I wished to inspect and performances I wished to guide visually.

Immediately after I began looking with a nearly normal FV, I reported (1/0–1/0):

The first thing I notice upon returning to a normal-size FV is the great dazzle causing eye blinking. There was no need for this during Stages 2–4, while my FV was restricted. I am aware of persistently engaging in a great deal of small excursion, up–down HMs, which I was unaware of during Stages 2–4 except at the very beginning of Stage 2, when the FV was first restricted. In short, I'm still behaving as though my FV were restricted. Whatever I accomplish by this head scanning, be it exploratory or performatory, could readily be accomplished with ocular scanning movements. These HM excursions, particularly in the vertical plane, are quite small in angular extent, which clearly suggests that I'm still attempting to get overlapping samples of optical information. With respect to the horizontal plane, the difference between the prism FV and the full field appears to be rather modest; with respect to the vertical dimension, on the other hand, that difference seems (and is) tremendous and accounts for several surprise effects. For example, it has been 3 1/2 weeks since I have seen certain parts of my body (viz., shoulders, upper arms, and chest). Most surprising though, is suddenly seeing parts of my body which I have not seen for the past 25 days (viz., my shoulders, upper arms, chest, and nose). Moreover, seeing my entire body without having to go through the novel kinds of head and body twists to which I have become accustomed is quite surprising. Even though I need not move my head now, I still persist in the HMs employed during Stages 2–4 (mostly 4) to see portions of my body which I can see perfectly well with a stationary head. The fact that a greater portion of the sky and horizon are visible now is no less surprising. They too are visible without the necessity of head-scanning (eye movements would more than suffice when the head is roughly in the primary position), yet I still bring my head up to foveate portions of the horizon and sky—as if still restricted by the FV of Stages 2–4.

I also noticed novel flow gradients while walking (1/0–1/4.5):

Plants, people, houses, fences, and so on are "flowing" by as I walk—as if I were moving in a train or car; the perceived flow gradient is quite smooth and symmetrical. This is while I walk and hold my head roughly in the primary position without purposely moving my head about. This "smooth world motion" phenomenon is most unmistakable and greatest in perceived velocity for objects and places closest to me and progressively less so for objects and places further and further away from me. Along the horizon there no longer is any of the flowing motion observed close by—all is stationary.

Dizziness due to large eye movements (1/1.5–1/6):

Extreme-excursion spontaneous saccades, as well as intentional eye jerks, cause dizziness but no perceived world or self instability. When my visual attention was "caught" peripherally during Stages 2–4, I also used to move my head in that direction, but now I'm beginning to make extreme excursions with my eyes only (in the direction of peripheral events). When I engage in those extreme eye movements, the feeling of that, in terms of haptic eye-muscle awareness of what my eyes are doing, is very strange, producing a light-headedness bordering on dizziness. But this has nothing to do with any visually perceived self-world motion or instability. The information is haptic. Today it is a rare and readily noticeable occasion when I engage in any eye movement of extreme excursion.

Orientation facilitated (1/11.5–1/11.5):

Perceptual and performatory orientation is facilitated during all activities due to a return to the normal FV. This is true for walking, swimming, bike-riding, diving, and so on. An activity like swimming, for example, proceeds more easily because I have a better chance to be geographically oriented. For a given eye–head–body posture, my immediate visual world is bigger, affording me more varied and detailed information about future possibilities or affordances for actions. I have a greater opportunity to discover, and act upon, a larger number of nested frames of reference, including a greater variety of visual horizons. As concerns the commonly accepted horizon, it too is effectively expanded now, affording me more opportunities for visual "anchoring" along a greater number of visible and distinctive horizon "points" (distinguishable places). In swimming, in virtually any direction, a very small right or left head-scanning movement now reveals the coastline. This was not the case during Stages 2–4, when I peered through prisms. Then the HM excursion had to be much larger, sometimes necessitating body twisting as well. Many of these combinations of eye–head–body movements have now "dropped out" for they are superfluous. What "cost" an extreme eye–head–body movement during Stages 2–4, now may require no more than a 40° HM.

And yet, I was strangely oblivious to body parts, places, and events in the periphery of my FV (1/11.5–1/11.5):

It's most curious, but today I'm mostly unaware, or surely not as aware as I was preexperimentally, of objects, places, and events in the peripheral portions of my FV. For example, it took me minutes to even notice that my arms and hands were in my FV while swimming. It's probably too strong to suggest that it seems as if I'm peripherally blind but peripheral attention—peripheral noticing of facts and events—is, to say the least, less effective. It appears that a significant shift (or dropping out) of visual attention has resulted due to the restriction of the size of the FV for 3 1/2 weeks. The evidence is that frequently today I have held my head in a given posture, foveating a place, call it "X"; then I head-scanned and foveated some other place or object, call it place "Y"; finally, I returned the head and eyes to their former posture (place "X"). And only now did I notice place "Y" peripherally—*a place of which I had previously been totally unaware; that is, place "Y" did not (consciously) exist for me until I foveated it; only then did it become visible (was it noticed) peripherally. In all these respects then, I'm acting as if I were still gazing through the FV-restricting prisms.*

With respect to visually guided actions, I reported (1/0–1/12):

Walking: Active downward head-scanning persists during walking despite the fact that I need not do so: Of course, the head-scanning I do now was formerly necessary in order to discover obstacles and avoid stumbling and falling. While walking down stairs from the house to the beach, I did not even notice that I actively head-scanned downward (to the chin-to-chest position) and [that] I continued doing so on the level beach. So head-scanning, which is [presumably] totally superfluous now, is going on quite as it has gone on during Stages 2–4. The haptic perception is that walking is a smoother process than during Stages 2–4.

(1/1.5–1/6):

I'm beginning to actively (consciously) inhibit small, obviously unnecessary, (primarily) up–down HMs during walking. I do so with some success.

(1/1.5–1/11.5):

I'm greatly surprised to see my hands and arms in the FV without having to engage in head-scanning. I swam on numerous occasions throughout the day and noticed, all of a sudden, my hands and arms in the water. During Stages 2–4, I could accomplish this only with premeditation but not while keeping my head and arms in a posture natural for swimming. The most surprising aspect is that I swam quite a long while before I noticed *or* discovered *that my hands were actually in my FV.*

(1/2–1/2.5):

Bicycle-riding: Looking at my feet without losing sight of the road was quite novel and perplexing. Even with a full FV sight of the horizon line appears to be a necessary condition for effective steering. I discovered this when I put my head in the chin-to-chest position; I lost my visual "lock" on the horizon and maneuvering in a straight line became difficult and then impossible. Turning my head back over my shoulder was no more, or less, difficult today than during Stages 2–4. Still, the opportunities for visually guided bike-riding behavior are more readily available now than during Stages 2–4, and the result is greater visual and hence performatory stability and self-assurance.

(1/2.5–1/2.5):

Wooden-racket tennis-like game proceeds smoothly: The only limitation is attributable to the weight of the helmet. Its presence makes throwing my head back rapidly difficult and leaping into the air painful because I come down first and the helmet follows, smashing back onto my head as I land. The suggestion is that I'm still greatly encumbered even though the helmet has truly become part of me.

(1/12–1/12):

Generally, any activity necessitating a great deal of HM is facilitated relative to Stages 2–4, now that I'm back to a normal-sized FV. This is true of any activity which required a great deal of head-scanning during Stages 2–4 such as ball-playing (throwing, catching, heading). With respect to throwing, for example, I could guide and initiate my movements almost equally well with the restricted field, but when it comes to following the trajectory of the released ball, the larger FV is an advantage, particularly since this trajectory contains important (visual) information for the next delivery. This information is seldom gotten with the restricted field. The situation is worse for an object coming toward one. Since the throw is not self-initiated, there is no advance information about its expected trajectory, and visually "intercepting" such a target is doomed to failure in the face of this lack of information. Activities not requiring much HM are much less influenced by the present difference in the size of the FV.

(2/16–2/30):

All is back to normal (last day of Stage 5). I am unaware of any perceptual or performatory novelties attributable to the restriction of the FV.

Discussion: Aftereffects of Restricting the Field of View

Three salient aftereffects were observed once my FV returned to normal size. As in the Tube Study, one of the main carry-over effects of which I was well aware was that I persisted in now apparently superfluous up–down HMs of small excursion. I did so even though there no longer was the danger that I would be deprived of end-point overlap of optical structure. Moreover, I was now free to reverse the previous process of substituting HMs for saccadic scanning but apparently, did not do so. When extreme-excursion saccades did carry the eyes beyond the previous limits of the restricted FV, I experienced dizziness. This was true when such saccades occurred spontaneously (i.e., when they were elicited in response to events in the periphery of my FV) and especially when intentional eye jerks were executed. The lightheadedness was exacerbated when I then maintained the eyes in that extreme posture.

Second, my perceived orientation to my environment, oriented locomotion, and visually guided skills seemed quickly improved, in spite of the fact that ostensibly unnecessary head-scanning persisted. The conscious noticing of places and body parts in the periphery was much less salient at first, seemingly requiring a relearning of attention, yet that relearning did not interfere with these improvements either. Generally, my opportunities for obtaining optic information useful in these activities were expanded.

Third, another carry-over effect from 25 days of living with a restricted FV appears to be that I was not consciously aware of peripherally available objects, body parts, and events. They were not visually noticed, almost as if I had learned to become functionally blind in those portions of the peripheral FV not available to ocular inspection during the FV restriction. Only after I foveated objects and body parts available to peripheral vision did I become aware of them by means of peripheral vision. What may be called a temporary *functional attention-blindness* or *attention-impairment*—possibly the result of disuse—was most striking for unmoving objects and body parts.[5]

The persistence of small HMs and the inattention to objects in the peripheral FV, though both the result of restriction of the FV, may not be independent phenomena. The length of time I persisted in making these small HMs may be correlated with the duration of the transitory functional attention-blindness. Continuing small HMs may not be functionally superfluous, given that my attention was trained for 3.5 weeks to vigilance within a restricted FV, and locked onto the HM system. As an adaptive mechanism, the observer should attempt to continue to insure *functional* overlap of optical information for any pair of head samples: He or she should persist in any routine that provides the time necessary to retrain or shift visual attention to peripherally located objects, body parts, and events. Further and more detailed controlled laboratory study is indicated to determine if, and to what extent, such a relationship exists.

[5]This interpretation may be applicable to Held and Bauer (1967, 1974) and Bauer and Held's (1975) finding that monkeys raised with a ruff (opaque shield) around the neck, which prevented sight of the limbs, seemed entirely unaware of the presence of their stationary limbs immediately upon removal of the ruff and groped for the manipulandum as if they were blind.

AFTEREFFECTS OF INCREASING THE WEIGHT AND SIZE OF THE OBSERVER'S FUNCTIONAL HEAD

Method, Results, and Discussion

For 30 days, or 424 waking hours, I had carried an additional weight of 3.8 kg (8 lbs., 6 oz.) on my head and had been subjected to an increase in the functional width and length of my head. The main aftereffects, upon removal of the helmet, were (*a*) General mobility, and mobility of the head in particular, were greatly enhanced; (*b*) at first, I was haptically hardly aware of "carrying" a head; and (*c*) my visually and haptically judged size of the head still showed the discrepancies described in Chapter 6, Table 6.1 and discussed thereafter. My direct report was as follows (1/0–4/64):

> *Both head mobility and general mobility are enormously enhanced. I am freed. Haptically, my head is perceived to be so light in weight that I'm hardly aware of it (i.e., of carrying a weight on my neck and shoulders). During the first day, my arms* feel *light, and during swimming, my arms and legs* felt *stronger; curiously, my neck or head did not share in this perceived increase in vigor.*

(1/0–3/45):

> *Visually and haptically judged size of the head: I continue to test all combinations in counterbalanced sequence three times daily, on awakening, at noon, and before retiring. The results are identical to those gotten during Stage 1.*

(4/46–4/63):

> *Both the visually and haptically judged size of the head is back to normal (preexperimental levels) regardless of the sequence of judging head size.*

SUMMARY

Using the results of Stages 4, 5, and 6 of the Prism Study as a paradigm, I discuss the perceptual and performatory aftereffects of having (*a*) up–down reversed my field of view (FV); (*b*) restricted my FV; and (*c*) increased the weight and size of my functional head with the helmet.

Three main aftereffects of up–down reversing the FV are detailed, beginning with the consequences of head movements and the seesaw effect. The perceived direction of the motion of the FV was congruent with preprism phenomenology. The rate of apparent world motion was very slight at first. It was more pronounced 50 minutes later, yet significantly less than with reversing prisms. I also experienced mild bodily instability but no nausea during brisk walking, suggesting that the preprism relationship between eye–head compensation was preserved and remained in readiness in spite of the reversal of compensatory eye movements during reversal. Thus, the adapted observer is *biperceptual* because he or she never relinquishes his or her preprism standard for differentiating the rate of self-movement from consequent environmental motion. Since this aftereffect seems to depend on a perceptual comparison with a retained preprism competence, I call it a *perceptual contrast effect.*

The aftereffects of visually guided actions are described next. They fell into two classes. First, I committed errors in the direction of head movements during eye–head pursuit. I call these errors of uncertainty and confusion *carry-over aftereffects.* Second, I was immediately competent in the activities that I had practiced while wearing prisms. I call these *persistence aftereffects.* Uncertainty and hesitation were experienced only with tasks that I had not managed to perform with adeptness with prisms (e.g., catching a ball).

Third, the aftereffects of simply having looked through the reversing prisms are discussed. Almost immediately, I judged the orientation of my head to be as it had been preexperimentally. At least 5 hours of visual inspection elapsed before I began to be (*see,* actually) perceptually, aesthetically, and emotionally comfortable in the new environment. I experienced a progressive decrease in the strangeness, unreality, bizarreness, and asymmetry of faces, expressions, and the natural environment. However, after 5 hours without the reversing prisms, I was already unable to remember what the contents of the reversed FV had been like, even though I had just spent over 200 hours looking through reversing prisms. For 2 days I observed a severe minification of objects and people and a spectacular compression of distances-from-self—what I collectively call the *Lilliput aftereffect;* only later did these effects disappear, returning objects and people to their remembered dimensions. Object minification and distance compression are considered contrast effects. Four related explanations are analyzed. I experienced two realities: a passive "gaze" and an active "locomotor" or "effort" distance. Exerting myself by walking, swimming, or cycling a specified distance appeared to produce a "correcting" influence on the phenomenally but passively viewed compressed distance. Eventually, the aftereffect disappeared when "gaze distance" was recalibrated to match "effort distance." I did this by visually perceiving the action.

After living with a restricted FV for 25 days, I returned to my normal FV. Yet, I persisted in making small up–down head movements. Moreover, I was frequently unaware of objects, body parts, and events that were actually present in my peripheral FV. Because of this transitory *functional attention-blindness,* I often had to first foveate the object or body part before I would notice its presence in the periphery. A third aftereffect was that geographic orientation and visually guided activities were nevertheless facilitated.

Increased head and body mobility followed removal of the helmet. The differences in judged head size, described in Chapter 6, persisted.

11

Theoretical Foci and Paradigms: Products and Processes of Adaptation

In this chapter I review the main descriptive, experimental, or theoretical contributions of seven influential researchers and theorists. The analysis is limited to two important and often inseparable issues. First, what is the end result of having worn transforming spectacles? It was Harris who asked this question in the following sense: "How does the adapted subject differ from one who has not adapted? [Harris, 1963a, p. 1, 1963b, p. 812, 1965, p. 419]." I will put this good question to Stratton, Kohler, Rock, and finally, to Harris himself. By *unadapted subject* I will most frequently mean an observer wearing spectacles who has not yet adapted; occasionally an observer who has never worn spectacles will be intended.

Given factual data and interpretations on the end-product of the adaptation process, the second issue arises: What are the mechanisms and–or preconditions for adaptation? More abstractly, this question becomes: Why does adaptation occur? Helmholtz, Held, and Howard were most concerned with the mechanisms by which adaptation succeeds or fails.

A few summarizing remarks about my own position on these two issues conclude the chapter. The information that at first confuses and misleads the observer, yet makes eventual adaptation possible, is also briefly described.

PRODUCT: HOW THE ADAPTED OBSERVER DIFFERS FROM THE UNADAPTED

Stratton: The Harmony Between Touch and Sight

In brief, Stratton believed that adaptation is the reestablishment of experiential harmony between touch and sight, and much more. He began his experiments in the dual hope of solving, on the one hand, the empirical problem of whether or not the inverted image was a necessary condition for seeing things in an upright position and on the other hand, he wanted to test the relative merits of the then extant projection and eye-movement theories. His theoretical notions came to focus upon the issue of the experienced relationship between touch and sight because "The inverted position of the retinal image is . . . not essential to 'upright vision,' for it is not essential to a harmony between touch and sight, which, in the final analysis, is the real meaning of upright vision [1897b, pp. 475–476]." In effect, Stratton operationalized the meaning of "upright vision." The adapted Stratton appears to have differed in the following six broad ways from the Stratton who had not adapted.

Touch–Sight Correspondence Achieved

It was not until 1899, two years following his justly famous experiments, that Stratton arrived at the firm theoretical view that the adapted spectacle-wearer differs from the one who has not adapted by experiencing a correspondence between touch and sight. Of both the 1896 and 1897 experiments, he said in 1899:

> The more recent investigation concerning touch and sight seems to indicate that the place in which any part of the body is persistently seen influences the localisation of the dermal and kindred sensations arising in that part. If one were to see his feet, for instance, in some direction different from their present visual position, he would in the end refer thither their kinaesthetic impressions also. This much, it seems to me was implied in the results of my experiments on inverted vision, reported not long ago . . . the results showed how tactual localisation is affected by disturbance of the normal visual directions merely, and indicated that sensations of touch and movement may come to be referred to an entirely new direction in sight . . . the experiments showed . . . that a discord between touch and sight which was a mere matter of direction would necessarily be transitory [p. 492].

Simply put, Stratton concluded that vision dominates and teaches touch—that tactually and kinesthetically experienced localization (position) and movement change in the direction of visually experienced localization and movement of body parts in the adapted observer. Yet, Stratton's position is inadequately represented unless one considers his description of the role of tactual, and particularly of visual, imagery in an evidently complex experiential process of reharmonizing touch and vision.

Novel Visual Memory Imagery

Second, it is clear that the adapted Stratton was, experientially, quite a different person: He was now equipped with novel and varied imagery, predominantly of visual origin. The imagery he had to contend with was either *visual or tactual* (haptic); it occurred with his *eye open or closed;* it related to, or "focused" either primarily upon parts of *the body* or on parts of *the external environment;* and, finally, his imagery featured often competing "views" *within or outside his circular field of view* (FV). The competition was of two sorts: First, preexperimental imagery competed with imagery established during inversion, and second, both of these forms of imagery competed against direct perceptions during inversion. The subject of such competition was the orientation or location of parts of his body or of parts of the environment. A careful reading of the log of Stratton's 87-hour experiment[1] reveals that he tried to keep account of 12 different kinds of imagery, occasionally commenting on how they interacted or what their relationship was to his perceptions of that moment in time. Thus, for example, on Day 7 Stratton reported:

> Seated by the open fire, I happened to rest my head on my hands in such a way that the fire shone directly on the top of my head. I closed my eyes, and the image of the fire remained true to the recent perception. But soon I noticed that I was representing the fire in pre-experimental terms, and I finally discovered that the change was caused by the growing sensations of warmth on the top of my head. My hair and scalp were persistently felt in their older position, no doubt because I never directly saw them in any other. And the old localization of the fire was the only one consistent with this old localization of the hair and scalp. But by passing my hands rapidly back and forth before my open eyes, ending the movement each time with a touch upon the top of my head, it was not difficult to produce a vivid localization of my scalp in harmony with the sight-perceptions. And with this change the old localization of the fire was suppressed [1897b, pp. 465–466].

[1]In his report of the 8-day experiment (1897b) Stratton defined his terms carefully and used them consistently. He said, "One has constantly to make a distinction between the appearance of an object as seen through the reversing lenses, and either the appearance it would have if the lenses were put on, or the appearance it would have had if the lenses were removed and normal vision restored. This appearance just described is called in the narrative the 'older,' the 'normal,' often the 'preexperimental' appearance of the object; while the appearance through lenses is called its 'newer' or 'later' appearance. Similar distinguishing terms have also to be used with references to the mere representation or idea of an object, as contrasted with its actual perception [1897b, p. 343]." By "representation or idea of an object," Stratton meant visual or haptic-kinesthetic imagery.

It seems evident from the next to last sentence that Stratton visually perceived the top of his head to be inverted relative to where he remembered or visualized or felt it to be. At the end of that day he said, "On removing the glasses, my visual images relapsed into their older form, with a constant interplay and accompaniment, however, of the new [1897b, p. 466]."

Head Visually Inverted

Third, the adapted Stratton perceived (and imaged) both the orientation and location of his body parts with respect to the perceived FV to be different and more stable than in the unadapted state. His head, especially, he judged visually to be inverted with respect to the trunk and located below his accustomed, preexperimental point of observation. For example, while eating, "the movements of my hands and of pieces of food across the visual field, constantly suggested that my mouth must lie between the line of sight and the new position of my legs [1897b, pp. 467–468]." Thus, based on visual evidence, Stratton localized his mouth where his forehead had been preexperimentally. And again:

> In other cases the re-localization of bodily parts that were beyond the reach of sight was brought about by the suggestive influence of such movements as I have just described, without any voluntary attention or visualization of the parts whatever. As I rocked in my chair, I found that by throwing my arms up through the field of sight into the visual region in which my shoulders, according to the old experience, were wont to be localized, the repeated feeling of the unimpeded motion of my hands through this region destroyed the old representation of my shoulders and back, and gave them a localization in harmony with the new visual experience, except that (as I noticed) my head seemed too deep-set in my shoulders—in fact, seemed buried in them almost up to my ears [1897b, p. 468, cf. Figure 9.2, this volume, p. 205].

Visual Field Appears "Normal" not "Erect"

Fourth, the adapted Stratton differed from the unadapted observer in that he acquired a visual familiarity with the appearance of the inverted FV. Thus he said on the fourth day, "During such active operations there was at times a surprising absence of incongruity in the appearance of things [1897b, p. 354]," and on Day 7, "When I began to pace rapidly up and down the room, I felt that I was more at home in the scene than ever before. There was perfect reality in my visual surrounding [1897b, p. 463]." The experience was compelling enough to lead to descriptions that have been widely misinterpreted; for example, on the last day of wearing spectacles he wrote, "As long as the new localization of my body was vivid, the general experience was harmonious, and everything was right side up [1897b, p. 469]." Nowhere does Stratton say that the orientation of his FV, relative to the orientation of his head, looked just as it had *before* he put on inverting lenses.[2]

Some Competent Action Achieved

It must be emphasized that Stratton's reports are primarily devoted to a careful and exhaustive description of his *experiences*. Quite unlike his more behavioristically oriented followers (e.g., Ewert and Wooster), Stratton was barely concerned with the issue of performatory indexes as measures of adaptation. Nevertheless, over the course of the second experiment in particular (87 hours of inversion), he achieved relative competence in many tasks required in daily life. Thus, for example, on the fifth day, "At breakfast, with the lenses on, the inappropriate hand was rarely used to pick up something to one side. The movement itself also was easier and less wayward; seldom was it in an entirely wrong direction [1897b, p. 355]."

"Swinging of the Scene" Ceases

Sixth and finally, the adapted Stratton differed in that he ceased to perceive the disturbing motions of the visual field (the "swinging of the scene") that initially accompanied his head movements (HMs). As early as the third day of wearing the inverting lenses he reported, "Head movements were still accompanied by a slight swinging of the scene, although in a markedly less degree than on the first day. The movement was referred more to the observer, so that it seemed to be more a moving survey of stationary objects [1897b, p. 349]." By the fifth day "the rocking seemed a harmonious and natural result of the rocking itself, and

[2]A simple and relatively reliable criterion that should be used to get at how the viewed scene appears to the spectacle-wearer is to ask the observer to first say whether whatever is being described is the same or different as compared with how it looked before looking through spectacles. The same–different judgment may be differentiated further with respect to the visually or otherwise perceived orientation and location of body parts *relative to* the phenomenal orientation or location of places in the FV. To date, there has appeared in every firsthand report (second- and third-party accounts being even more contradictory) some linguistic ambiguity, some confounding of description of observation with theoretical leaning, and some observations that simply cannot be interpreted because no frame of reference is provided as a guideline. If such a same–different criterion is applied, then it may be said that no one has yet claimed that there was any "flipping over" (either sudden or gradual) of the perceived FV, whatever "flipping over" might mean. The appearance through inverting or reversing spectacles is at first "strange," "bizarre," "inverted," "different," and comes to seem "normal," "upright," "erect," but not with respect to the *remembered* prespectacle appearance.

not, as formerly, a shifting of the scene, unnatural, and therefore suggestive of illusion [1897b, p. 356].''

Upon rereading Stratton's detailed account I find it virtually impossible to dismiss Walls' suggestion that Stratton was an eidetiker (Walls, 1951, p. 90). Imagery, particularly visual imagery, was either actively and deliberately practiced and-or obtruded itself upon Stratton throughout the experiment, making it the most salient experiential feature of his study.

Kohler: "Correcting" Vision

The studies of Kohler and his associates described the process and product of phenomenal and behavioral adaptation in everyday living situations. In Ivo Kohler's opinion it is the physical dimension of things that has a tendency to become visually "correct" by a process he called "restructuring" of vision, which again becomes correct veridical perception (Kohler, 1964, p. 127). The conclusion of Kohler's associate, Kottenhoff, implies an emphasis on behavioral readjustment. He asked: "What is correct seeing with reversing spectacles and in what sense does seeing (visual perception) change?" His answer is that a person sees correctly as soon as he or she has learned that he or she no longer needs to verify obstacles via touch but instead can maneuver past these objects, without touching them, on the basis of visual and kinesthetic impressions (Vorstellungen).

Kohler arrived at the view that the observer who has adapted to up-down reversal[3] [4] differs from the unadapted observer in two main

[3]The first observations of looking through up-down reversing prisms were apparently made in the 1880s by Roberto Ardigò at the University of Padova (cited in Giannitrapani, 1958). He used a right-angle glass prism with the hypotenuse face perpendicular to the line of gravity. The results were published in 1886, 10 years before Stratton's inversion experiment was presented at the International Congress of Psychology at Munich (August 4-7, 1896) and 19 years after Helmholtz's description of looking through a displacing prism, which Ardigò had read. His observations have gone virtually unnoticed by psychologists, probably because he was a philosopher, wrote in Italian, and his descriptions were quite brief and received but little circulation in the *Opere Filosofiche*. The following translation, graciously provided by Professor Fabio Metelli of the University of Padova, is based on a later (1897?) edition of the *Opere Filosofiche,* but the relevant material is, according to Ardigò, identical to that in the 1886 edition:

> *Fifth Series.* Several years ago, I repeatedly performed an experiment I imagined to solve the problem originated by the fact that the images of objects on the retina are reversed. I put on my eyes [the context suggests that the device attached to his head] a prism of glass whose section is a right-angled triangle, properly mounted, directed in such a way that the side corresponding to the hypotenuse is the upper one and

ways. He says, first, that the adapted observer achieves correct (upright) vision in that things again appear upright after perceptual errors are eliminated; second, the adapted observer achieves correct (errorless) behavior.

Perceptions Become Correct

Stratton wondered and presumably hoped that if one gazed through inverting lenses long enough, the perceived world would somehow reinvert or become upright, or flip right side up again in spite of "vision without inversion of the retinal image." Curiously, Kohler's interpretation of his own results is more faithful to Stratton's original expectation than is Stratton's. I contend that it is unclear what either Stratton's expectation or Kohler's interpretation mean, and it is therefore important to consider both the intended meaning of Kohler's claim

---

> horizontal; this way, it reflects into the eye the images of the objects reversed, and therefore they are upright on the retina. Consequently, as I expected, the objects appeared to me reversed. But, little by little, putting together the images of the objects I saw with those of my hands and feet, I was orienting them and I ended with seeing upright. On the contrary putting away the apparatus, things at first appeared reversed to the free eye . . . [1897 ?, p. 441].

Following Ardigò, no other observations with up-down reversing prisms were reported for the next four decades. According to Kottenhoff (1961, p. 41), up-down reversing prisms were built into spectacle frames in W. Stern's Hamburg University laboratory in 1927. The FV was greatly restricted, however, and sundry reflections, probably created by binocular disparity of the two prisms, interfered with controlled observations. In 1928, Erismann began with experiments at the University of Innsbruck by using a mirror carried below the observer's nose. This equipment was not usable except in the laboratory. It was not until 1947 that an observer, von Kundratitz by name, designed a mirror system that could be used outside the laboratory. It was worn like a visor, parallel to the ground and attached to the head above the eyes. (The device described in the Introduction is modeled after this design.) Kundratitz' experiment lasted 6 days. It was followed by similar, long-term studies in the real world by Marte (one 9-day study in 1947 and another, lasting 10 days, in 1950), by Scheffler (a 5-day study in 1954), by Kottenhoff (14 days in 1954) and an 11-day monocular exposure to up-down reversal by Fjelstadt, also in 1954 (Kottenhoff, 1961, pp. 41–60). The first right-left reversing experiments (Kottenhoff, 1961) were conducted in Kohler's laboratory by Grill (in 1951), by Kohler himself as the observer (in 1953), and then by Kottenhoff (in 1954). Kottenhoff's study of 71 days is the longest such adaptation study on record. Papert also wore right-left reversing prisms attached to the head in 1953 (Taylor, 1962). These studies were long preceded by so-called *mirror-drawing* experiments, for example, by Starch (1910) and Siipola (1935); their main interest was trial and error motor-learning, however.

[4]I am here not concerned with Kohler's important research with displacing prisms, colored spectacles, "situational" aftereffects, half-prisms, two-toned spectacles, or with the theoretical conceptions that deal with those results (cf. Kohler, 1951, 1956, 1962, 1964, 1966, Chapter 16, pp. 616–655).

and the evidence that he offers to support it. Indeed, what seemed expecially important to me after my own experience with gazing through up-down reversing prisms and after rereading Kohler was describing one's observations without linguistic ambiguity, without allowing theoretical preconceptions to guide the description of observations, and without mixing inferences with direct observations. Using such descriptive words as "upright vision," and "seeing upright" or describing the orientation of objects as becoming *visually correct* is confusing or misleading, as I hope to show.

In Kohler's studies all of the observers wore a mirror, attached like a visor-cap to the forehead. They thus had to maintain their eyes in an extreme, cast-upward posture to intercept light reflected from the mirror. Their up-down reversed visual field "measured approximately 40° × 80° from side to side [Kohler, 1964, p. 31]." The first observer, von Kundratitz, wore the mirror for 6 days. The second subject, Marte by name, spent 9 days, and then 3.5 years later, 10 days, as an observer (this latter study was filmed). Kohler reported these bewildering observations–claims, beginning with Kundratitz:

> At first, this subject saw everything inverted. . . . During all this time, however, his perceptions were only sporadically right side up; things appeared right side up only when they were simultaneously touched, when a plumb line was used, or when they happened to be in the subject's immediate vicinity [1964, p. 31; originally in 1951, p. 17].

Of Marte's 9-day exposure, Kohler wrote:

> Correct veridical vision was achieved by subject M. after wearing the experimental spectacles for nine days. . . . After four or five days, however, his vision also underwent a remarkable change: it seemed as if the verticality dimension had "gotten lost." To illustrate: two adjacent heads, one upright, the other inverted, were *both* perceived as upright. Gradually, more and more objects appeared right side up [1964, p. 32; originally in 1951, p. 17].

Finally, Kohler related these observations from the filmed experiment:

> When the subject (M. in this case) was permitted to reach for and touch an object in his immediate vicinity, a new integration immediately took place; the object, first seen as inverted, now suddenly appeared to be right side up. [The experience of this "reinversion" was somewhat similar to Schroeder's, 1858, well-known stair illusion.] The same result was obtained when the subject touched the object with a stick. In both cases, the subject's hands were the first objects reported seen in an upright position. Simultaneous sensations of touch thus appear to be one of the determining factors of the phenomenon. Another factor seems to be the experience of gravitational pull. When the subject was presented with a weight attached to the end of a line, he correctly perceived the relative position of the weight (to the line) as soon

> as he took the end of the line in his hand; and once the pendulum was seen correctly, the perception of more distant objects also became veridical. When the subject experienced a strong gravitational force by driving uphill in a car, the landscape righted itself perceptually. Familiarity with objects proved to be a third determining factor involved in veridical vision. A candle, at first seen in an inverted position, wick downward, was seen right side up as soon as it was lit. The same effect was observed when the object was a burning cigarette: in this instance, it was the direction of the smoke that indicated to the subject which part of the visual world was "up" and caused the percept to correct itself [1964, p. 33; originally in 1951, p. 19].

Another procedure was this:

> . . . let the subject read; if he read an M as W, then we knew at once that his vision was inverted. . . . In this investigation we found that after five days the subject's adaptation had progressed to a point where perceptual errors hardly ever occurred [1964, p. 34; originally in 1951, p. 19].

The Trap of Upright Vision: How to Avoid Ambiguous Descriptions

I propose that there are four interrelated areas of confusion that make it difficult—for spectacle-wearers and experimenters alike—to distinguish between their observations and inferences and that it is these confusions that encourage verbal ambiguity when one is labeling perceptions while looking through reversing or inverting spectacles. I also propose four rules to prevent such ambiguities:

1. To achieve clear verbal descriptions of one's perceptions, it is necessary to distinguish, as did Stratton, between appearances before and during spectacle-wearing and to relate one's descriptions to this *dual temporal frame of reference.* This rule should help us avoid confusing "familiarity" and "naturalness" of appearance with direction or orientation attributions labeled *right side up* or *right way 'round.*
2. Consistent descriptions also depend on the use of a *relative spatial frame of reference,* which necessitates the recognition of the perceptual reciprocity between the observer and his environment, naturally including the relative location and orientation of perceived body parts and objects. This rule may help future researchers avoid meaningless assertions about, for example, the "upright" or "reversed" orientations of objects, devoid of a reference to either the spatial relationship to the surrounding environmental context or to the observer's point of observation.
3. To render a consistent description, one must distinguish between the perception of the direction and orientation, *relative to gravity,* of both objects and body parts.

4. Accurate relational descriptions can profit from a distinction between the *simultaneous and successive perception* of body-part and object context. Since the relative orientation of what is visually perceived remains constant, the availability of sky or earth for simultaneous perceptual comparison as a guide to the orientation of the viewed object remains very important to verbal pronouncements about perceived "uprightness." For example, the trunk, not the crown, of a tree remains closer to and "faces" the ground. In fact, to date no one has claimed that anyone gets confused about this sort of basic relationship, provided that the visual information for it was attended to and simultaneously available within the restricted FV.

I propose that the verbalizations of perceived "uprightness" of an object are frequently utterances about perceived familiarity when the FV contains no simultaneous optical information specifying the geographic context for the relative orientation of the object with respect to the ground or sky. I also suggest that all of Kohler's observations reported previously in this volume could have been free of ambiguity if these four simple, but hard to apply, rules had been employed. I offer one example. To report that of "two adjacent heads, one upright, the other inverted, *both* were perceived as upright [Kohler, 1964, p. 32; originally in 1951, p. 17]" violates at least the first two rules and results in an ambiguous, contradictory, or meaningless description of one's perceptions. By applying the rules that I have suggested, on the other hand, an observer might say, without ambiguity:

> *The head of the person with the cigarette in his mouth is oriented just the way I judge mine to be (i.e., the top of his head looks closer to the ground than his chin and so does mine); the other person's chin is closer to the ground than the top of his head. However, neither seems strange or bizarre to me; they both look natural and somehow familiar in that the one without the cigarette looks the way I remember (other people's) heads used to look before I began wearing spectacles and the way I used to perceive the orientation of my own head.*

What does Kohler mean by asserting that adaptation entails a change in visual perception? The reader of his reports—such as I—may disagree with Kohler's interpretation or be frustrated by the ambiguity of the descriptions or arrive at the conclusion that the data cannot be interpreted. No matter. Kohler cannot be dismissed because he has reemphasized the importance of distinguishing between phenomenal and behavioral adaptation and he cautioned against the behavioristic fallacy that observable, performatory output is a sufficient substitute for—or an inclusive basis for inferring—changes over time in the perceptual experiences of the spectacle-wearer (Kohler, 1956, p. 409). This fact remains a solid contribution of the up–down reversal studies carried out at Innsbruck: Spectacle-wearers experienced visual perceptual changes. And if there is a change in the way things look—as surely there was—then that change may, by definition, be called a visual change (cf. Rock, 1966, p. 133). Moreover, even if it were the case that such changes in visual experience did not affect the accuracy of pointing or reaching, that presumed fact would not constitute evidence against the occurrence of a visual change. If anything, the difficulty in describing, without ambiguity, these phenomenal changes speaks for their veracity. One simply cannot ignore such a multitude of descriptions in the face of their perplexing similarity to phenomena with which everyone is familiar. That is, phenomenal adaptation, as described by Kohler's subjects, appears to be a change in "visual perception," at least in the sense in which a never-before-seen room or a new town to which one moves or a new face begins to become familiar and appear different than before—perhaps by virtue of the observer noticing (perceptually learning) details and relationships previously "not there perceptually" or simply "not attended to." If such a similarity holds true, then what Kohler's observers are describing are, indeed, "changes in visual perception" or more appropriately, complex changes.

Overt Behavior Becomes Correct

Agreement as to what constitutes "correct" behavior (i.e., competent action), unlike claims about "upright vision" or "correct seeing," is readily secured. Thus, in the following excerpt no confusion results because both evidence and interpretation are meaningfully related. Kohler said:

> At first, this subject . . . could not grasp objects without making errors, was extremely unsure of himself, and had to be escorted at all times. After three days, marked improvement was noted in all respects. On the fourth day, the subject went on a bicycle trip; on the last day he went on a skiing excursion. . . . During a simulated fencing match the subject parried all blows correctly [1964, p. 31].

Rock: New Memory Images

Rock echoes an important concern of both Stratton and Kohler, namely, that adaptation is a change in appearances, a perceptual change in the way things look through spectacles. In brief, to Rock, adaptation is the reorientation of the perceptual frame of reference, mediated by the acquisition of new memory images. In his indispensable book, *The Nature of Perceptual Adaptation,* he focuses on what he regards as the problem of perception: how things look in the private world of sensory appearances (1966, p. viii and p. 269). Rock sets this analysis within an ingenious theoretical framework in which he argues that the adapted observer differs from the unadapted one in that the former has acquired visual memories of the specific character of the distorted image, establishing an altered coordinate system in the neural substrate. Thus, "Adaptation entails a shift in an already established coordinate system [1966, p. 254; also cf. 1975, p. 180]." Two questions now arise in Rock's analysis, namely, "Why is this shift necessary and how is it possible?". First, the shift is necessary because memories of the specific character of the normal retinal images have been established in the past; it is because of these memories that things look distorted when one first gazes through prisms (1966, p. 268). Second, the shift in the established coordinate system is possible because the specific character of the new distorted retinal images becomes associated with veridical information about actual spatial properties of objects (i.e., the former becomes a sign of the latter) (1966, p. 269). The functions of the altered coordinate system are to facilitate egocentric localization and orientation, now represented in memory traces, and to facilitate the recalibration of the visual and haptic systems, similarly mediated by memory images. The acquisition of new traces in the new (seen) orientation similarly accounts for the observer coming to recognize familiar objects, print, and faces, and for judging, for example, an inverted scene as "familiar" or "normal" (1966, p. 64).

I prefer to characterize these perceptual changes as a process of differentiating newly available features in the optic array, combined with a superordinate process of discovering newly available optical invariants. Yet, the visual system, broadly construed, must somehow keep track of such perceptual gains and the advantages of perceptual learning over time. To postulate, as Rock does, some form of laying down of memory traces that can be recovered or used as a basis of comparison or as a "resonance bank" thus seems required by the evidence. No theorist other than Rock has spelled out, with comparable specificity and detail, a proposal that can help us understand such phenomena. Indeed, Rock's formulations seem to me to have particular relevance to accounting for the perceptual learning of the spectacle-wearer. Koffka's question, "Why do things look as they do?" is quite as legitimate when applied to the adapting spectacle-wearer: Things do look different when one first gazes through spectacles and the appearance of much that is viewed does change. Some notions, rather similar in form to Rock's seem to me to be necessary to make sense of what he calls, properly, perceptual adaptation or changes in visual perception.[5]

Harris: The Proprioceptive Change Hypothesis

According to Harris, the end-product of adaptation "consists of changes in the position sense for various parts of the body [1965, p. 419]."[6] The adapted subject differs from the one who has not adapted in that the felt location of body parts seen through spectacles comes to coincide with the seen location of those body parts; that is, parts of the body relative to other parts have undergone changes to correspond with the direction of the stable visual information available to the spectacle-wearer. Harris' main thesis expands Stratton's main 1899 conclusion that, during adaptation, tactually and kinesthetically experienced localization and movement is attributed or referred to in the direction of the newly visually experienced localization and movements of body parts (cf. Stratton, 1899, p. 492, quoted on p. 262).

The evidence mustered by Harris appears convincing in support of the contention that when visual information and so-called *proprioceptive* (i.e., haptic-, kinesthetic-, or felt-position) information conflict, the felt position of body parts shifts in the direction of its seen position rather than the reverse.[7] However, the heart of the matter is whether adapta-

[5]This conclusion remains valid, I believe, even if one were to disagree with some of the terminology used by Rock and even if one were to take issue with some theoretical particulars in his proposals, for example, that "traces congruent with the new stimuli *take the place of* the original traces [1966, p. 251; italics mine]." If old memory traces become supplanted by new ones, how could the adapted spectacle-wearer easily recognize faces, places, words, etc. not seen since before donning the spectacles? It seems more likely that new correspondence rules relating the old to the new are established. Other theoretical particulars may also be challenged without impairing the basic integrity of Rock's proposal. For example, the principle of selection of the appropriate memory trace, or the claim that traces "enrich or supplement that which could otherwise be perceived on the basis of the stimulus alone [1966, p. 257]," or the postulate that "memory traces of speed or direction of image displacement (of stationary objects) different from that in which the image now displaces [1966, p. 99]" are laid down, presumably for every magnitude and direction of each HM. Such a process would place a tremendous burden of reliance on brain time and brain space.

[6]I wonder to what degree the limiting of the FV led to an emphasis on the felt position of body parts in adaptation, given the greatly increased frequency of head and body movements demanded when moving about with a restricted FV and given the more limited visual information the observer now has for limb location.

[7]The dominance of optic information over haptic information in the perceptual adaptation to the curvature of contours was demonstrated by Gibson (1933). Hay, Pick, and Ikeda (1965) reported a displacement in the felt location of the seen hand through prisms in

tion "is" or "consists of" such shifts in the felt location of body parts or whether felt position changes are mere (incidental) accompaniments to many forms of adaptation that are initiated, directed, and completed through and by the visual system.

At issue is whether the felt position changes proposed by Harris are either a necessary or sufficient condition to account for two widely substantiated classes of changes in (all long-term) adaptation situations: achieving competent visuomotor action and experiencing phenomenal changes in visual perception. I believe that felt position changes cannot explain many of these well-documented facts.

My reason for devoting an uncommon amount of space to the proprioceptive change hypothesis is that, in spite of its widespread acceptance, I think it is important to show that the hypothesis contains contradictory claims and unsupported assumptions that are challengeable. Seven are embedded in the discussion of how well the hypothesis handles the facts of the adaptation of (*a*) perception and (*b*) action.

First, Harris appears to have accepted a false dichotomy, courtesy of George Berkeley, that there is a win–lose relationship between touch and vision. Harris illustrates his belief in this dichotomy:

> There are two ways to eliminate this discrepancy between the seen and felt locations of the hand [seen through displacing prisms]. One way . . . is to shift visual perception to match the (veridical) proprioceptive perception of the hand. The other possibility is to adjust the felt location of the hand to match its visually perceived location [1963a, p. 13; also cf. 1965, p. 421].

Clearly, Harris has rendered an important service by emphasizing the dominance of vision and the malleability of haptics. "When vision and proprioception disagree, it seems to be proprioception that changes [1963c, p. 2137]." However, his acceptance of the dichotomy itself—much like the false heredity–environment dichotomy—assumes that a

---

the direction of the hand's seen location; they named this immediate effect *visual capture*, after Tastevin's (1937) observations and designation (also, cf. Scholl, 1926). Ryan and Ryan (1940) also emphasized the great stability of vision relative to other "senses." Rock and Victor (1964), too, showed the relative lability of haptic shape judgments when in competition with nonveridical visual information. Since Harris, the interest in the experimental confirmation of the dominance of visual over haptic and kinesthetic information has grown and since Hay, Pick, and Ikeda's report the further elucidation of the *visual capture* phenomenon has burgeoned (e.g., Easton, 1976; Easton & Falzett, 1978; Easton & Moran, 1978; Kelso & Frekany, 1978; Kinney & Luria, 1970; Lackner & Zabkar, 1977; McDonnell & Abraham, 1978; McDonnell & Duffett, 1972; Miller, 1972; Over, 1966; Posner, Nissen, & Klein, 1976; Rock, 1966; Rock & Harris, 1967; Singer & Day, 1969; Warren & Cleaves; 1971; Welch, Widawski, Harrington, & Warren, 1979).

single explanatory principle can subsume the great complexity and multiplicity of adaptation phenomena and their different rates and degrees of completeness. (I contend that whether adaptation can be explained exclusively or even primarily by recourse to the touch-vision dichotomy, however, remains both an empirical and theoretical question.) That it is unrealistic to make this assumption is reflected in the fact that over the years Harris has found it necessary to broaden the meaning of his proprioceptive hypothesis. Originally, his pivotal terms, *position sense* and *felt position,* appeared to refer to only an afferently felt position (i.e., the haptically or kinesthetically appreciated sense of position of a limb) (1963a). Later he expanded these terms to mean the registration within the central nervous system of eye position and head position (1964, 1965). If this registration is postulated to direct bodily movements, then the hypothesis becomes indistinguishable from Held's correlation storage notion, as Howard (1970, p. 348) has pointed out. (Because Harris posits that *felt position* need not necessarily be "sensory," that is, consciously noticed, but may be "registered" without awareness [1965, p. 420], direct empirical support for this assumption is not readily obtainable.) Note, moreover, that when Harris expanded his hypothesis to include *registered position* of a body part, his concept of *a change in the felt eye position* comes dangerously close to being indistinguishable from what Helmholtz meant by *a change in the direction of gaze:* a change in the efference that is presumed to register and direct eye movements.[8] The point is that it is unclear how Harris operationally defines his central concept that the observer undergoes a change in the felt position of body parts, and consequently, it is unclear how to test the validity of the proprioceptive change hypothesis.

[8]In his latest expansion, Harris has renamed as the *straight-ahead shift* (1974) a variety of what seem to me to be bona fide, short-term perceptual effects and aftereffects of adaptation. Some of these had previously been identified aptly as the *immediate correction effect* (Rock, Goldberg, & Mack, 1966). Judgments of the subjective visual straight ahead (or up or down) are naturally part of any adaptation situation, and no benefit accrues from lumping them together and treating them as a special phenomenon. Indeed, the many complexities reviewed by Harris emphasize, rather, that there are many distinct ways of judging one's orientation in an enclosed laboratory environment after donning spectacles and that there are many visually guided actions that are, to various degrees, contingent on these perceptual phenomena. Relabeling is no substitute for careful description. Finally, to call judgments that are demonstrably dependent on visual perception a *cognitive* effect is misleading (cf. Uhlarik, 1973). In reading this article, I was left with the impression that any change that does not have a felt position change as its end-product is not considered genuine adaptation by Harris. If so, we are in danger of defining facts out of existence before we have a chance to get them right.

Proprioceptive Change and Visual Perception

The most important difficulty, however, with Harris' hypothesis, expanded or otherwise, is that it cannot account for the phenomenal changes in visual perception experienced by the observer during adaptation or for the end product of perceptual adaptation.

Spectacle-wearers, particularly those gazing through inverting or reversing spectacles, are at first unable to recognize individual letters or to read, yet achieve competence in reading; they fail to recognize facial expressions or a particular person, yet eventually both become familiar; they describe many events and entire scenes in their FV as "bizarre," "uncanny," "strange," yet later they experience and describe these same events and scenes as "symmetrical," "aesthetically pleasing," "natural," etc. (cf. Chapter 9). The observer's full description of such changes in phenomenal appearance may be called *phenomenal changes* or *visual changes* or *changes in visual perception* or *visual system changes*. Harris, however, asserts that no change in (pictorial) visual perception takes place during adaptation (1965, p. 433). In support of his hypothesis, Harris posits a hypothetical experiment to describe the pictorial perception of an observer who has worn right-left reversing spectacles for some time:

> But still his pictorial visual perception remains unchanged. The letters on the blackboard and the license plates on cars look just the same as they did when he first put on reversing goggles. The only difference is that he now feels the right side of his body to be on the same side as the curve of the backward R that he sees . . . he says the curve is "on my right" [1965, p. 435].

But Harris' is an inaccurate description of the facts; neither letters nor numbers "look just the same" throughout prism exposure. Moreover, I believe that the *end-product* of perceptual adaptation cannot be accurately specified unless one provides an accurate account of its *processes*. Upon donning spectacles, an observer is unable to decipher license plate numbers-letters without prolonged attention and effort. Progressively, he or she gains more facility. Above all, I contend that if the orientation and location of distinctive parts of letters and numbers relative to the observer's body parts are influenced at all, they are influenced by the *seen* confusions and the *visually* perceived apparent location and orientation of body parts, not by their barely noticed, felt, or otherwise "registered" positions. I believe it is the *seen* locations of the body parts that are optically prepotent for the observer, and consequently, it is the more perceptually demanding source of confusion and, eventually, the source of consistent judgments. Harris, however, asserts that the only difference in pictorial perception during adaptation is the felt position of the observer's body relative to the seen letters. His own descriptions of how changes in the felt or registered position of *any* body part account for the visual-perceptual changes in the phenomenal experience of a spectacle-gazer is either unclear and-or unsupported. Indeed, Harris argues for the stability and dominance of visual perception and yet maintains that judgments are made on the basis of the position sense that he considers vaguer and more variable, which is an unresolved contradiction.

The difficulty of the proprioceptive hypothesis in clarifying the *relationship* between optic and haptic-kinesthetic information in adaptation becomes further evident when Harris insists that phenomenal changes in adaptation are neither visual nor "in the visual system." After lucidly describing some of Kohler's linguistically inconsistent descriptions of reading mirror-reversed writing and ego-relative statements about the seen location of objects containing the writing (1965, p. 432–433), Harris concludes: "Adaptation to reversal consists of a change in proprioceptive perception of parts of the body. There is *no* visual change; *S*'s visual perceptions after he has adapted are identical to those when he first put on reversing spectacles and saw all writing as mirror writing [1963a, p. 46; also cf. 1965, p. 433]." This conclusion, however, does not follow from the evidence. There is, I believe, a genuine change in which the visual system participates but not in the sense in which either Kohler assumed (a return to "correct" seeing) or in the sense in which Harris denies there is. The facts are that immediately upon donning inverting or reversing spectacles, the observer is unable or hardly able to read normally oriented print, let alone script. It is also a fact that one end-product of looking at print long enough is that observers will again be able to read it. No one is the old-fashioned, experienced typesetter's equal when it comes to reading inverted print. Harris, too, acknowledges that reading mirror writing becomes easier with practice (1963a, p. 47). The facts agreed upon, the question again arises: What sort of change *is* learning to read in a novel orientation? I believe a valid answer is that after much looking, noticing, attending, and, I dare say, discovering the distinctive features of inverted or reversed letters-numbers by processes of visual-perceptual learning, the observer begins to distinguish and read again. Since pictorial perception *has* become experientially different for the adapted observer, we may well infer that perceptual learning is a change in the functioning-operating characteristics of the visual system, perhaps of the kind suggested by Rock.

Harris is right, of course, in saying that a visual change does not occur in the misguided sense of expecting "things (eventually) to flip over again (cf. Chapter 9)''; agreed, the linguistically careful, adapted spectacle-wearer would *not* say, ''The print now looks precisely the way that I remember print looked when I learned to read as a child or before I donned these spectacles.'' Yet, Harris seems to maintain that the observer's visual perceptions after he or she has adapted are identical to those made when he or she first puts on reversing spectacles, a claim clearly contrary to the evidence.

The second challenge is this: Harris uses two assumptions as a test of the validity of any interpretation that proposes that adaptation consists of a visual or visuomotor change. First, Harris believes that in order to correctly infer a ''genuine'' visual change, the spectacle-wearer's pictorial perception after adaptation would have to be indistinguishable from his or her pictorial perception prior to donning spectacles. That is, at the experiential level, the observer would have to report that, following the process of adaptation, he cannot distinguish the orientation and appearance of, for example, print from its preexperimental appearance: It looks the same. However, no one has ever explicitly reported such experiential data, once findings such as Kohler's are stripped of linguistic ambiguity. Therefore, it is unacceptable to use this criterion to judge the validity of hypotheses that do not explicitly claim altered visual perception in the restricted sense assumed by Harris. The kind of flexibility in visual experiences and functions that *can* be expected have been amply documented in this book and are especially evident in the direct reports of the long-term spectacle-wearers. Second, Harris argues that his required experiential change in pictorial perception would imply anatomical-functional ''changes in retina–cortex connections [Harris, 1974, p. 461]'' and since none occur, no genuine visual adaptation has occurred in the adapted spectacle-wearer. Again, the particular narrow sense of *visual change*—the ''rewiring'' of retinal–cortical connections in an adult human—has not been accepted as a reasonable criterion for inferring visual adaptation. (Stratton abandoned the idea once his results were in and Walls, 1951, successfully dismantled it.) Ultimately, however, whether or not, and where in the brain, structural and–or functional changes are hypothesized as a result of learning to read inverted print or coming to recognize a smile for a smile instead of a frown remains an empirical question. Who doubts that the experienced typesetter's *visual* nervous system is not distinctively different from that of the beginning apprentice in visual memories, pattern recognition capability, and so on? As we have seen, Rock (1966) is the theorist who speaks most clearly to that issue.

The third source of confusion embedded in the proprioceptive hypothesis is that felt position changes are doing double duty: They are occasionally presumed to be both the end-product of adaptation and its basis. Thus, Harris concludes from his reading of Stratton's reports "... that proprioceptive changes, far from being temporary and trivial, become more and more extensive as adaptation progresses and are directly responsible for the 'correct' perceptual judgments that ultimately emerge [1965, p. 434; similarly, 1963a, p. 40]." Harris' interpretation of Stratton's data either contradicts Harris' own hypothesis or points up an inherent confusion. If the visual system is dominant, as Harris contends, how can the nondominant and relatively imprecise position sense be "directly responsible" for altering the position sense? To add to the confusion, Harris later writes, "Although the proprioceptive change interpretation does not specify any particular process or precondition for change, it is tempting to assume that adaptation results from a discrepancy between proprioceptive and visual information [1965, p. 440]." Several sentences later, Harris admits that "On the other hand, there is no logical necessity that proprioceptive inputs be used at all by the mechanism that recalibrates the position sense [1965, p. 440]." These disparate and unresolved claims make it difficult to interpret clearly his central concept, changes in felt position. Moreover, from the standpoint of building a testable model, it seems to me necessary to explicitly postulate the processes that yield the end-product of adaptation before arriving at a confident conclusion as to the nature of the end-product. I believe I have shown that the source of the proprioceptive changes discussed by Harris is the variable, and invariant, transformed optical information imposed on the spectacle-wearer. Such information is, I believe, the principal basis for, and directs the course of, the felt position changes emphasized by Harris.

Fourth, a closely related assumption made by Harris is that vision is a constant standard to which the felt position of body parts accommodates itself (1965, p. 441). Can Harris mean that the optical information the observer is exposed to while looking through prisms is unchanging? Hardly, because as the observer reaches away from the body, the apparent degree of displacement of the arm increases with its distance from the body as Ogle's (1951, 1952) analysis has made clear (to say nothing of the optical "earthquakes" produced by HMs during reversal or inversion). Yet, Harris' assumption is consistent with his position on the inflexibility and dominance of the adult visual system. The difficulty arises because he is aware of the evidence indicating that proprioceptive shifts are variable throughout the course of adaptation (1963a, p. 40, 1965, p. 439). The paradox is this: How can an inflexible visual system give rise to such proprioceptive variation? As I have demonstrated throughout this book, the fact is that the *optical* information the observer is obliged to subject himself-herself to during bodily movements is exceedingly variable, and the visual system, with its memory and cognitive apparatus "behind" it, may be presumed to be anything but "constant" in its effort to make sense out of extreme changes—to extract the meaningful invariants within this optical flux.

Finally, I will reinspect how the proprioceptive hypothesis handles the facts of a universal perceptual phenomenon of spectacle-wearing: the visual instability created by HMs. Harris believes that the apparent movements of the visual field, produced by movements of the head or body during the wearing of inverting goggles, are more closely related to proprioceptive arm adaptation than to purely intravisual phenomena (1965, p. 431). He claims that "whenever Stratton saw the world as stationary, he misperceived the direction in which his head was moving [1963a, p. 67, also cf. 1965, p. 431]." As supporting evidence, he employs the following quotation from Stratton (1897b): "Movements of the head or of the body . . . seemed to be toward that side on which objects entered the visual field, and not toward the opposite side, as the pre-experimental representation of the movement would have required [p. 358]." Stratton's observation cannot serve to draw the conclusion Harris draws: Nothing is said about perceiving the world as *stationary* or *misperceiving* the direction of his own HM. Stratton is simply describing the visually perceived direction of his HM and comparing that direct visual perception with the (visual?) image (representation) remembered from prespectacle days (cf. Footnote 1). Moreover, Stratton correctly perceived and remembered that his HM was in the opposite direction from the way it used to be. The full quotation bears this out:

> Movements of the head or of the body, *which shifted the field of view, seemed now to be in entire keeping with the visual changes thus produced; the motion* seemed to be toward that side on which objects entered the visual field, and not toward the opposite side, as the pre-experimental representation of the movement would have required [1897b, p. 358, italics mine].

As expected, Harris interprets adaptation to "illusory movements of the visual field" as "a kinesthetic change, which would stabilize visual perception without any change in the neural mechanism that normally takes head movements into account to yield a stationary visual world; only the felt movement of the head, the input to this mechanism changes [1965, p. 431]." Here, then, is the fifth difficulty implicit in the proprioceptive hypothesis: It seems that Harris' statement that *kinesthetic* change can "stabilize visual perception" implies that the dominant and stable visual system becomes the beneficiary of a stable visual world because of changes in the felt movements of the head. If that is what

Harris means, he implies an interpretation in favor of kinesthetic dominance and capture: quite the opposite of what the proprioceptive change hypothesis implies under other circumstances. But how can a kinesthetic change still the fierce optical perturbations that accompany head and body movements? Moreover, if only the kinesthetic input of the mechanism that normally takes HMs into account changes but the neural mechanism remains unaltered, of what use is the input? By what mechanism does the hypothesized kinesthetic input express its influence then? It is unlikely that Harris would have come to these conclusions, or indeed to his main view, had he had an opportunity to wear reversing or inverting spectacles and observe their effects directly. As I have shown in Chapter 7, to understand how the spectacle-wearer conquers visual instability requires that one consider a host of facts: visual and vestibular control of compensatory eye movements as well as visual, vestibular, kinesthetic, and cerebellar control of HMs. Neither the evidence nor the interpretation offered by Harris can satisfy the complex facts.

Proprioceptive Change and Action

To an observer wearing inverting, reversing, tilting, or displacing spectacles, objects and body parts appear to be in portions of visual space where they are not. As a consequence, observers are at first incompetent in every manner (e.g., mispointing in the direction of the optical transformation), yet observers achieve varying degrees of competence in many of these actions. After removing the spectacles, observers either mispoint in the direction opposite to the transformation or, I believe, they perform competently depending on the completeness of performatory adaptation achieved while still wearing spectacles (cf. Chapter 10).

As was the case for perceptual changes, I will endeavor to show that the proprioceptive change hypothesis cannot account for much of the competent action achieved during adaptation. It must be noted that, minimally, there is consensus that arm-pointing with *displacing* prisms with a fixed head entails a change in the felt position of the pointing arm (Dodwell, 1970, p. 174). However, even though I will analyze the more complex cases of inversion and reversal, the main arguments are transferable to pointing with displacing prisms.

In his attempt to account for the behavioral success of Stratton's adjustment to "inverted vision," Harris says:

> Proprioceptive changes... account for the behavioral aspects of Stratton's adjustment to inverted vision.... If the felt locations and movements of his hands and feet

> came to agree with their seen locations and movements, he would have no trouble reaching for or kicking things, whereas before adapting he had to move the limb in a direction that felt wrong [1965, p. 429].

This account cannot, it seems to me, explain competent action in adaptation. If the *seen* location of objects and body parts is objectively wrong when the observer looks through prisms, as it surely is, and if the observer merely comes to *feel* his or her body parts where he or she sees them—in the objectively wrong location—coming to reach correctly would not be possible. It seems to me that the complex coordinated actions of daily life cannot be executed competently unless they are preceded by accurate *visual* perception as to the *relative* location of objects and the body parts used in action. Harris seems not to think so because in another discussion of Stratton's and Kohler's inversion and reversal experiments, he says, "I think that subjects in these experiments *end up* not with correct visual perception, but with mistaken perception of where the various parts of their bodies are and which way they are moving [Harris, 1966, p. 3, italics mine]." Agreed, "correct vision" is linguistic confusion. But Harris seems to imply that spectacle-wearers, who admittedly end up getting around successfully, also end up with a *mistaken* proprioceptive and kinesthetic perception of the location and the direction of movement of their own body parts. I do not understand how such mistaken perceptions can lead to or be compatible with competent action. This description also seems incompatible with visual capture evidence. Furthermore, Harris contends that "the major changes take place *within* the nonvisual sense that registers positions and movements [1966, p. 19]," *within* the position sense. It seems to me that the proprioceptive hypothesis does not clarify how any change that is confined to one (non-visual) perceptual system can mediate competent (visually guided) actions.

Two further challengeable assumptions—sixth and seventh on my list—are implicit in these interpretations by Harris. He supposes, quite appropriately, that at first Stratton was faced with a discrepancy between the seen and felt location and movements of his body parts. This assumption is borne out by the geometry of the situations as well as by the reports of other observers. However, Harris assumes that there are just two ways to eliminate this discrepancy: shift visual perception to match the (veridical?) proprioceptive perception of the hand or adjust the felt location of the hand to match its visually perceived location (1963, p. 13, 1965, p. 421). If, as Harris proposes, the visual system and visual perception are not changeable, then the only way to resolve the discrepancy is for the relevant limb(s) to come to feel in the objectively wrong location: where they are *seen* to be. The puzzle in accounting for correct reaching, kicking, or pointing then becomes: How can a limb be moved as if it were in its actual location if it is felt or "registered" in the wrong location? To put it another way, accept the proposition that the felt position of a body part changes "in the direction of the visual information," as Harris and others appear to believe (e.g., Rierdan & Wapner, 1967, p. 62). What has the observer accomplished? With right–left reversing prisms his or her right (pointing) arm feels to be on the left side of the body, provided it is visible. If, as Harris appears to believe, this constitutes the sufficient condition for correct pointing, the observer should not be able to point properly if he or she now both sees and feels the arm where it is not. The observer simply cannot point correctly at an object that is seen to be where it is not with an arm that is seen and felt to be where it is not. At best, an observer can point at the *apparent* object, toward a place where it is not. To act competently again, I contend, the observer makes use of *visual* information about the true spatial *relationship* between the *seen* arm and *seen* object.

The point is, of course, that mere agreement between touch and vision by no means insures correct or competent action, no matter how normal the "feel" of limbs. Another solution is called for: There has to be another way to eliminate the discrepancy between the seen and haptically registered position of body parts. Neither vision nor visual perception nor visual information can be thought of as the inflexible standard with which felt positions of body parts come to agree. Nor can it be assumed that changes in felt position direct the high-precision accuracy of many an action under conditions of optical transformation.

The solution awaits challenging the a priori validity of one final assumption: that the discrepancy between the seen and felt location of body parts constitutes the information for correct pointing (Harris, 1965, p. 440) and that this discrepancy must be eliminated in order for competent action to occur. Specifically, Harris seems to assume that correct pointing necessitates feeling the arm where it is seen (i.e., that a *perceptual change* in the felt position of the adapted arm [1965, p. 424] is responsible for correct motor output rather than a perceptual change in the *seen* relationship between the object and the pointing arm relative to other body parts). Harris is right, I believe, in supposing *that* changes in the felt (i.e., the haptically or kinesthetically registered) position of body parts, frequently *result* from seeing them located and moving in a direction where they are not. Yet, the real question is whether such perceptual changes in the felt position of the arm are sufficient to explain correct pointing. I contend that correct pointing must proceed on the basis of optical information and changes in the visual perception of the relationship between self and places in the environment. Perceptual changes in the *felt* position of body parts can, at best, be an *accompaniment* to learning to point correctly or to any other form of coming to act competently (cf. Day & Singer, 1967, p. 319).

As an example, take an observer attempting to point correctly at an object near the ground while wearing up–down reversing spectacles. If adaptation consisted exclusively of coming to feel the arm where the observer sees it, then he or she could never come to point correctly because at first, he or she would point skyward toward the virtual image of the object when intending to point toward the ground: The observer points in the direction in which the eyes are pointing. Yet, that movement *looks* as if it had been in the direction of the ground because as the observer moves the arm geographically upward, it visually appears to enter the top of the FV and to move downward. Thus, the observer cannot insure correct pointing just because he or she (erroneously) *feels* the skyward directed arm to be pointing downward, even if a seen–felt discrepancy no longer exists. Correct pointing, as any other competent action, has to be achieved on some other basis. Naturally, pointing must proceed according to the facts in the world, not merely according to perceived changes in the location of body parts, be these changes "haptic," or "visual," or "cognitive."

One of the end-products of adaptation may incorporate a felt position change, but competent action is not likely to be *achieved by* changes in the felt position of body parts. Examples such as writing legibly without that action either looking or feeling right when seen through reversing spectacles underscores the point (cf. Chapter 9). I argue that the reason for coming to act competently is because of the resolution of quite another discrepancy than the one suggested by Harris. The main discrepancy with which the spectacle-wearer is confronted is between *visual* and *visual* information, not between proprioceptive and visual information. The observer is faced with optical information that at first misleads and confuses him, yet contains enough optical invariance to adapt in many ways, with competent action being eventually possible. Thus the critical class of discrepancies for the spectacle-wearer is the visual–visual. Haptic–visual discrepancies are directed by the resolution of visual–visual discrepancies but are incidental to these and dependent on their prior resolution (cf. Chapters 7–9). Harris' belief, that adaptation occurs in the control system for hand position rather than either the visual or oculomotor systems (Carpenter, 1977, p. 266), is partly based on the finding that observers mispoint to auditory targets once the prisms are removed. However, if you assume or show experimentally that the visual system monitors auditory space (e.g., Bower, 1977; Pick, 1974), then the visual or oculomotor systems are still viable candidates for the site of adaptation. This conclusion becomes even more likely when one considers that hand position is normally controlled by the visual system. (Carpenter has thought about and modeled the control mechanisms for hand position [1977, p. 266].)

In this context, Harris reported that pointing with the adapted hand seen through the displacing prism at a visual, auditory, and "straight ahead" target yielded changes that compensated for the displacement (1963a,b, 1965). While pointing straight ahead or at the ground, observers kept their eyes closed. Harris took this finding as support of the view that such mispointing is the result of a change in the felt position of the adapted hand. This interpretation has been generally accepted. However, a very different interpretation can account for these results: *vision-based* action. Harris precedes his explanation by an attempt to dismiss a view that does not rely on inferring a felt position change. He writes, ". . . one might suppose that adaptation affects only the correlation between behavior and *vision*. However, such terms as 'changes in hand–eye coordination' and 'changes in visually guided behavior' prove misleading. They imply that adaptation is confined to visual targets [1963b, p. 813]." But there is no such implied restriction on what modality visually guided behavior responds to, or controls, or to what use visual guidance is put. Furthermore, Harris and others seem to assume that tasks that do not permit the observer to make use of direct optical information (e.g., pointing in the dark) somehow remove the visual system as an agent of control (e.g., Hardt, Held, & Steinbach, 1971, p. 230; Harris, 1963b, 1966, p. 19). Such a claim assumes that the visual system cannot or does not control and guide behavior such as pointing in the dark or when the eyes are closed. This presumption ignores a widely reported fact of phenomenological experience: a person's visualized and schema-represented cognitive knowledge of his or her orientation and of his or her body layout relative to the visually remembered layout of the environment. It also ignores the evidence from the laboratory that shows that visual information improves doing new visual tasks (cf., Pick, 1974). Indeed, my discussion of *vision-based* guidance and the results of the pointing study (cf. Chapter 8) indicate that the direction of positioning of the eyes in the head affects the direction of ballistic arm movements intended for the target, even when the eyes are then shut.[9]

An analysis of aftereffects of the adaptation of perception and action would follow a similar course. For example, the proprioceptive

[9]I hypothesize that recordings of positionings of the eyes when closed and in the dark during and shortly after exposure to optical transforming spectacles will reveal that, just prior to initiating an arm movement to point at an imagined external target, any body part,

hypothesis cannot account for the Lilliput aftereffect: the minification of objects and compression of distance I observed. Similarly, the performatory persistence aftereffects, for instance reaching, require different explanatory principles (cf. Chapter 10). In this regard, there is one final assumption that should be rethought. It is frequently used to discredit Helmholtz's direction of gaze hypothesis: A visually controlled adaptation is supposed to transfer to the limb not used in the pointing task during exposure. A pointing task is probably inappropriate to test a hypothesized "visual change" of this sort, however (cf. Dodwell, 1970, Chapter 8).

In conclusion, I agree with Harris when he says that "the belief in the primacy of touch is so ingrained that experimental results are sometimes flagrantly misinterpreted in order to support it [1965, p. 441]." But danger is not past. The touch-vision *dichotomy* is so ingrained that it is hard not to misinterpret experimental results in favor of one or the other extreme. Indeed, an alternative for which evidence exists has been ignored. Harris' emphasis has been to "turn around" the Berkeleyan notion of the primacy of touch, as echoed by Carr's interpretation of the Stratton experiments. "It is the visual system that is disrupted and then reorganized so as to conform to touch . . . [Carr, 1925, p. 141, quoted in Harris, 1965, p. 441]." Harris, on the contrary, concludes, "Vision seems to be largely inflexible, whereas the position sense is remarkably labile [1965, p. 441]." Let me offer a reinterpretation, especially applicable to the findings of all long-term studies to optical inversion and reversal.

---

or at a sound source, the observer's eyes will be deviated in the direction of the optical transformation. Indeed, Bower has observed that even blind babies turn their eyes toward a sound source and track their hands with unseeing eyes, and that sighted babies tested in the dark behave the same way (1977, p. 95). Moreover, I hypothesize that shortly after looking through the spectacles, the following actions will be in the direction of the deviated eye posture: Pointing at an imaginary target, straight ahead with the body midline or straight ahead with the remembered geographic layout as reference; pointing at other body parts; and at a sound source. Mispointing is predicted for these immediate effects. As an end-product of having adapted, substantially more correct pointing would be expected; yet, the eyes should be deviated as before. If this is so, and there is favorable suggestive evidence (Kalil & Freedman, 1966; McLaughlin & Webster, 1967), then this inference seems warranted: The observer has achieved a new interpretation of eye position: a meaning change. Pointing the eyes in one direction is tantamount to looking in another, a constant magnitude removed. Kornheiser summarized the contention nicely: "stimulation of a given retinal locus that . . . corresponded to a location of 10 degrees to the left would, after adaptation, correspond to a location 20 degrees to the left [1976, p. 801]." In my terms, the observer is now pointing in line with his or her line of foveation, not fixation. The aftereffect of having adapted less than completely should bring pointing errors in the direction opposite to the initial effects. Again, the direction of the pointing arm should provide an approximate index of eye deviation.

For now, I will purposely couch it in Berkeley-Carr-Harris terms: During adaptation, it is the visual system that is disrupted and then reorganized so as to comform to the demands of the observer's ecology for consistent perception and competent action in order to direct both; rather incidentally, the haptic-kinesthetic system conforms first to the disruption and then to the reorganization of the visual system. If the word "reorganized" is understood to mean that the observer begins to act on the basis of optical invariants that continue to specify the whereabouts of things veridically (cf. Chapters 7 and 8), then we have achieved a fair approximation of what I believe goes on in adaptation. To reiterate: Harris believes that a proprioceptive shift is the primary end-product of the adaptation process. I think it is only one insufficient accompaniment of the adaptation process: The observer first has to resolve the visual-visual discrepancies. Changes in the *seen* locations and movements of body parts and things in the environment precede, and consequently help determine, changes in the felt position of body parts. But that is far from all that goes on: The actual positions and movements of body parts during actions change drastically, including the eyes, head, arms, legs, and the body itself (cf. hybrid action). As I have shown (Chapters 7-9), it is not the case that the observer wearing reversing spectacles points and moves his or her eyes, head, arms, and legs in the self-same manner as before donning the prisms. To say that the observer's felt position of body part changes as the end-product is an incomplete description of the complex facts. The observer reorganizes totally what he or she does, not just what he or she perceives (himself-herself) to be doing.

If pressed to make some oversimplified statements, I would say this: Touch does not educate vision, as Berkeley thought. Vision does not merely educate touch, as Harris thinks. Occasionally, touch educates touch and with special effort and attention (to haptic information) can be employed to guide vision. Most typically, however, vision educates vision and, in the bargain, touch; thus is touch successful.

Summary and Conclusions

The proprioceptive change hypothesis contains several puzzles, confusions, apparent contradictions, and unsupported assumptions. Several of them are affected by the difficulty that the central construct—that adaptation consists of "proprioceptive" or "felt position changes"—is not clearly (operationally) defined, and hence it is unclear what the hypothesis intends or how to test its validity. Seven interrelated assumptions were discussed and challanged:

1. A single principle—the touch-vision dichotomy—can explain a multitude of demonstrably complex phenomena.

2. "Genuine" visual adaptation must entail two changes: Pictorial perception after having adapted must be indistinguishable from normal preadaptation, and anatomical-functional changes in retina-cortex connections would have to occur.
3. A testable model for specifying the end-product of adaptation is possible without making explicit the process(es) that produce that end-product, yet proprioceptive changes in the position of body parts are occasionally presumed to be both the end-product and the source of adaptation.
4. Visual perception is a *constant* standard to which proprioception accommodates itself.
5. Kinesthetic changes are said to both stabilize visual perception during HMs and be subject to visual dominance.
6. There are only two ways to eliminate the discrepancy between the seen and felt position of body parts: Vision aligns itself to touch, or vice versa.
7. The discrepancy between the seen and felt position of body parts constitutes the information for correct action (pointing) and must be eliminated before adaptation can occur.

A review of the evidence and the arguments suggests these qualifications of the proprioceptive change hypothesis. First, the hypothesis is insufficient to describe the facts, particularly of the process of adaptation to long-term inversion or reversal. It can account, at least in part, for the rapid and incomplete adaptation to and aftereffects of mild (displacement) distortions (Dodwell, 1970, p. 160). Since the hypothesis does not purport to account for the process of adaptation but only for some of its end-products, it may seem unacceptable to make this a criterion for assessing its validity or generality. However, my contention has been that a sufficient description of adaptation phenomena cannot be arrived at by any model that does not specify the route by which its end-products were acquired. Second, rather than adaptation *being* a change in the felt position of body parts, one of the changes that may be *entailed in* adaptation may be a change in the felt position of body parts in congruence with their visually perceived location. As I have shown throughout this book, the primary difference in end-products of adaptation is that the *seen* location and orientation of body parts and the *seen* location and orientation of objects and events have become perceptually consistent and they enable the observer to act competently again. Third, no changes in the felt or registered position of body parts can account for the (visual perceptual learning) changes that enable the observer to become someone who can read again, recognize faces and their smiles, and understand the (visual) meanings of myriad events, including his or her own actions. A structural change in the visual system is not required by any interpretation of adaptation phenomena. One must act upon the fruits of *visual* perceptual learning, however, to do justice to the facts of phenomenal visual experience. Fourth, the evidence and analysis from my own and other long-term experiments suggest that many forms of adaptation exist and that changes in the felt or registered position of body parts is not a *sufficient* condition to account for the end-product of *any* of these adaptations—be they to the motions of the FV generated by HMs (directed by the compensatory eye movement control systems), changes in many actions (directed by the saccadic, vergence, and pursuit systems), or changes in the appearances of things and events (directed by visual memory images and visual–cognitive schemas).

As I have shown, the fluctuations in proprioceptive changes during the course of adaptation are created by the perturbations in the observer's inconsistent use of now novel and misleading optical information and now old, veridical invariants that steer the course of action right. These changes in the felt position of body parts are engendered, moreover, now by novel and disturbing sights of the still or moving self and now again by newly achieved consistent sights of the orientation and location of body parts. Ultimately, relativity speaks: Sight does not revolve about touch nor touch about sight, but both, complexly about themselves and one another. The gravitational attraction of sight is more forceful, hence touch is more affected by sight than vice versa. Sight is more self-sufficient and self-referential, yet in need of its servant touch to give it expression. Touch is in service, even when not apparent.

PROCESS: THE MECHANISMS AND PRECONDITIONS FOR ADAPTATION

Helmholtz: The Change of Gaze Hypothesis

In a nutshell, Helmholtz believed that adaptation to displacing prisms is a change in the judgment of the direction of gaze. He was the first to offer a careful description of the effects of pointing at an object during and after gazing briefly through laterally displacing prisms.[10] At

[10]Helmholtz's study was followed by Wundt (1898), Wooster (1923), Scholl (1925, 1926), Gibson (1933), Kohler (1964: a 124-day study done in 1951), Taylor (1962), Harris (1963a), Held and Rekosh (1963), Pick and Hay (1964), and others. In these experiments wedge prisms were attached to an observer's head. Displacement studies, with the prisms attached to one or both eyes, were carried out by Taylor (1962) in 1959, by Festinger *et al.* (1967), and by Slotnick (1967, 1969). Numerous displacement studies in which the wedge prisms were not attached to the observer have been carried out in Held's laboratory (e.g., Held & Gottlieb, 1958).

first, the observer misreaches in the direction of the apex of the prism; gradually, either with or without immediate visual guidance, he or she manages to touch the desired object. Upon removing the prism, if the observer regards the object and then closes the eyes, he or she again misreaches, but now in the direction of the base of the prism (1962, Vol. III, p. 246). Helmholtz was also the first to suggest an explanation of these observations in terms of the underlying mechanism. Of both the eventual correct reaching and the subsequent aftereffect, Helmholtz said, "Here it is not the muscular feeling of the hand that is at fault or the judgment of its position, but the judgment of the direction of gaze (Beurtheilung der Blickrichtung) [1962, Vol. III, p. 246, originally in 1867, Vol. I, pp. 601–602; and then in 1910, Vol. III, pp. 206–207]." What did Helmholtz mean by his critical term "Beurtheilung," translated as "judgment," and how is the judgment of the direction of gaze accomplished? To begin with, Helmholtz believed that knowledge of visual direction is not so much a function of the positions actually assumed by the eyes, as of the central impulse of innervation or effort of will (later labeled *efference* by von Holst) applied in the adjustment of the eyes. Moreover, the appreciation of the position of the eyes in the head and of the head with regard to the body is extremely uncertain, according to Helmholtz, and the adjustment of the eyes requires continuous control of the amount of innervation (1962, Vol. III, pp. 244 and 250). The result of the effort of will that is applied to maintain the eyes deviated from their primary position, assuming a fixed head, in order to foveate an object located in front of the nose is a "change of position of objects on the visual globe for the new position of the eye [1962, Vol. III, p. 246]." The variations of the image thus produced "are being continually utilized to regulate the proper relation between the impulse of will and its effect [1962, Vol. III, p. 246]."

The judgment of the direction of gaze, therefore, is determined by the reciprocal relation between a central efferent command, which controls ocular position, and the optical image information yielded thereby (corresponding to what von Holst later called *reafference*). I also read Helmholtz to mean that the optical image information can, in turn, modify the central effort of will. One can but surmise that the "Beurtheilung" (i.e., judgment) is a process of unconscious inference. What Helmholtz's proposal amounts to, in simple English, is that a person knows where he or she is looking because he or she knows where the gaze is cast while simultaneously knowing where he or she is located with respect to the places and objects surrounding him or her. The spectacle-wearer has to learn that when he or she sees an object clearly, he or she is actually casting the gaze to one side of it by a consistent amount in a given direction. It is the judgment of this new consistency that provides for eventual correct reaching! In that sense, seeing is dependent on knowing. Mispointing immediately after removal of the prisms, however, may be ascribed to the observer continuing to act on the basis of this newly acquired consistency.

My notion is that if the old and new consistent relations between the direction in which the observer points the eyes and the direction in which he or she foveates become well learned rules, then he or she should be able to point competently without a prism, with a prism, and after removal of the prism: a bit like being able to alternately drive a car from the left side in the USA and from the right side in England without hesitation—without negative transfer. The fact that the two systems can coexist has been shown by Taylor (1962). My own evidence also indicates that an observer can become biperceptual and biperformatory (cf. Chapter 10).

Held: Adaptation Is a Change in Sensorimotor Coordination

Held and his co-workers have wrought significant methodological innovations in the measurement of adaptation and stimulated a wide wave front of ingenious experimentation. On the theoretical side, Held's interest has been to define the change of state that is produced in the central nervous system as a result of the adaptation process and to specify the site or sites at which adaptation occurs. Held developed the view that the mechanism underlying adaptation is a recorrelation of motor output and sensory feedback signals, based on a comparative correlation between outflow and sensory input (reafferent) information. In his process description of adaptation, "Active movement with its accompanying sensory feedback is an essential condition for adaptation *under circumstances in which no other important source of error information is available* [1968a, pp. 57–58, italics mine]."

The Correlation Storage Model

Held's model is roughly as faithful to Helmholtz's intent as Kohler's view of adaptation is to Stratton's. Another important precursor to Held is von Holst who also took his cue from Helmholtz. The basic constituent ideas for von Holst's model may be found in Helmholtz (especially 1910, Vol. III, p. 205). Von Holst and Mittelstaedt (1950) and von Holst (1954) refined, expanded, and made explicit Helmholtz's ideas on the relationship between the effort of will and resultant optical input. Their reafference principle is meant to account for an animal's ability to distinguish between its own movements and motions in the environment that are not generated by the animal's movements (see Chapter 8).

Held has modified and extended von Holst's model in an attempt to account for prolonged modifications of perception (Hein & Held, 1962; Held, 1961). Held's model "assumes that commands to the musculature (efferent neural signals) are monitored by an internal memory storage which also received the concurrent feedback from the movement-produced stimulation of distance receptors. These two paired inputs are then assumed to be correlated (associated) in the memory storage. An important feature of this coupling of output with feedback signals is the dependence of sensory feedback upon bodily movement [1968a, p. 58]." The observer does two things at once: He or she tells the muscles to do something and tells the sensory system what the motor system is about to do (1968b, pp. 55–56)—the role of the corollary discharge (Sperry, 1950; Teuber, 1960).

The model is attractive because the description it offers is likewise intended for normal, everyday sensorimotor coordination as well as for visuomotor adaptation to rearrangements, especially those involving simple input transformations. This is so because Held assumes that the normal phenomenal stability of the environment insures that "any particular efferent signal (movement) should always be accompanied by a feedback signal having certain unique properties [1968a, p. 58]"; he further assumes that rearrangements "alter the relation between particular values of efferent and feedback signals but do not change their one-to-one correspondence [1968a, p. 58]."

Is Active Movement Necessary for Adaptation?

Briefly, Held's answer to the question of the necessity for active movement is yes, provided no other error information is available. The active–passive distinction[11] figures importantly in Held's model because it predicts that adaptation requires active (i.e., self-produced) movement. Several theorists challenged the early contention of Held and his

[11]Helmholtz was one of the pioneers who contrasted "purely passive observations" with voluntary, active movements of the body in his discussion "Concerning the Perceptions in General." He said, for example, "the tests we employ by voluntary movements of the body are of the greatest importance in strengthening our conviction of the correctness of the perceptions of our senses [1962, Vol. III, p. 29]." Stratton was the first spectacle-wearer to emphasize that active movements vis-à-vis passive observations yield superior adaptation (i.e., harmony of the localization by sight and by touch or motor perceptions (1897b, p. 356). Scholl concluded that active movements were necessary for prism adaptation (1926, p. 299). As early as 1828, J. F. Fries distinguished between "active" (intentional) and "passive" habits (cited in Kohler, 1964, p. 137).

co-workers that executing self-produced movements was a *necessary* condition for achieving adaptation (e.g., Held, 1965; Held & Gottlieb, 1958; Held & Hein, 1958, 1963). The consensus now is that only a more moderate conclusion is firmly established: Active movement is both a *sufficient condition* and typically a more potent means for producing adaptation than being moved passively (e.g., Howard, 1970, pp. 337–352; Howard & Templeton, 1966, p. 394; Howard, Craske, & Templeton, 1965; Pick & Hay, 1965; Singer & Day, 1966; Templeton, Howard, & Lowman, 1966; Wallach, Kravitz, & Landauer, 1963). While the spirit of Held's idea was thus exonerated, its letter could not be because, I believe, it rests on this unconfirmed assumption: that the central nervous system has available "equivalent visual stimulation and information about bodily movements of either kinesthetic or labyrinthine origin [Held & Mikaelian, 1964, p. 685],"[12] whether the organism moves actively or is being moved passively. To sustain this claim requires equating or demonstrating the equivalence of the "active" and "passive" group on many variables. Two of these are critical: (*a*) The kind and amount of optical information and (*b*) the attention the observers pay to the available optical information.[13] For example, a subject who is wheeled about without moving does not have access to the same (movement-correlated) optical information as one freely walking (Held & Bossom, 1961) or one pulling a gondola containing a passive kitten (Held & Hein, 1963).[14] The active subject has sight of the moving limbs as they enter the FV, whereas the passive observer does not have sight of his or her own body in relation to the optically displaced contents of the FV. Moreover, the probability that passive observers do or can maintain attention on the optical displacement is likely to be more limited than for an active observer, who must remain alert to avoid obstacles such as corridor walls (cf. Held & Bossom, 1961).

Held has qualified his original contention: Active movement is a necessary condition for adaptation "under circumstances in which no

[12]Kinesthetic information is clearly different for the subject propelling himself–herself in a wheelchair (Held & Mikaelian, 1964) or for the observer being pushed while standing on a dolly (Held & Bossom, 1961), as compared to the freely walking observer; the passive observer is also deprived of the discrepancy between visual and kinesthetic information experienced by the active observer. Their respective points of observation also differ.

[13]An everyday example makes the point simply: Being driven in a car along an unfamiliar route is quite unlike operating the car. The passenger is less likely to pay attention or to remember what route to take were he called upon to drive the same route afterward.

[14]An additional problem was that the active group practiced the dependent variable during exposure for anywhere from 6–63 hours, whereas the passive group did not for anywhere from 9–126 hours.

other important source of error information is available [1968a, p. 58]." The "active-passive" controversy may need to be reconsidered in this light. Clarification of the qualification would prove helpful, however, in reanalyzing past experiments and in designing new studies to test the modified proposition. Such a reconsideration also should be alert to Held's view that self-produced movement, with its concurrent visual feedback, is particularly relevant for the (neonatal) development of visually guided behavior (Held & Bauer, 1967; Held & Bossom, 1961). Finally, it is important not to lose sight of Held's important contribution: The theoretical emphasis and empirical demonstration that active interaction with the natural ecology of organisms maximizes the acquisition of competent action, even when major obstacles are introduced.

Howard: The Sites and Conditions for Visuomotor Adaptation

Howard's contributions to the study of visual-motor adaptation to optical distortion have been characterized by (*a*) offering insightful critical appraisal of others' work (especially Howard, 1968; Howard & Templeton, 1966); (*b*) executing ingenious experiments (e.g., Howard *et al.*, 1965) to give empirical support to his theoretical analyses (e.g., Howard, 1970, 1971, 1973, 1974, 1978; Howard & Templeton, 1966); and, subsequently, (*c*) introducing a highly articulated descriptive notation by means of a flow diagram (see Figure 11.1, adapted from Howard, 1971, p. 249: cf. 1974, p. 310). This chart illustrates the many potential sites at which recalibration-adaptation to optical displacement can occur (Howard, 1971, 1974, 1978). Potentially, the diagram is useful for pinpointing the complex relationships between incoming information and the observer's outward directed effort that can occur while a spectacle-wearer performs. In this regard, Howard hypothesized that the sites of adaptation to prismatic displacement were the joints moved during exposure, but his experiments were interpreted as consonant with the hypothesis that adaptation tends to be associated with a joint that remains stationary during exposure (Howard, Anstis, & Lucia, 1974). The facts are complex because of the great combination of potentially influential variables bearing on this issue (cf. Chapter 2). It seems to me that we need to distinguish between body parts that are stationary, those that are moving, or those that have moved but have come to rest again. Moreover, experimenters need to systematically vary these independent variables as well as the variable of whether the observer was given the opportunity to view any given body part before, during, and after exposure to the optical transformation. Whether the movement was initiated

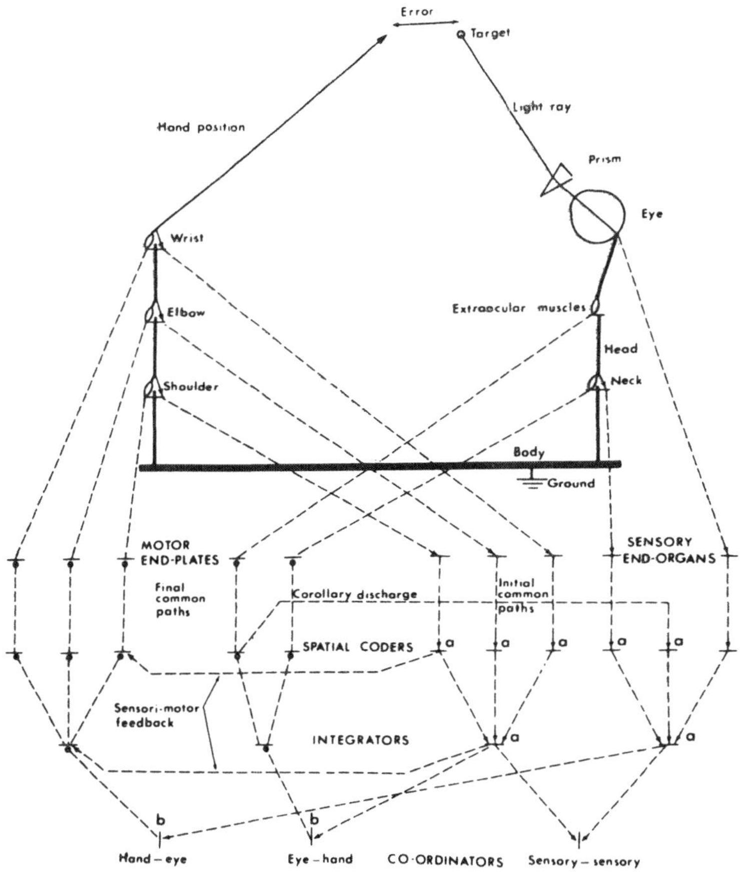

FIGURE 11.1. Flow chart for the visual-motor system. In the upper half of the diagram, basic structural components of the eye–hand coordination system are drawn in lines of medium thickness (the instantaneous position of the hand and the light ray from target to eye and retina are also considered to be structural components—lighter lines). The body (extra thick line) is considered to be fixed to the ground. Components are linked by articulations; the following symbols are used:

position-sensitive receptors

muscular elements

In the central and lower parts of the figure, neural elements are drawn in interrupted lines; junctions represent neural coding processes; arrows depict inputs to sensory elements; and filled circles depict inputs to motor elements. Sites of lability according to Harris are marked "a"; those according to Held are marked "b." (Adapted from Howard, 1971, p. 249. Medical Department, British Council: *British Medical Bulletin.* Used by permission.)

by the observer or the body part was passively transported is also of interest. The sequencing of movements may also provide quite different information to the observer. Many dozen combinations of conditions are feasible and provide ample opportunity for important parametric study.

The second issue of evident concern to Howard was to specify, as Held did before him, the conditions under which the visual-motor system develops or adapts to novel inputs. His position is more general than Held's and is that:

> Sensorimotor behavior will develop and change in response to properly displayed *discordance*, including (a) intersensory discordance, or an unusual special association of stimuli in different modalities, (b) sensory-motor discordance, or unusual association between motor innervation and consequent sensory inputs (reafference) [Howard, 1974, p. 312].

Howard's most recent conclusion is that:

> Animals seek out covariance functions within modalities, and between different modalities, as well as between corollary motor discharges and reafference. The perceptual-motor system will surely correlate what it can in order to reduce uncertainty, to economize on coding, and to coordinate action. Once such covariance functions have been detected and stored by the animal, any persistent discrepancy in current stimulation will be discordant with respect to these stored schemata, and the system will adjust itself accordingly [1978, p. 301].

SUMMARY AND CONCLUSIONS

Some of the main descriptive, experimental, and theoretical contributions of Stratton, Kohler, Rock, Harris, Helmholtz, Held, and Howard are presented. Helmholtz and Stratton, the pioneers, as well as all others, have made significant and lasting contributions to our understanding of adaptation phenomena: of the flexibility of the human person in the face of imposed disturbing optical transformations. The diversity of facts, methods, and theoretical conceptualizations is a testament to the complexity of the phenomena under study and to the conclusion that no single model suffices to account for the wealth of complex facts.[15] Some concluding statements about my own views on the two main issues of this chapter now follow.

[15]The work of many diligent and creative researchers in this vibrant field (e.g., Brouchon, Cannon, Epstein, Hamilton, Paillard, and Taub) was neither discussed nor cited because of space-time limitations.

Product: How the Adapted Observer Differs from the Unadapted

The adapted observer appears to differ from the unadapted observer in several main respects. After some 200 hours of living with reversing prisms, an observer once again experiences visual stability of the perturbed environment. This is true for a wide range of rates of head movements (HMs). Moreover, the adapted observer has acquired what may be called another "personality" (i.e., he or she has the dual facility to be perceptually and emotionally comfortable and to act competently both with and without transforming prisms). The adapted observer is thus a very different creature from the unadapted observer—somewhat like someone with a second language or a novel set of skills that can only be directly displayed under special circumstances (cf. state-dependent learning and recall). The observer becomes what I call *biperceptual* and *biperformatory*. At present, very little hard evidence is available on how much perceptual or visuomotor learning remains, once the long-term wearing of prisms is over. I suspect that retention or savings scores would be comparable in most respects to similarly practiced skills in typical learning situations not involving the use of optical transformations. The perceptual change that occurs within the observer during prism-wearing, for example, is itself a process of perceptual learning. This process ultimately results in the acquisition of new visual schemas and images composed of the observer's novel memory traces, which correspond to the new transformed sights. If that were not so, how could someone who looks through reversing prisms after not having done so for a full year still experience an immediate sense of "Oh, I remember that" familiarity with the scene viewed? (My own observations; also cf. McLaughlin & Webster, 1967, p. 43; Taylor, 1962, p. 204.) Or how, indeed, could an observer suffer "only a slight and momentary negative transfer effect on the progress of the (visuomotor) tasks performed [Snyder & Snyder, 1957, p. 30; similarly, Peterson & Peterson, 1938, p. 19]" after two years of not wearing inverting spectacles? Or, how could an observer read with some success print he had learned to read while wearing prisms when he looked through them again? Or, why would an observer experience inordinate difficulty in recognizing someone whom he had only seen while wearing reversing prisms once he removed them (author's observation)? In general, the adapted observer is capable of living in both worlds, under both sets of information conditions and behavioral requirements with roughly equal comfort and competence.

Process: The Preconditions and Mechanisms for Adaptation

How does an observer arrive at these end-products of adaptation? One answer is that the observer satisfies the unique adapting requirements imposed by the transforming spectacles. These are the *preconditions* for achieving consistent perception and competent action. To get at the *mechanisms* of adaptation, I next inquire as to what it is that adapts in adaptation. It is likely that the observer learns to perform the unique eye-head-body movement combinations now necessary for successful action and that repeating them influences the visual system to change its control parameters for eye-head-body movements. There may, indeed, be as many distinct forms of adaptation as there are distinct control sites. The means of obtaining adaptation is, of course, the information the observer uses. I will briefly say what the nature of that information is. How the perceptuo-motor systems use the optically transformed information is still unclear.

To What Does the Prism-Wearer Have to Adapt in the Process of Adaptation?

In our paradigm case, the observer achieves consistent perception and competent action when he or she satisfies the unique adapting requirements imposed by the optical reversal transformation. The most basic of these is this optical invariant: the visually detectable discrepancy between the apparent and actual direction of places, objects, people, events, and parts of the observer's body. Perceptual, cognitive, aesthetic-emotional, and performatory consequences follow from this optical constant. Thus, the immediate effects of donning reversing prisms are that the observer's visual world and seen self are disoriented and that he or she acts incompetently. The latter results from a new functional visuomotor invariant: The prism-wearer is obliged to position and move the eyes in the direction opposite to the head and hands in order to look and reach accurately toward intended places. (In Chapter 3 I elaborate on the demands transformed light places upon the prism-wearer. In Chapters 7–9 I then show how the observer copes with these adapting requirements.) To be sure, the observer may also adapt to the transformed optical information that confronts him. Even though adaptation is also to the discrepancy between the transformed field of view and haptic-kinesthetic information, changes in the *seen* position and movements of body parts appear to precede and control changes in the felt appreciation of body parts.

What Adapts in Adaptation?

I believe that the visuomotor control mechanisms, which direct every form of eye movement (EM) and eye-head-body movement combination, change their control parameters. For example, to maintain fixation, compensatory EMs now have to move opposite to the direction of the head. Similarly, a ground-skyward eye-head (-arm) pursuit now requires that the eyes move groundward to maintain fixation while the head (and arms) must be directed to move in the opposite direction: skyward. Thus, the control mechanisms that originally controlled the observer's compensatory EMs and coordinated his or her upward eye-head (-arm) movements to pursue the same events is maladaptive as soon as the observer dons reversing prisms. A new, unique, and separate set of motor signals must be issued by existing or newly developing visuomotor control mechanisms for the eyes and, shortly after, for the head and other body parts to affect successful action. This view is distinct from Held and Freedman's (1963) position, for example. They have characterized the end-product of adaptation as follows: "Full and exact adaptation to a rearrangement represents a change in state of the relevant sensorimotor control system such that the input-output or stimulus-response relation becomes *identical* to that which existed prior to the arrangement [p. 457, italics mine]." As I have shown (cf. Chapter 9 for details) this interpretation cannot be literally correct because, for example, continued successful fixation of a target during a HM requires a reversal in direction of the compensating EM. Similarly, successful eye-head-arm pursuit necessitates that the direction of the head and arm movement be controlled by motor impulses that send them in the direction opposite to that in which EMs proceed. Thus, the adapting requirements impose radical changes on the sensorimotor control systems and the input-output and output-output relations they mediate in competent action. Consistent perception and competent action depend on learning families of rule-abiding correlations between input-input relations. Such correlations make possible approximations to accurate action and result in constant input-output relations before the smooth working together of the observer's motor and visual systems resumes. At one level, at least, adaptation appears to consist of changes in the motor programs that control EMs, EM-HMs, HM-EMs, and various combinations of eye-limb and eye-head-limb movements. Whether adaptation occurs, its rate and its degree of completeness appear to be a function of the nature of the control (systems) recruited to perform a given task: holding a fixation, saccading, optical compensation, optokinetic or vestibular nystagmus, smooth pursuit, or the coordinated combination of several of these in rapid succession.

What is the Information the Prism-Wearer Uses to Adapt?[16]

My emphasis in this book has been to analyze the nature of optical information. It is this information that serves to make eventual adaptation in long-term everyday situations possible, even though it is this same information that is responsible for the disorienting effects experienced by the observer immediately after he or she dons transforming prisms. In general, I am impressed by the great dependence of action on the immediate optical information confronting the observer and by the extent to which misinformed perception directs incompetent action.

Adaptations are changes toward perceiving more consistently. The observer is forced to discover new invariances (consistencies of optical structure) in the optical information seen through prisms. Thus, adaptation consists of an observer attending to new, distinctive features of his or her optically reversed body parts, objects, events, facial expressions, print, and pictorial displays. For example, the visually unique dynamic optical events during object motion take on new meaning, and the new parameters of rate and direction of seen motion become the new standard. Similarly, visually unique symmetry relations simply become the new standard of aesthetic acceptability.

Adaptations are also changes toward performing with increased competence. Action is directed by optical information that contains the facts as they exist in the observer's ecology. Thus, to adapt, an observer guides his or her actions according to the optical invariants that continue to specify the true state of affairs of the ecology, quite irrespective of the imposed transformation. For example, even though lowering the head provides optical information *during* the movement that makes it appear as if the observer raised the head, ground becomes eventually visible. Noticing such visual discrepancies tells the observer that the direction of seen motion during the HM was opposite to what it appeared to be. After many repetitions of attending to the optical motions during a downward HM, not only does the observer expect to see ground before

[16]Several early variants of the view that adaptation occurs when the observer has (a sufficient amount of) information for the nature of the transformation may be found in Coren, 1966; Freedman, 1968; Howard *et al.*, 1965; McLaughlin, Rifkin, & Webster, 1966; Rock, 1966; Wallach, 1968; Weinstein, Sersen, & Weinstein, 1964; and Wohlwill, 1966. The most frequent emphasis of this "information hypothesis" has been how the observer resolves the discrepancy between visual and haptic-kinesthetic information for the position of the pointing arm (cf. Welch, 1978, p. 24).

it appears in the field of view, but the direction of the optical motions now looks appropriate to the actual direction of the observer's HM. Such perceptual changes in the meaning of information direct action toward competence. Thus, the observer is confronted with two kinds of contradictory optical information, which begin to compete for his or her attention and compete as the guide to bodily movements. To adapt, the prism-wearer must resolve these conflicts between new prism-produced invariants—visual information that confuses and misleads his or her action—and old preprism invariants—visual information that remains untouched by the transformation. Competent action can be expected of the prism-wearer as soon as his or her understanding of the visual meaning of the direction of bodily movement during the movement is congruent once again with the actual location of the moving limb at the termination of the movement: The discrepancy between two kinds of visual information is eliminated, and contradictory optical information ceases to be contradictory. An almost cognitive, though clearly visually acquired understanding, is gained in what events signify and what one's actions mean. The process toward the adaptation of action is uneven, however, following complex metamorphoses, which I have described as hybrid action patterns: unique concatenations in reaching and twisting movements used for eating, for example. In conclusion, during the course of living in a world transformed, the observer's initial fears become calmed, he or she finds the discomforts quite tolerable, the strange sights fade and become common, and ineptness changes to competency.

12

Practical Applications: Sleep and Space Travel

What are some of the benefits of the study of adaptation to optical transformation? What practical use can be made of the knowledge that a human being is extremely flexible in situations that place diverse and conflicting demands upon his visual, gravity-orienting, haptic-kinesthetic, and auditory systems? In addition to the answers we have gleaned so far in this book, this and other research suggests that during sleep, the human being processes information obtained during waking hours and that such processing permits him or her to utilize this information upon awakening. Second, we can utilize, in the study of space travel, the knowledge gained that the visual system is of primary importance to the human being forced to adapt to new surroundings. I will briefly explore these two extensions and applications of our understanding gained from living in a world transformed, even though there are others to choose from, including living under water.[1]

PRISM ADAPTATION AND SLEEP

Sleeping, following exposure to the prismatic transformation, appeared to: (*a*) Inhibit the nausea created by head and body movements;

[1]Welch has ably reviewed adaptation to underwater distortion (1978, Chapter 12).

(*b*) "consolidate" gains in perceptual learning (e.g., orientation); and (*c*) improve action. Thus, on Day 1 of the Prism Study, I reported that the nausea that accompanied head movements had disappeared after the first period of sleep (see Chapter 7). I also observed:

> *After 6 hours of wearing the prisms, I was tremendously debilitated. I slept for 4 hours. Visual imagery upon awakening was consistent with my perceptions while wearing prisms: For example, I had the impression that I was viewing the scene while my head was suspended upside down on my shoulders.*

On Day 1, I further reported the following apparent facilitation effects:

> *After taking a 4-hour nap, I am able to walk with noticeably more confidence and success. It's as if I had practiced walking for the past 4 hours rather than sleeping. For the first time it is possible to walk on a paved road without losing my balance while freely moving my head from right to left (cf. Appendix A, Table A8.2).*

On the morning of Day 2 of Stage 3, 13 hours after donning the reversing prisms, I reported:

> *After last night's sleep, my gross performatory capabilities have markedly improved; my extreme instability has greatly decreased, and so on. This morning I'm going about the house looking for my slippers. This I would have regarded yesterday as an impracticable waste of concentrated effort.*

Moreover, on Day 5 of Stage 3, after about 60 hours of adaptation, I reported an apparent sleep-contingent consolidation:

> *It's quite definite that following every sleep period, beginning with the afternoon nap of the first day of Stage 3, there is a* dramatic *improvement in all motor activities that [I] have engaged in prior to that sleep period. It's as if some consolidation of competence were going on during every sleep period.*

I believe that active, possibly rapid-eye-movement (REM)-related, *perceptual learning* and *motoric practice* during sleep account for a large proportion of the observed improvements. Clearly, the Prism Study does not allow the conclusion that ongoing processes during sleeping, rather than resting as such, are functionally related to the described changes. Nevertheless, the kind and magnitude of gains experienced suggest to me an active dual process of (*a*) *sleep-contingent refinements in perceptual learning* combined with (*b*) *sleep-contingent consolidation of competent action.*[2]

[2]Following these sleep-related observations during the Prism Study, I conducted a follow-up pilot study at Cornell during the winter–spring of 1971–72. Its purpose was to

That processes during sleep inhibit nausea has not been unequivocally demonstrated. Yet, it is possible that during sleep the conflict is further resolved between vestibular control mechanisms, which attempt to drive compensatory EMs as always, and visual control mechanisms, which are responsible for the reversal in direction of the new compensatory EMs. If this conflict is indeed partly responsible for the nausea the observer experiences, then its resolution during sleep should preclude

---

test the possibility that processes during sleeping enhance competent action more than continued practice. These tasks included walking a straight line, ball-catching, pointing, setting up the figures on a chess board, writing letters and words after seeing them for three seconds, drawing continuously visible familiar and unique figures, drawing connecting lines between squares placed in all orientations, and others. The magnitude of the difference in the number of confusions, errors, and in the latencies after a night's sleep were uniformly and considerably greater than after continued practice. The data appear to point to the conclusion that time spent sleeping results in substantially greater gains in adaptation (performatory competence) than a practice trial. Nevertheless, no unequivocal conclusion is permissible because these observations failed to include a control for rest rather than sleep after original learning and because not as much total time intervened between the original learning and final testing for observers who continued (massed) practice relative to the observers who slept after original learning.

A second pilot study conducted at Cornell during the winter following the Prism Study explored the *dream content* after a day of adapting to up–down reversing prisms. Three observers wore the prisms while undergoing a wide battery of perceptuomotor tests in this double-blind study. The aim was to see if dream content was related to the visually perceived orientation and location of the prism-wearer's head during the waking state. Observers were awakened by a signal during REM sleep, asked if they had dreamt and if so, to simply describe the content of the dream in as much detail as possible. Observers spoke into a tape recorder. The REM recording technician, who was unaware of the purpose of the study, remained in the adjoining room. On the next morning the experimenter (I), after listening and then allowing the observer to listen to the taped report, interviewed each as to what had been dreamt and asked each to provide more detail where possible. The observer was then told the purpose of the study and the empirical hypotheses I hoped to explore. The results, and especially any interpretation of them, were tentative at best. All three observers spontaneously reported looking or being looked at through a narrow, rectangular window: phenomenally the shape of the restricted field of view seen during the day. Their reports were also sprinkled with events *suggestive of* observing and being observed by people who "walked" on a ceiling and suggestive of a *difference* in the way in which the head of the *subject of the dream* (not necessarily the dreaming observer) was oriented vis-à-vis the head of others in the dream. These reports must be viewed with skepticism until more evidence is collected within a more refined research hypothesis and with more stringent controls (e.g., for the restriction of the field of view) and within a design that allows for the following: (*a*) Comparison between asking specific questions of the observer versus open-ended dream reporting; (*b*) alerting the observer to specific questions that will be asked versus not priming him or her to subsequent dream reports; (*c*) dream reports of observers who move about actively and perform prior to sleeping versus those of observers who gaze through the prisms passively for equivalent periods of time.

further nausea upon awakening. The finding by Lenzi, Pompeiano, and Satoh (1969) that the production of depressed nystagmus was significantly associated with REM sleep indicates at least the possibility of modulation of vestibular control of EMs during sleep. The report by two Russian cosmonauts, that the vertigo they experienced during space flight improved so greatly after sleep that they were able to carry out their intended program (Sjöberg, 1970), lends further support to the supposition that vestibular control parameters are modified by (REM) sleep.

The finding that the prism-wearer soon recognizes people he or she has seen only while looking through the spectacles (cf. Chapter 9), indicates that he or she established a set of visual memories cognate with the new sights. Consequently, we should expect that such newly established memory traces are at least "protected" by sleep, as Jenkins and Dallenbach (1924) first showed. Recent evidence reveals an important qualification. Sleep acts to prevent, rather than protect, memory consolidation if the new (verbal) material has not been transferred from short-term to long-term memory before its onset. Sleep does appear to promote retention of memory traces that have passed through the first critical stage of consolidation (Feinberg & Evarts, 1969, pp. 339–340). The weight of the evidence appears to favor the conclusion that REM sleep is directly and adaptively involved in information processing for learning, memory, and cognitive functions, but it is still debated (e.g., Greenberg & Pearlman, 1974; McGrath & Cohen, 1978; Moruzzi, 1966; Shapiro, 1967).

Although my data from the Prism Study and the follow-up pilot are not conclusive, it is probable that sleeping, which follows complex actions during transformation, improves these actions. Future experiments are needed to establish whether motor memories are consolidated by sleep, whether competing control tendencies are inhibited, or both. That changes in the functions of the motor cortex, vestibular system, and in compensatory EMs occur during sleep has been reported by Lenzi *et al.* (1969). Moreover, the finding that changes in cerebellar function occur during sleep has been documented (e.g., Pompeiano, 1974) and lends some credence to the notion that modification toward smoother control can be a sleep function. Furthermore, McGinty and Siegel found that "In neurons associated with motor behavior, REMS discharge patterns closely resemble those in waking, indicating an expression during REMS of normal movement patterns [1977, p. 154]." It may therefore not be too farfetched to suggest that learned adjustments are motorically "rehearsed" during REM sleep. Such activity may represent preparation for subsequent behavior based on such rehearsal and storage. REM sleep may even function to selectively inhibit or erase the perceptuomotor conflict created in the waking state and thus enhance adaptation.

The finding that deprivation of REM sleep does not impair subsequent recall and learning (e.g., Chernik (1972)) in no way allows the conclusion that sleep cannot aid the process of consolidation, integration, or refinement of perceptual and motor schemas. Even the Greenberg, Horowitz, and Pearlman (1972) finding that REM-deprived subjects increased the smoothness of tracing a Porteus Maze by more than control subjects is not conclusive; both groups had already had one previous uninterrupted night during which the major portion of adaptation to inversion could well have occurred. Moreover, whether or not deprivation of REM sleep impairs the recall or relearning of *complex* verbal, perceptual, and motor tasks is quite a separate and little-studied question. Furthermore, to the extent that the immediate effects of living with radically transforming spectacles is stressful—and it undoubtedly is—dreaming may ameliorate such stress and thereby aid postsleep performance indirectly. Indeed, Greenberg, Pillard, and Pearlman (1972) have offered evidence that implies such a stress-reduction role for REM sleep.

Several studies have appeared that bear on the question of whether distorted visual input affects REM sleep. Zimmerman, Stoyva, & Metcalf (1970) reported increases in total REM time, EM profusion, and decreases in the latency (time from sleep onset to onset of the first REM episode) for subjects wearing up-down reversing goggles. Allen, Oswald, Lewis, & Tagney (1972) failed to confirm these findings in a more rigorous experiment, which used a right-left reversal transformation. Two further experiments by Prévost, De Koninck, Barry, & Broughton (1974) and Prévost, De Koninck, & Proulx (1975) tend to confirm Zimmerman *et al.* (1970); they found an increase in the percentage of REM sleep. The most recent series of five experiments by Zimmerman, Stoyva, & Reite (1978) employ exacting controls for several confounding variables not considered in their first (1970) study. Once systematic effects, due to insufficient time to adapt to the new sleeping quarters of the laboratory and to simply being confined to a laboratory setting during (prism) adaptation were accounted for, these results remained: Adaptation to reversal or inversion does not reliably alter REM sleep time, percent, latency, or the number of rapid EMs during REM periods. That REM sleep aids perceptual and performatory adaptation to reversal has, of course, not been directly demonstrated by these studies. Nevertheless, a review of the literature by McGrath and Cohen (1978) led to the general conclusion that REM sleep facilitates adaptive waking behavior by aiding consolidation and retrieval of presleep learning and prepares the organism for subsequent learning.

PRISM ADAPTATION AND SPACE TRAVEL: VISUAL WEIGHTLESSNESS TRAINING

A vast and complex research literature exists that deals with the effects of weightlessness on maintaining perceptual and performatory skills.[3] My aim is to comment on just one related issue: the relationship between the nausea experienced by observers during bodily movements immediately after donning inverting or reversing spectacles and the motion sickness[4] and vertigo experienced during weightlessness. Astronauts typically experience symptoms of motion sickness in space. During Skylab flights, for example, the effects lasted for 3–5 days (Graybiel, Miller, & Homick, 1974).

My main point is that gravitational information has long been assumed to be most prepotent in directing orienting behavior (e.g., Gibson & Mowrer, 1938; Kellogg, 1971) and that it is time to rethink the evidence by starting with the supposition that the phylogenetically younger visual system is more capable and more vital to all forms of visually guided behavior than has been supposed heretofore.[5] The peripheral visual system, especially, appears to control orientation in the immediate visual surround, as suggested by the Tube Study, which restricted the field of view (cf. Chapter 4). The visual system is also capable of exerting an "override" over vestibularly controlled compensatory EMs, as I have shown (cf. Chapter 7). Evidence of this nature leads me to proffer this suggestion: Expend more effort in space-related

[3]For example, Agadzhanyan, 1971; Bergstedt, 1966; Brown, 1961; Chkaidze, 1966; Flaherty, 1961; Gurovskiy, 1967; Hanrahan and Bushnell, 1960; Johnston, Dietlein, & Berry, 1975; Loftus, 1963; Pirie, 1961; Sells and Berry, 1961; Shillinger, Baumgarten, & Baldrighi, 1973; Simons, Walk, & Sears, 1965; Stahle, 1968; Yuganov, Gorshkov, Kasyan, Bryanov, Kolosov, Kopanev, Lebedev, Popov, & Solodovnic, 1966.

[4]Motion sickness is inducible by a large number of circumstances in which the person is actually moved or perceives himself-herself to be moving in unfamiliar ways. Real or apparent motion of portions of the environment is typically present. The resultant effects are equally varied in number and include the perception of cold or flushing, actual sweating, increased salivation, dizziness, pallor, headache, yawning, drowsiness, sleepiness, stomach awareness, epigastric discomfort, nausea, and finally, vomiting. In addition to many autonomic effects, the observer may experience a blurring of vision, bodily instability, and considerable apprehension (cf. Johnson & Jongkees, 1974).

[5]My argument does not deny the importance of cognitive or personality factors in rendering an observer more susceptible to motion sickness (e.g., Collins & Lentz, 1977; Lentz & Collins, 1977; Long, Ambler, & Guedry, 1975; Reason, 1969).

research programs to find out how visual training may help prevent the nausea and motion sickness generated by weightlessness by preadapting space travelers using what I will call *visual weightlessness training*.

We have seen that an observer adapts to the nausea and vertigo created by inverting and reversing spectacles (cf. Chapter 7), and that REM sleep appears to aid this process. Indications are, furthermore, that an observer becomes biperformatory, provided he or she adapts fully and thus suffers no major aftereffects of nausea or vertigo (cf. Chapter 10). This capacity to function interchangeably under perceptual conflict and under quite opposite conditions of demand is evidently acquired and maintained by a modifiable visual–vestibular system. Indeed, other perceptual systems appear to adapt to the unique requirements for competent action demanded by the visual system.

Some specific proposals follow from the above considerations. Expose matched groups to the nausea that attends HMs and locomotion while wearing up–down reversing or inverting spectacles. Adapt observers until their experienced nausea and vertigo have subsided. Then put these observers through centrifuge training or parabolic flight.[6] Two kinds of serial adaptation groups should also be trained: those that adapt first to reversal, then inversion, or vice versa and those that adapt to the same transformation twice with an intervening rest period before they return to the normal world. Then compare the adapted, serially adapted, and unadapted groups under conditions of parabolic flight and centrifugation in various orientations on all measures of experienced well-being and skillful action. Prediction: Fully adapted, and serially adapted observers, especially, should perform with less discomfort and incapacity then unadapted or "vestibularly" trained observers. The narrowing of the field of view will be a critical variable and must be held constant scrupulously. It may be possible to create an approximately normal size field of view for reversal or inversion with fiber optics. Such a technological breakthrough would make visual weightlessness training even more useful.

Trainees should have the transforming system attached to the head and engage in active and natural head–body–locomotion movements during all phases of training. Held's evidence is rather clear: Active performance maximizes coping with the unique adapting requirements imposed by any form of transformation or visuomotor conflict and hence

[6]Short-term weightlessness is produced by flying an aircraft in Keplerian parabolic trajectory because then the gravitational force of earth is counterbalanced by the centrifugal force of the aircraft (cf. Graybiel & Miller, 1976; Howard & Templeton, 1966, Chapter 16).

augments full adaptation (cf. Chapter 11, Appendix A, Table A7.3). Nevertheless, some benefit may be derived from visual weightlessness training or pre- and posttraining with a panoramic screen on which up–down reversed, inverted, and normal scenes are presented in motion films that simulate real flight, docking, and landing conditions *from the point of observation* of the viewer (cf. Parker, 1971; Parker, Schaefer, & Cohen, 1972). I believe that a program that utilizes these training procedures would be of substantial benefit in decreasing the nausea, motion sickness, and weightlessness sickness experienced by astronauts. Cinematographic displays on a panoramic screen, showing simulated scenes of the observer floating under conditions that he or she is likely to encounter, may also prove useful for positive transfer of training in preparation for space travel (cf. Brown, 1976). Note that motion sickness should be more severe when very experienced pilots of aircraft, helicopters, etc. who have conquered its symptoms are suddenly exposed to a simulator in which they have no active control over correlating displayed motion information with their own bodily adjustments. Note also that part of the strategy of this approach is to purposely maximize the conflict between visual and vestibular information in order to recruit the maximum control that the visual system is capable of exerting over the vestibular system. Suppression, inhibition, or takeover of function by the visual system in milder conflict situations is expected to be made more likely by this "shaping" procedure. Naturally, severely conflicting stimulation (e.g., HMs away from the axis of acceleration producing motion sickness) may represent overstimulation that cannot be accommodated by any perceptual systems concerned.

The principle proposed is simple: Provide *visual* perceptual learning opportunities for potential space travelers. The prediction is that the visual system of those so trained will learn "rules of governance" for the other gravity-orienting systems and will come to override or control them. Indeed, the newly integrated cooperation of these systems will be practiced during such training. The ideal outcome is a minimum of time lost in "switchover" to the new system for coping with weightlessness. This should be particularly true of serially trained subjects. The optically reversing–inverting-prism training should be extended to the underwater environment because gravitational information is attenuated there. This suggestion follows from my assumption that the maximally flexible observer is least likely to be incapacitated by novel or emergency conditions he or she might encounter because he or she has a wider repertoire of capacities from which to choose. Finally, visual reversal–inversion adaptation should be combined with *concurrent*, standard, centrifuge-training techniques. Group comparisons will show whether benefits accrue. My hunch is that something analogous to bilingual language training will occur: Training to criterion will take considerably longer, but the products should be greater flexibility and, hopefully, greater imperviousness to weightlessness sickness.

The unfamiliar combinations of visuo-vestibular stimulation, to which, especially, aircraft and spacecraft travel subject both operator and occupant, produce disorientation, vertigo, motion sickness, nausea, and performance degradation.[7] My aim is not to review this complex literature, which seems to me to emphasize the importance of vestibular factors, because others have already done so skillfully several times (e.g., Clark, 1970; Graybiel, 1972, 1974; Guedry, 1965a; 1974). Rather my aim is to argue that my evidence, as well as my cursory reading of the cited literature, suggests that more attention should be paid to the powerful role of the visual system in the analysis of motion sickness and other untoward effects accompanying disorientation here on earth and in space. (Indeed, I believe that vision weightlessness training of recruits for space travel, whether such training is done on earth or in space, may prove more beneficial than either vestibular training or attempts to control motion sickness with drugs.[8] Undesirable side effects could be avoided, at least.) I will cite two examples of human visual control over vestibularly induced disorientation and motion sickness in support of my contention.

First, spectacle-transformation studies have recently been recognized as instances where researchers create conflicts between visual and vestibular input that are closely related to the conflict suffered by the space traveler. Yet, an incorrect assumption has been made about this common and critical condition: "In many sensory rearrangement experiments, visual information has been altered optically... while proprioceptive and labyrinthine sensory input remained unmodified [Guedry, 1965b, p. 459]." Evidence such as the reversal of compensatory EMs (cf. Chapter 7) allows us to infer that neither (neck-muscle) proprioceptive nor labyrinthine sensory input remains unmodified by the

[7]The following are just examples of a vast literature of documented circumstances that have produced such effects: Ambler and Guedry, 1966; Berry and Homick, 1973; Clark and Stewart, 1967; Clark and Stewart, 1973; Cohen, 1976; Cohen, 1977; Dowd, 1973; Graybiel and Knepton, 1976; Graybiel and Lackner, 1977; Grose, 1967; Guedry, 1968; Lackner, 1976; Melvill Jones, 1970; Pitblado and Mirabile, 1977; Potvin, Sadoff, & Billingham, 1977; Ryback, Rudd, Matz, & Jennings, 1970; Spector, 1974.

[8]For example, Benson, 1969; Benson and Brand, 1968; Brand, 1969, 1970; Giurgea, Moeyersoons, & Evraerd, 1967; Graybiel, Knepton, & Shaw, 1976; Graybiel, Wood, Knepton, Hoche, & Perkins, 1975; Green, 1973; Johnson, Money, & Graybiel, 1976; Medoff, 1970; Wood, 1966; Wood and Graybiel, 1970.

transformed visual input; rather, optical information appears to control and modulate both the haptic and vestibular information the observer utilizes in action. For those instances in which motion sickness is due to a mismatch between information from visual, vestibular, and other perceptual systems, optical motion information may suffice to inhibit the discomforts and disturbances that accompany motion sickness.

Second, experienced seafarers, divers, circus performers, ballet dancers, ice skaters and, most recently, flying personnel are known to be relatively impervious to the vertigo and nausea (properly a combination of moving, being moved, and motion sickness) typically suffered by the novice. I contend that unaffected persons are immune not by virtue of habituation (as demonstrated by Dodge, 1923a and defined by Thorpe, 1963) but because these individuals have learned various techniques of visually anchoring or stabilizing the self (principally the eyes and–or the head) to a fixed place in their visible environment. Moreover, the successful execution of these complex visuomotor behaviors functions to provide central inhibition of the disturbing *consequences* of vestibular signals. These signals may well be indistinguishable for the novice as well as for the experienced individual. The following exemplifies my contention. Visual "spotting" during multiple pirouettes and fouettés of ballet dancers entails fixating a stationary object by keeping the head immobile for as long as possible during these rapid turns of the body. The head is then whipped around rapidly, covering an arc of approximately 360° to regain visual fixation with an again stationary head. The head and eyes leave the place of fixation for the shortest possible time by keeping the head stationary for the longest possible time. Since each 360°-turn can be executed in less than one second by an experienced ballet dancer, an angular velocity of the head may be in excess of 500°/sec and decelerate at about $2000°/sec^2$ within a one-quarter turn (Osterhammel, Terkildsen, & Zilstorff, 1970). The fact that ballet dancers do not experience vertigo or nausea during or after such turns (Collins, 1966; Tschiassny, 1957), even though they elicit powerful vestibular stimulation, indicates that visual information, when utilized by this fixation technique, overrides and prevents vestibularly induced loss of balance or illness. To assume that this kind of visual control merely constitutes a form of vestibular habituation (e.g., Guedry, 1965b; Pfaltz, 1977) may not be warranted (cf. Collins, 1968, 1974). Indeed, the fact that ballet dancers' nystagmic threshold responses to angular acceleration are normal in the dark but greatly raised when in the presence of optic fixation (Dix & Hood, 1969) calls a vestibular habituation explanation into serious question; thresholds should also be raised in darkness to allow that inference. Although dancers experience vertigo during the early stages of training (Osterhammel *et al.*, 1970), careful observations are needed before we can decide whether and to what extent such vertigo should be attributed to true habituation or to inexact and inconsistent use of the spotting technique—and of consequent ineffective use of the stabilizing optical information. Indeed, to reach an appropriate conclusion, we need a comparison with experienced dancers who purposely introduce variations in the length of time they keep their head stationary during a turn, the rate at which they decelerate their head, and the degree to which they over- or undershoot the fixation object. Care must be exercised in applying conclusions about the visuo-vestibular responsiveness of subjects rotated passively in a chair to subjects who engage in a complex, integrated (visuo-vestibular-reticular-cerebellar) action consisting of active eye fixation and active turning of the body while exercising finely tuned control over the neck musculature to accelerate and decelerate the head.

This much seems clear: The more visual information an observer can get about the environment, the more veridical are his or her judgments about the relationship of his or her own orientation to the surround. Moreover, the greater the observer's opportunity to perform under visual guidance, the more skillful his or her actions.

SUMMARY

In this chapter I emphasize two practical extensions of data gleaned from living in a world transformed. In the first section I deal with the likely role of rapid-eye-movement (REM) sleep in inhibiting future nausea and other symptoms of motion sickness; with the possible function of REM sleep in consolidating new perceptual learning; and with the suggestion that new motor memories are "rehearsed," and that such "motoric practice" improves future competent action.

In the second section I urge a new emphasis on the role of visual information in the control of motion sickness experienced under zero-gravity conditions. First, I argue that learning to adapt to the demands of an optically transformed world can prepare a person for some of the adaptation processes he or she must undergo during space travel. Secondly, I argue that the visual system is a better guide to understanding adaptation to optical transformation and to the effects of space travel than even the vestibular system, the generally acknowledged gravity-orienting system. In particular, I contend that "nausea-adaptation," preparing an astronaut for the loss of gravity, can best be affected not through vestibular training but through what I call *visual weightlessness training*. Repeated exposure to real-world adaptation with up-down reversing and-or inverting prisms is especially recommended. The feasibility of visual training for space travel, in particular the visual control of motion sickness in space, is suggested by the remarkable flexibility of the visual system, the demonstrated power of optical information (especially as used by peripheral vision to direct all forms of visually guided action), and the evident plasticity of the vestibular system, as exemplified by the reversal of compensatory EMs. All three factors argue in favor of a new emphasis in the preadaptation of future space travelers. Indeed, the very effort of learning to learn to adapt to various forms of conflicting demands should yield some positive transfer.

Human flexibility is remarkable. Knowing this with greater certitude, we need fear the unknown less. Knowing that we can conquer the radically different gives us hope that we can transform the unknown to the familiar.

A

Appendix: Long-Term Adaptation to Up–Down Reversal: Observer's Direct Reports

The following tables feature descriptions of my observations of the immediate effects, gradual modifications, final accomplishments, and aftereffects, taken from the protocol of the Prism Study.

CONSEQUENCES OF HEAD AND BODY MOVEMENTS (STAGE 3)

Table A7.1: World Motion with Scotopic Illumination
Table A7.2: Judgments of the Slant of the Ground
Table A7.3: Being Driven and Driving a Car
Table A7.4: Knowledge of Location and Orientation of Objects Relative to Self
Table A7.5: Judging the Size and Distance from Self of Objects
Table A7.6: Inverting the Up–Down Reversal and Size and Distance Judgments

VISUALLY GUIDED ACTIONS (STAGE 3)

Table A8.1: Ability to Remain Oriented
Table A8.2: Walking

PERCEPTION OF THE SELF AND EVENTS (STAGE 3)

AFTEREFFECTS OF UP–DOWN REVERSING THE FIELD OF VIEW (FV) (STAGE 4)

CONSEQUENCES OF HEAD MOVEMENTS (HMs) AND BODY MOVEMENTS[1]

Table A7.1. World Motion with Scotopic Illumination

(12/164–13/178)[2 3]

Global world motion in very dark room very noticeable in contrast to daytime observation: Under conditions of very low [scotopic] levels of illumination

[1]All tables are presented consecutively, as if they were text.
[2]See Footnote 1 in Chapter 7, p. 112.
[3]All table entries are taken from Dolezal (1976). No quotation marks are used.

(moonlight through closed shutters) . . . very slow up-down and onto-the-shoulder-tilt HMs produced tremendous perceived world motion comparable to Day 1 levels. In daylight . . . comparable rates of HM (particularly up-down HMs) have ceased to reveal a noticeable "world motion" component. Day 13. . . . I can barely make out objects painted white and of the size of my head in a mirror. Very slow up-down HMs (1-1.5 seconds for an excursion going from extreme head thrown back to the chin-to-chest position) produce a marked world motion.

Table A7.2. Judgments of the Slant of the Ground

(3/41-11/146)

When I push my chin as close against my chest as possible and bend forward, the ground beneath my feet and behind me becomes visible. As I do this, the cement floor behind my feet rises against the sky as if it were a movable plastic loading platform, the slant of which can be changed. The floor behind me is seen to rise, and now describes a parallel line with the line of gravity, and visually I am standing perpendicular to this floor—in the same orientation as I know the real concrete floor to be oriented. Now, not only does the ground behind me slant upward, but the ground in front of me (of which only 2-3 feet, including my feet, are visible) opens into an abyss. Now when I walk backward, in crab fashion, visually I'm walking up a slope. Haptically, however, this walk is as effortless as walking downhill.

Table A7.3. Being Driven and Driving a Car

(10/125-10/128.5)

Being driven: *Being a passanger in a car going up and down a curvy mountain road produced severe nausea, vertigo, and generally motion (being moved) sickness. The experience is quite similar to what I experienced 9 days ago while moving my head up and down; what is similar about the result of up-down HMs on Day 1 and being driven in a car now is that now, as then, I seem to be provided with information that I am moving, or that I am being moved, without having initiated these movements and that I am moving with totally unaccustomed suddenness, jerkiness, and rapidity. Now, as then, the (visual) information seems to tell me that I am moving, or being moved, in such a fashion that, even if I tried, I could not initiate, or carry out, such movements. Now, as then, closing my eyes stops the vertigo and nausea subsides gradually. There is an important difference, however: Nine days ago the visual information causing perceived global self-world upheaval seemed to be directly responsible for experiencing nausea and vertigo. Today, however, two factors seem to produce my experience of nausea and vertigo. The first and lesser of the two factors is that, even though the speed of the car was between 15-35 km/hour, places and objects nearby appeared to be zipping by at at least 2-3 times that rate of speed . . . while the trees only a few yards away were zipping by at a blinding rate of speed, the mountains in the distance moved along quite slowly. . . . The second factor seemingly responsible for vertigo and nausea I experienced . . . trees, rocks, street signs, especially those close to me, but not the mountains in the background, appeared to jerk about quite a bit and most disconcertingly* [and] *was particularly severe and disturbing (to my head and stomach) when brakes were put on or gears were shifted (i.e., when a* change *in the rate of forward progress was introduced) because then my head came forward and then snapped back involuntarily. Vertigo and imminent throwing up were by far greatest and highly correlated with this involuntary head activity. Conscious anticipation and "correction" for any change in the prevailing rate of speed of the car was unsuccessful, though I tried all sorts of maneuvers. . . . The information contained in this complex situation of being driven in a car seemed to be made up of two movement components, specifying to 3:5 to 4:5 observer movement (rather, self being jerked, joggled, and bounced in highly uncommon ways I could not anticipate, counteract, or control) and 1:5 to 2:5 world motion. The visual and haptic information seems to say: "There you are, being joggled about, incapable of making allowances for it . . ." We drove for 45 minutes, stopped for 20 minutes for tea, drove for 20 more minutes, stopped for 1.5 hours for lunch and drove another 35 minutes (100 minutes of being driven and 110 minutes of rest). There was* no *remission or perceived decrease in any effect described during any of the driving periods. Indeed, when I finally got out of the car (after going* down *the mountain for 35 minutes rather than up it), I felt very sick—quite as awful as I had after sitting in the car for less than a minute initially.*

(10/128.5–10/129)

Driving the same car: *10 minutes after I stepped out of the car I had been driven in, I sat behind the steering wheel myself to drive it on the straight, even, paved road of the village. I got into the car (this was difficult) but as concerns instrument reading, operating the clutch, and shifting, releasing the handbrake, etc., that gave me no trouble at all. In fact, as unbelievable as that sounds, shifting was smoother and more accurate than it had been 20 days earlier when I drove the car for the first time without helmet or prisms (stick-shift Mercedes 170V). The one thing I was quite unsure about was how much room I had to spare on either side of the bumpers—I still overestimate the distance between self and obstacles such as cars, people, dropoffs, or fences. For about 2 minutes, the owner provided me with knowledge of results as to the real distance (on the right and left sides of the car) to obstacles and after that, I felt quite comfortable, backing up and pulling into parking spaces, turning 360°, etc. All maneuvers were executed with a high degree of accuracy. Most importantly, I did not experience even a hint of vertigo or nausea. It must be noted that I drove on a straightaway and did so slowly (10–25 km/hr.). Still, I am convinced that driving is in several vital ways radically different from being driven. Note that the flow gradients ("zipping by" of nearby places) and focal joggling were just as noticeable but suddenly didn't bother me. Being prepared for action and acting, as in shifting gears or breaking or accelerating, did carry different consequences than being witness to, or victim of, these actions when performed by someone else. Apparently, I anticipated or preadjusted for the head coming forward and then snapping back while shifting gears, etc. This simply did not happen when I was driving and in control. . . . If I had no FV restriction, I feel quite confident that with a few hours of practice I could drive safely back to Athens, over the mountain road.*

Table A7.4. Knowledge of Location and Orientation of Objects Relative to Self

(4/48.5–4/48.5)

Maintaining the visual horizon in the FV optimizes orientation. Keeping the head in the chin-to-chest position or slightly tilted favors perceptual and performatory disorientation. . . . Viewing an object in the vertical plane maximizes accurate object-orientation judgments and the ability to perform consistently (if not accurately). When objects are located off to the right or left side (in the coronal plane) and–or when my head is tilted, all orientation judgments and actions toward that object become highly variable.

(5/62–5/62)

Example 1 *supporting above claim: I saw chess men being set up and a game played. I was totally lost as to who was doing what, how, and why. I was facing the chess board from a novel direction and my head was inclined toward one shoulder. When I finally stepped behind one of the players, I began to make sense of the entire situation.*

(5/66–5/66)

Example 2: *A young woman was sitting diagonally across a table on my left. My head was inclined to my right, hers to my left. A large, bare cross dangled from her neck. I tried to figure out which way a figure of Jesus would have to be placed upon that cross if my task were to visualize, or draw, or carve that figure. I could not. I also couldn't figure out which way his eyes or nose or mouth would be facing* either *relative to the ground or relative to me. I mean, I could have determined these things only if I had shifted myself directly opposite the young woman. Once I did so, the problem was solved.*

(5/67–5/67)

Example 3: *As I'm walking down a narrow mountain path, two people have come up the mountain, passing close by. Even though I know that they are coming toward me (I see their faces), the instant they pass by, I am totally unable to say, or point, in which direction they disappeared. My head is slightly tilted onto my shoulder as I make this observation.*

Table A7.5. Judging the Size and Distance from Self of Objects

(1/0–3/37)

Visual overestimation of distance from self and underestimation of the size of objects: Visually, the railing of the balcony is much further away from me and lower than I remember it to be. The table, too, looks as if it's the height of the distance between the ground and my knee. When I actually come in contact with it, I experience surprise because the table actually reaches a good 8 in. above my knee and the balcony railing 12 in. above my knee. Thus, there is a substantial discrepancy between visually and haptically perceived height [which disappeared by Day 6, 72 hours].

(1/1–3/37)

The perception of the visual cliff is greatly enhanced in walking down *stairs. I remember the stairs to be much shallower in depth than they appear now.*

(3/40.5–5/70)

Height–depth-distance estimates appear to be a function of head posture: The perceived size of objects off the ground seems to be a direct function of head posture. For example, I'm standing on the veranda with the railing on my right. As I assume, respectively, 3 successive head postures—head thrown back, head in primary position, and head in the chin-to-chest position—the railing is perceived to be very low (about 1.5 feet off the ground), 2 feet, and finally 3 feet high, respectively. Three feet is its actual height. The balcony railing is perceived to "rise" as I lower my head from the "head up" to the "chin-to-chest" position. [Effect ceased by Day 6, 72 hours.]

(4/46.5–4/46.5)

Perceived layout ("distance" along the ground or "distance" from self) appears to be a function of head posture. Any given place along the ground appears closest to me when my head is in the chin-to-chest position, further off when my head is in the primary position, and furthest away from me when my head is in the up (thrown back) position.

Table A7.6. Inverting the Up–Down Reversal and Size and Distance Judgments

(11/145–11/145)

For the first time since I've put on these prisms, I'm putting my head between my legs. I'm standing on the beach and will be looking at 50 yards of beach and the sea beyond. What I behold is entirely unlikely. I am about 30 yards away from a well-known woman and child playing in the sand, but visually (phenomenally) they are about 5 steps from me, and they appear very tiny. The whole scene has the aspect of irreality or surreality about it. It would take me about 5 giant steps to get to the shoreline and another 10 steps to reach the horizon. It's as if I were peeping through a hole in a weird device in a circus—gazing upon a minified, shrunken world in which I'm the only giant—as if I had suddenly been thrust into Swift's Lilliput.

VISUALLY GUIDED ACTIONS

Table A8.1. Ability to Remain Oriented

(1/0.5–8/105)

Whenever my head is in the chin-to-chest position and I turn my head to the right or left as I'm beginning to take a few steps, my feet, . . . which are in my FV . . . and then my body . . . "follow automatically"—as if mechanically yoked to the direction and extent of the HM. . . . On Day 2, 20 hours, while attempting to walk the length of the 20-foot balcony while my eyes were closed, *the same thing happened. . . . If I move my head to the right or left while it remains in the chin-to-chest position, I am unable to move in any direction for more than 3 steps before I have to stop, realign my head, body, and feet and raise my head in order to reorient. This turns out to be a laborious, failure-prone procedure which takes much time.*

(2/14–2/20) and (3/37–5/57)

I managed to walk a short distance . . . 4–5 steps . . . while my head was in the chin-to-chest position without becoming totally disoriented. I had to keep my head as motionless as possible, though, in order not to veer off in the direction of the HM.

(6/75–8/105)

I can traverse treacherous paths which require direct visual guidance of my feet. In spite of this improvement, I still must be careful not to engage in right–left or onto-the-shoulder tilt HMs while in the chin-to-chest position, lest my feet again "follow" in the direction of that HM.

(4/43–13/175)

To get into the 18-foot boat is tremendously difficult because in order to hoist myself up and in, I need to have my head in the chin-to-chest position much of the time. This engenders terrible orientation difficulties. I simply do not know where I am with respect to the boat or where its relevant parts are. I finally managed to tumble into the boat. Rowing itself was no problem. Finding the place where I had launched the boat was difficult because of the swaying of the boat on fair-size waves. People and objects along the shore swayed and bobbed up and down most unobligingly and tenaciously. I had to resort to the use of mnemonics (number of houses from one end of the beach) to guide the boat to the general vicinity of its launching place. Getting out of the boat was most difficult. The problem is not one of knowing where up or down is as much as of finding out and acting upon *where I was relative to a particular place in the world and, in turn, getting to know the relationship of that place to others. Boarding and getting out of a 40-foot boat in fairly heavy sea 9 days later produced equally devastating disorientation, and I was equally incompetent (see Figure 7.1b).*

Table A8.2. Walking

(1/0–1/0)

The first few steps I took using visual guidance were like the first (toddling) steps of an infant—tremendously shaky. These steps were awkward, difficult, and didn't feel *right; there was nothing familiar about walking.*

(1/0–1/22)

In walking with my head in the chin-to-chest position just the 15–20 feet on the balcony, I lost my orientation totally and there were several occasions on which I almost fell to the ground, simply not knowing what to do or how to do it. In these cases I guided my steps visually.

(1/0.5–1/12)

Trying to walk is truly a Catch-22 *situation. If I maintain my head in the sagittal plane and in the chin-to-chest position, my FV includes my ankles, my feet, and a few feet of ground underfoot, extending the width of the balcony I'm on. Keeping my head in this posture has the advantage of revealing the terrain underfoot and preventing stumbling over obstacles. But the disadvantages are that I am paralyzingly disoriented in the sense of not knowing which way I'm facing relative to any place or object around me and not knowing where I'm going. If I maintain my head in the primary position, on the other hand, neither my legs nor the ground underfoot is visible and walking is much easier. However, I will not know when I might knock into, or stumble over, obstacles. The obvious solution is to engage in up–down head scanning between these two head postures. Unfortunately, such HMs are hardly useful because they result in loss of balance, nausea, vertigo, and disconcerting global movement of the visual world.*

(1/2.5–1/2.5)

I notice a substantial improvement in my ability to walk a straight line after walking only about 40 feet. It is mostly due to the fact that I do not visually guide my feet now. I simply look down to make sure no obstacle is in the way; then I raise my head to the primary position. Now no part of my feet or body are in the FV. I orient myself by choosing a place on the horizon and using it as a visual "anchor".

(1/2.5–1/12)

At this time I am totally unable to walk down *stairs or an incline by myself. My progress down stairs is painfully slow, extremely hazardous, and difficult. I could not have accomplished it without holding fast to the hand of a companion, for I often lost my balance. I was quite confused about the direction of the gradient of the ground underfoot—at times the earth seemed to come up toward me and at times the distance to the ground seemed much greater than it ought to have been, given* my *known (remembered) height. HM-produced world–self instability may be responsible.*

(1/2.5–9/120)

Walking down *stairs or down an incline is perceived to be far more dangerous than walking* up *that same terrain.*

(1/12–1/12)

As this morning, late tonight I swayed like an intoxicated person while walking and once again needed someone to hold my arm. I was quite tired.

(2/14–2/20)

For the first time I was able to walk down *6–8 steps without help. To be sure, I used a walking stick for balance and support.*

(2/20–4/51)

For the first time I went down the entire stairway (50 stairs and 20 yards of mountain path) by myself (with walking stick), but I relied heavily on the now usual procedure: keeping my eyes on the horizon and simply standing still after each step or two to head-scan downward, preparing for the next step. Once on the beach with more or less level sand, I walked successfully while continuously *head-scanning up and down. However, I was careful not to get my feet into the FV for that still causes disorientation. As long as I keep the horizon in the FV—even though it isn't a stable horizon—I retain orientation and am able to walk effectively.*

(2/22–3/37)

Walking on the straightaway *was a bit like swimming today in that, at times, I appeared to be walking uphill and then downhill. . . . Walking "uphill" seemed correlated with the "head-thrown-back" position and phenomenally, walking downhill with head postures around the primary position. Moreover, when I stand on the beach with my head cocked back and eyes up and a person is walking* away *from me, he appears to be walking up a rather steep slope; when someone* approaches *me, he appears to be walking down toward me—down a "sandfall." It looks precarious, indeed, for them. Only when my head and eyes are in the primary position does the slope of the ground appear to be level or at a slight decline.*

(3/37–3/37)

This is the first time I've been able to walk up *stairs by* alternating *steps (i.e., one footstep per step). I have not been able to do this while going* down *a set of stairs.*

(4/48–15/193)

Walking in unfamiliar surrounding much less smooth and efficient than in familiar ones: I've just climbed some unfamiliar stairs. They are of the same description as those I walk frequently. Yet both climbing up and coming down these stairs seemed extremely hazardous and most discomforting by comparison with the familiar stairs. 20 hours later I again walked on unfamiliar territory but very similar to the path I take several times daily. In order not to come to harm, I had to exercise uncommon amounts of vigilance and slow down greatly. I was shakier, and my performance was poorer. A full 10 days later: Even today I experience similar difficulties though the nature of the terrain may be virtually identical. In familiar surroundings walking now proceeds almost automatically and errorlessly and visual guidance is no longer a conscious effort which requires great concentration. Quite the reverse is the case for unfamiliar territory. Hence, visual guidance is maximally involved, I'm more hesitant, errors abound, danger information is more apparent, and so on.

(4/55–4/55)

On the whole, my almost absolute dependence to keep the horizon in the FV has decreased, making up–down HM during walking less precarious.

(5/57–5/57)

I've abandoned the use of my walking stick.

(6/73–6/73)

I'm more sure-footed than ever before. For the first time I've successfully alternated feet going down *the last 6 of the 50 stairs. This was unthinkable even yesterday; yet this morning I did it fairly naturally and briskly. This radical improvement again came after a period of sleep.*

(7/83.5–7/83.5)

After sleeping, walking is very smooth this morning. I'm able to carry my share of equipment down to the beach for the first time. Until now I needed my hands free to balance myself.

(9/113.5–9/113.5)

For the first time I've successfully alternated steps in walking down *all 50 stairs. My balance was precarious, and haptically, it felt unfamiliar, uncomfortable, and somehow "wrong."*

(11/141–11/141)

Carrying heavy suitcases up and down wet and slippery mule trails poses no problem.

(12/153–12/153)

Alternating feet while walking down stairs and slopes is not perceived as dangerous and feels comfortable for the first time. When I tried not *to alternate steps this was perceived as "boring," as unnecessary relative to my ability to maintain balance and orientation; moreover, haptically, it felt uncomfortable and awkward.*

(13/170–13/170)

Beginning today (on the paved straightaway), walking has changed from a wide-stanced, cumbersome mode to a comfortable, relaxed mode: I had not been aware of it, but during Stage 3, I have apparently been walking the way astronauts do, as if packed down with heavy gear and encumbered by inflexible or bulky clothing. Whether this was done to gain better balance I do not know. Today this has suddenly changed, so I am told by several people in the household. Moreover, I noticed the difference in walking, though I could not place it. Once others had described their observations though, I knew they were correct in their descriptions. It appears that today I have begun to walk the way I did before putting on reversing prisms . . . today I began forgetting and had to remind myself that I am wearing reversing spectacles. The family with whom I'm living and who have known me anywhere from 2 months to 6 years all have said to me, "You don't appear to me to be different than you were in Stage 2, or no different than at any other time." Of course that's an overstatement, though I am approaching a "no difference between now and Stage 2 performance state" with respect to gross motor activities.

(13/173–13/173)

Mountain-climbing along a narrow, steep mule trail very trying: The main problem with this 1.5 hour climb was compounded by the heat of the day and the exertion, which caused profuse perspiration, which, in turn, produced a great deal of fogging of the prisms. In climbing uphill I behaved, or at least felt, like a blind man who had had too much to drink. Keeping my eyes on the "horizon" was virtually impossible, as the terrain was unbelievably rocky, slippery, and treacherous. . . . to survive I kept my head in the chin-to-chest position while moving forward a few steps, then stopped, raised my head to get my global bearing and lowered the head again to get my focal bearing—to avoid falling over a rock or falling into a hole. Nevertheless, I stumbled countless times and took some mild falls.

(15/200–15/200)

On the whole, walking is still not quite as smooth or stable as during Stage 2, when only the FV was restricted.

Table A8.3. Sitting Down in a Chair

(1/1–4/51)

It's a relatively simple task now to visually locate and get into the general vicinity of the chair on which I plan to sit, but once I manage to come to stand directly in front of it, facing its sitting surface, it is simply impossible to visually direct myself to sit upon it. Once I put my head in the chin-to-chest position, I'm again disoriented. Is the chair on my right or left? Am I facing it, or is it on my side? Where am I relative to its sitting surface? I just did what I did not visually anticipate I would do—I sat next *to the chair!*

(4/51–10/135)

Sitting down on a chair is decidely one of the most difficult and frustrating tasks I face daily. Getting to the chair is the first problem. Usually, I wind up standing next to the chair. Once I put my head in the chin-to-chest position to locate the sitting surface, I'm instantly confused as to which way my legs are facing, which way my body is twisted, indeed, which way my head is turned. Perhaps, as a consequence, I don't know which way the chair is facing and what I need to do not to sit next to it on the ground, as I have repeatedly done. If I follow my "visual commands," I would wind up on the floor or possibly with my head on the sitting surface of the chair. I have to look up, find some stable and–or familiar point (i.e., place or object), orient myself relative to the chair and the chair relative to that place. Then I need to make a note of how I'm facing relative to the way the chosen place and the chair are facing. Still, I need to approach the sitting surface of the chair head on, turn 180°, grasp hold of its armrests and slowly lower myself into it. I have frequently sat next to a chair rather than on it, or [once] on the lap of an astonished moviegoer rather than next to her.

(15/210–15/210)

Trying to sit in a chair still causes some disorientation, interfering with unhesitating performance.

Table A8.4. Bicycle-Riding

(2/20–2/20)

I just rode a bicycle fairly successfully for the first time with prisms on. I needed to apply the same strategy I apply while walking (viz., select a place of reference on the horizon and head toward it). The instant I put my head in the chin-to-chest position or threw my head back, I lost orientation and fell off. Riding without visual guidance did not work, in short. My ability to orient myself relative to the bicycle [and to get on it] was much poorer than my ability to ride it, once mounted.

(3/37–4/51)

I just rode the bicycle for about 1.5 miles. I was successful within limitations. Doing turns was the most difficult part. Now, after the ride, which has exhausted me, I don't walk well at all, being very unsteady on my feet, and I have some orientation difficulties. Riding down the street on your head is an inane kind of experience with all sorts of goings on above and underneath you—it's hard to say which. What your feet and arms are doing seems to be irrelevant. It's hardly noticed. And that is reinforced by the fact that as long as the road is smooth everything goes very well. When I hit a bumpy stretch of road, my visual world became a jerky mass of places and events which couldn't be differentiated. Moreover, the jerky world-joggling was direct information for my own instability in a fluctuating surround. That compounded the problem of steering. This time, when I put my head in the chin-to-chest position (and now had my pedaling feet and the front wheel of the bicycle in the FV), I did not become immediately disoriented, as I had on all previous occasions in this circumstance. Of course, I had to look up again after no more than about 1 second to [draw a bead] on the horizon and to continue going straight. I was able to successfully complete only one wide turn out of 8 trials. I also succeeded steering with one hand.

(5/65–15/193)

Cycling progressively improved and in all essential respects began to approach my cycling competence of Day 1 of Stage 2. Nevertheless, there are no changes in things like perceived joggling about of the world when I ride over rough terrain. . . . The same is true for riding a mule over rough terrain. Maintaining my head in the chin-to-chest position for more than about 3 seconds is also still impossible for it causes disorientation. . . . My own feet—in contradistinction to watching someone else pedal—seem to be moving clockwise rather than counterclockwise.

Table A8.5. Swimming and Water-Skiing

(1/3–2/15.5)

Breaststroke: *Visually I was greatly tempted to take a dive, but I kept my head in the thrown back position consciously and the horizon in the FV. This afforded orientation because when the FV was filled with water, I had no information for where I was relative to the shoreline. The haptic (muscular) appreciation of swimming was quite natural. As concerns HM-correlated stomach discomfort, lightheadedness, and so on, all these are much less noticeable and troublesome while swimming or walking in water than while walking on land.*

(2/15.5–4/45)

Breaststroke: *The sea is calm. Swimming is the most comfortable of all activities. When I maintain my head in the primary position, I'm swimming in a level medium. In swimming* out to sea *my head is cocked back a bit and the horizon line consists of a margin of water. Given this head posture, I appear to be swimming up a slight incline. If I throw my head back even more, I appear to be swimming up a steep mountain of water. I am scaling, by swimming, a wall of water which appears about to descend. The water appears to be flowing, fairly rapidly, toward my mouth and eyes. But this is not altogether a discomforting sight. Haptically, swimming with my head cocked back seems clearly more strenuous than when I keep my head in the primary position because I* see *myself swimming up into the descending waterfall. The slope of this waterfall appears steepest when my eyes are in the "up" rather than in the "primary" position. Swimming* toward shore, *on the other hand, is somewhat like swimming downward but the steepness of the slope is not as great as swimming toward the sea–sky horizon . . . and has to do with the lack of a FV-filling, homogeneous horizon in the latter case. The people and umbrellas on the beach, the houses and the mountain in the background provide ample information to comparatively judge the slope of the water surface, it seems. When waves . . . fill the FV, I am unable to see the horizon and quickly become disoriented . . . and can no longer swim along a straight path.*

(5/60–5/60)

Crawl: *Rapidly alternated tilting of the head from right to left produces immediate disorientation. The global self–world upheaval created is so disconcerting that I must return to a breaststroke (with relatively immobile head) after about 10 meters.*

(7/85–7/85)

Backstroke *in toward shore: My head is in the chin-to-chest position and visually I'm swimming–sliding down this FV-filling waterfall. Sometimes there is a hint that it will descend on me. The steepness of the slope of this apparent waterfall seems to be a direct function of head posture.*

(12/155–12/155)

Crawl: *Neither up–down nor onto-the-shoulder tilt HMs during this stroke bother me any more. This is probably because I now perceptually attribute a large component of the perceived world motion to my own HMs. Thus, even though I'm aware of rapid HMs, they are perceived either as causing relatively little global world instability or they are perceived to be unrelated to this world instability.*

(13/168–13/168)

Breaststroke as smooth and comfortable as during Stage 2. Water-skiing: *Reversing prisms no obstacle to efficient water-skiing: I skied on 2 skis, though until 5 years ago I was used to slalom skiing (exclusively on 1 ski). I had not been on skis in 5 years. Initially, I experienced orientation problems while in the water on my back, head in chin-to-chest position, trying to put on skis. They had straps which came across the arch of the foot, something I had never put on before. On the second try, putting on the skis went smoothly. I got up out of the water on the first try and was pulled about 1000 yards before I started to do skiing tricks and was downed by a medium-sized wave. Again, the trick was to keep my eyes on the horizon. This was sufficient for general orientation. . . .* [*however*] *the portion of the world which I focused on was joggling and jerking about fiercely. When I had a visual "bead" on the horizon, my feet and skis were not in the FV. On several occasions, I lowered my head to the chin-to-chest position. The instant I lost the horizon and had the skis in the FV, the perceived flow gradients proved most disturbing. There I was, back to Day 1 of Stage 3 or worse, if worse can be imagined. The flow gradient was incredibly fast, apparently 8–10 times the actual speed I was traveling (about 20 mph), and if I had continued to keep my head in the chin-to-chest position, I would undoubtedly have taken a bad fall.*

Table A8.6. Dressing Myself

(1/2.5–8/105)

Getting into slippers: Not the least factor contributing to disorientation when my head is in the chin-to-chest position is the perception that my feet are facing me, that is, my toes are pointing toward my stomach or forehead at the level of the ground. And this is the way to get into my slippers—this is absurdly correct, though not visually. When I raise my head a few degrees all that is visible is the ground and my slippers, which point the way they ought to in order to get into them—toe portion pointing away *from my midsection. But this is a perceptual contradiction! I am perplexed and need to sort it out. I turn 180°, and now both my feet and my slippers are pointing* toward *me! This is absurd. In order to get into my slippers, I need to turn them so that* visually *their toe portion face the toes of my feet to get into them. However, when I regard this arrangement, I again walk around the slippers because visually the meaning of toes and slippers pointing toward each other does not afford getting into them. Note that right and left are (apparently) reversed—tough not optically—when I perceive my feet to be pointing* toward *my midsection.*

(1/12–8/105)

Front–back reversal of clothing: I just discovered that I put my underwear wrong way 'round this morning. I did the same with my bathing suit this afternoon.

(2/13–9/120)

Up–down reversal of occluding mask: Last night I put my light-occluding mask on reversed, that is, I felt the patch which belongs below each eye and alongside the bridge of the nose to shut out light with my fingers and promptly put the mask on in such a way that the patches were pointing toward my forehead instead of the ground, as they should have, if placed correctly. On Nights 4–8 I tried very conscientiously to put on the mask correctly. This was done in total darkness. Each time I discovered, upon later checking the placement of the mask haptically, that I had up–down reversed the mask while putting it on. Does this mean I haptically perceive my nose (head?) as up–down reversed?

(8/105–15/200)

The tips of my slippers still *appear to point toward my forehead (at ground level), and I still struggle to get into them. I still put undershorts and undershirts on front–back reversed. Two differences are of note, though. These things don't happen as frequently as they used to and when I notice them, I have less difficulty correcting the problem rather than repeating what I want to avoid, as I did initially. On Day 14 I decided that the most effective and least laborious procedure for putting on shoes or underwear correctly is to* memorize *the item's relative orientation to myself when this action was carried out correctly. Thus, I have simply memorized that when I look down and my toes are pointing toward the toe portion of the slippers to go ahead and get into them. Note that such visual mnemonics would not have worked in the early days of prism-wearing. Then I was literally paralyzed from carrying out actions contrary to visual information, even if these actions would have been competent relative to the true state of affairs.*

Table A8.7. Fine Motor Coordination

(1/1–4/55)

Any task requiring careful visual guidance and precise performatory coordination is horrendously strenuous, requiring great concentration, calculation, and the ability to persist despite continual frustration resulting from utter failure.

(2/20–4/45)

The most serious difficulty now is not engendered by gross bodily activities such as walking but by such seemingly trivial tasks as operating my portable tape recorder or opening a "toolbox" (a cardboard carton) to get at a screwdriver. (This will remain true for the rest of Stage 3.) If the screwdriver is on the end of the box actually closest to my midsection, I invariably reach toward the opposite end of the box and there my hand will remain "glued" because *visually, I'm trying to raise it*—[*it is*] *seemingly held down by some force I'm unable to overpower.*

(9/120–9/120)

For the first time it's relatively easy to change batteries in the portable tape recorder; though I have done this daily, it was always a frustrating chore. I inevitably put the positive end of the battery where the negative belongs, and vice versa, visually convinced I was doing the correct thing as I was carrying out the action. *Only afterward did I notice the error. Today I perform correctly.*

(15/200–15/206)

Fine motor coordination is somewhat improved (e.g., taking the tape recorder apart, changing its batteries, looking for tools in boxes, and generally performing tricky mechanical tasks all have become smoother, less error-prone, and require less concentration). Yet, none of these activities can be performed with the same nonchalance, speed, or exactitude as at any time during Stage 2.

Table A8.8. Playing Soccer

(2/20–12/200)

Ball-throwing accurate, catching totally impossible. . . . Trying to find and pursue a floating ball, which landed on the water surface, either by walking or swimming, was simply a fiasco for when I put my head down—even if I had the ball in the FV—I was disoriented and had difficulty (motorically) deciding which way the ball was relative to me. If any portion of the horizon was in the FV, I did not experience this difficulty. (N.B.: Visual "horizon-guidance" for other activities.)

(5/62–5/69)

My effectiveness was limited to kicking the ball away defensively, roughly in the direction of the other goal. Once I put my head in the chin-to-chest position to accomplish the kick, I became disoriented, kicking other players without being aware of it and generally losing balance after the kick and falling down. On the whole, sustained, coordinated, visual following of the ball or dribbling was impossible. Once lost from the FV, I needed to scan extensively and often fruitlessly for quite a while to visually find the ball again.

Table A8.9. Eating with the Unpracticed Hand: Transfer of Training

(1/14–1/14)

I used my left hand 3 times on the first day of Stage 3, attempting to cut some food. I was totally unsuccessful. In the interest of gathering information on transfer of training, I will now only use my right hand while eating. . . . In all other activities, I shall use my left hand as is customary for a right-handed person.

(13/169–13/169)

At lunch I began eating with the left hand, which I had kept to my side while eating these past 12 days (155 waking, plus 114 sleeping, hours) in order to establish whether what the right hand had laboriously acquired during that time had somehow "transferred" to the left hand. It appears it has (engaging in other activities "generalized"). Anyway, eating with the left hand today—holding the fork, spearing food, pouring liquids, scooping soup, and cutting meat—was quite competent and comparable in every respect to using the right hand (except for the first 10 seconds or so). . . . Hand movements were not quite as quick but very precise. . . . It may be relevant that preexperimentally I could handle eating utensils equally well in either hand, having held the fork in my left hand most of my life. . . . It must be recalled that when I began eating, using my right hand to spear food from the plate and so on, I was totally disoriented, pushing the fork into the plate and expecting to see the fork rise, was unable to find the intended target on the plate, etc.

Table A8.10. Judgments of Distance-from-Self

(4/48–6/60)

I consistently misjudge distances from self (from toes, hips, knees, elbows, shoulders) to objects by 1–1.5 feet. This is true particularly for obstacles I'm approaching, say a wall, a door, a chair, people sitting or standing, or the edge of a sidewalk. Visually, I have quite a distance to go before collision, but the next instant, to my unpleasant surprise, I knock into these obstacles or slip off the edge of the sidewalk.

(14/185–14/185)

Even in places maximally familiar to me, I continue to knock into the table on the veranda, convinced I will clear it by at least 1 foot. The bruises on my thighs have taught me nothing. In unfamiliar places, I reach out and thus avoid colliding with objects, but in familiar surrounding, where I move with greater mobility and speed, I do collide.

Table A8.11. Sound, Smell, and Temperature Localization

(1/0.5–7/87)

Sound localization *is quite accurate in the right–left plane if measured by a quick head- and body-turning and facing [of] the source rather than by pointing. This is true for many kinds of stationary and moving sound sources (radio, voice, steamboat, plane, bird). Pointing is more accurate when the sound source is at the level of my midsection than when it emanates from the ground or above head level.*

(6/82–6/82)

Smell Localization: *A case of nosmic "capture": The visual-system information dominated nosmic-system information. It is late evening. I was just walking by a wall which was covered with flowers called "night glory"—they are tightly closed during the day and open up during the night. They were in full bloom, giving off a powerful aroma. I walked toward the wall, stretched my neck, and threw my head back in order to get my nose into a particular bushel. It turns out that there I was, the flowers actually about chest high, close to my nose had I not, under visual guidance, stretched my neck and thrown my head back to get my nose "closer." Instead of bringing my nose closer to the flowers—using nosmic information—I removed it further—using visual information.*

(7/97–7/97)

You not only hear things where you see them; you also smell things where you see them. Today I again went by the night-glory flower bush. Despite the fact that my nose was right in the thick of the flowers, I threw my head back vigorously in order to "locate" them nosmically. The visual information was apparently more powerful or compelling than the nosmic information.

(12/164–12/164)

Temperature Localization: *When food was touched to my lips, I experienced surprise and judged my mouth to be* above *my eyes—where my forehead had once been. However, when I was in danger of being burned, I experienced no surprise or apprehension; I simply drew back. Shortly after my observation on the apparent direction of smoke from a cigarette, I asked a companion to move the burning cigarette close to various body parts. When the cigarette came close to my lips the information was unequivocal: Though I still judged the top of my head to be closer to the ground than my chin, I localized my lips below my eyes and drew my head back. To be sure, this was happening* outside *my FV, and I had no active part in getting the information.*

Table A8.12. A Novel Point of Observation

(11/147–11/147)

I must adopt new habits of exploratory eye–head–body scanning and performance to gain available information about facts and events in the world and to act upon that information. It is not clear whether perceived head location is directly involved, but one thing is certain: It is quite impossible to receive optical information from the same place in the world while engaging in the same kinds of exploratory eye–head–body scanning movements and engaging in the same kind of performatory actions with and without reversing prisms on. For example, while reading the instrument dials of my tape recorder, I cannot hold the recorder in the same way I used to and simply glance down (employing the same eye–head movement combination I used to) because if I do, I will see nothing. Now, instead of holding the recorder close to my chest, I have to hold it at arm's length, put my head in the chin-to-chest position, and position the eyes up *in the head to read the [instrument] dials. [Similarly,] to see the contents of the trunk of a car . . . to place anything in the trunk . . . to shake hands with a person seated in a car . . . I must . . . go to my knees and bring my head in such a position that light from these previously occluded or invisible places can now enter my eyes. . . . These are real changes which will never change.*

PERCEPTION OF THE SELF AND OF EVENTS

Table A9.1. World-Relative Observations

(3/32–10/138)

Walking of other persons . . . seems to be quite comparable to the information given in a nonreversing situation by people on a dancefloor performing modern, exotic–sensual dances. The exaggerated up–down movements of head and body, the throwing out and rubbery sucking in of body parts, say the chest and belly, the heaving of hips and shoulders, and so on. The head of a person when walking normally describes a sinusoidal wave, rather than a straight line. What one perceives with reversing prisms on is roughly what one perceives when watching another person walk when the only part of his body visible is his head—if that person moves behind a high, occluding hedge. As I'm sitting here, people's heads are rising above and falling below the horizon line (the sea–sky dividing line) as they are walking by. Moreover, the difference between a man's walk and a woman's walk is much more apparent and exaggerated than without reversing prisms. . . . On the whole, women walk with greater elasticity and rubberiness than men. Men walk with fewer undulations and more muscularly, it appears.

(10/138–10/138)

As I'm sitting at the dinner table at the restaurant, the very quick walking, jogging, and running movements of the waiters and waitresses, as they are coming toward me, may be described as rubbery, spongy, half-galloping movements that one ordinarily notices in slow-motion photography . . . it appears slowed down somewhat . . . like what one detects in slow-motion sequences of people running (e.g., the film Elvira Madigan*).*

Table A9.2. Visual Imagery with Closed Eyes

(1/3–4/56)

When I close my eyes, I inescapably visualize the scene as I saw it just a moment ago when my eyes were open. The experience is comparable to a vivid afterimage. This "visualizing" includes the ability to describe the relationship of the beach to the sea and sky. Most important, I judge the scene to be identical to the scene viewed through reversing prisms except in immediacy of vividness. No part of this imagery included any part of my body. It's as if I were looking at a picture without awareness of the orientation or location of my own body parts. No matter how hard I try, I cannot imagine, "image," or conjure up any image or visual idea of how the world looked [during Stage 2], just 3 short hours ago.

(1/6–1/6)

After a 4-hour nap, following the first 6 hours of wearing prisms, I awoke and experienced the first vivid imagery of my head being oriented *upside down. Even though I wore an occluding mask, the experience was rather similar to looking through the prisms. The imaged* location *of my head, on the other hand, is indeterminate. I am not sure whether my head is at the level of my shoulders or just above the ground. The upside-down orientation of the head was uninfluenced by this uncertainty as to the imaged location of the head. I am not certain that a haptic component wasn't part of this (visual) imagery.*

(4/56–5/81)

It's midnight. I'm enveloped in total darkness. I take a few steps. The visual imagery and the haptic appreciation which accompany this walk are unequivocal: I'm walk-

ing with my head up–down reversed. The top of my head is virtually touching where I know the ground to be. Moreover, I'm quite unsteady as I walk, particularly when I move my head up or down or right or left. When I maintain my head in the chin-to-chest position and move my head to the right or left, I veer off into the direction of the head movement (cf: the apparent yoke of head–leg-movement direction, Table A8.1).

(14/185–14/185)

No instances of visual imagery have occurred since Day 5.

AFTEREFFECTS OF UP–DOWN REVERSING THE FIELD OF VIEW

Table A10.1. Judgments of the Slant of the Ground

(2/15.5–3/33.5)

Visually, the ocean bottom slopes downward and away from me, regardless of whether I'm facing landward or seaward and independent of head or body posture. This effect makes its appearance when the nonreversing prisms are submerged in the water and when they are parallel to the shoreline. (When I view the bottom of the ocean while the prisms are perpendicular to the shoreline, the slant of the ocean floor is judged veridically.) . . . When facing seaward, the judged direction of [the] *slant of the ocean floor corresponds to the facts, but I overestimate the magnitude (gradient) of this slope. Thus, in taking a step, my foot makes contact well before visually anticipated. In spite of the fact that the visual information, while facing toward shore, was "The ocean floor is slanting away from you and the water is getting deeper," the haptic information from active touch with my chin, my hands, or legs was "It's getting shallower". This discrepancy repeatedly produced surprise and toe-stubbing. One full hour of continuous observations of this nature produced no change. Now, while inverting my head today (Stage 4, Day 2), I judged the direction and magnitude of the slope of the ocean floor veridically. The above effect persists, though it became slightly attenuated during another full hour of observations the next day.*

(3/33.5–3/33.5)

Substituting a regular diving mask (the "backup system" with a FV of the same size) destroys the effect. Both direction and magnitude of slant of the ocean floor are perceived veridically.

(3/34.5–3/34.5)

Upon substituting the reversing prisms for nonreversing prisms for a while, I observed that I could not detect any change in these underwater slant observations, that is, the effects are identical whether I'm wearing reversing or nonreversing prisms.

Table A10.2. Judgments of the Visual and Haptic Size of Objects

(1/9–1/9)

During the first 3 days of wearing reversing prisms, the railing on the balcony here was visually judged to be quite low—at about knee level. When I approached it and made bodily contact, I was astonished to find that the railing actually reached just below my belt—its actual height. That's a 12-inch discrepancy, which caused surprise. I made the very same observation just now, during Stage 4.

Table A10.3. Distance-Compression Aftereffect and Adulthood Judgments of Distances Observer Experienced during Childhood

(1/1.5–1/4.5)

I experienced a striking similarity between the aftereffect of distance compression and adult distance judgments I [chanced to] compare with my memories of distance judgments which I had experienced 18 years earlier as a 9–12-year-old. The most striking and dumbfounding experience I had in visiting my home city, Salzburg, Austria, for the first time in 18 years (before initiating the spectacle experiment) *was that all the places which were well known to me then were, or appeared, shrunken. Specifically, . . . the distance between the inner city and the house where I lived . . . seemed then to be perceptually and motorically very great—it took terribly long to walk those four bus stops. This summer, I walked it in under 10 minutes, and the distance seemed quite short. The length of the block on which the apartment house stands seemed great in those days, both perceptually, that is, just standing there and gazing from one street corner to the other, and motorically, that is, walking or running the length of the block required quite a bit of exertion. This summer, however, this block seemed, perceptually* and *motorically, very short. The park in which I used to play as a child was huge—a virtual jungle. This summer it seemed but a small spot of grass with a few trees on it. I recall that running the circumference of the park was a feat if one did it without stopping to catch one's breath. That the performatory distance could even have seemed that great seemed most improbable this summer. Finally, the height of each individual stair in the house in which I lived, leading up to the second floor (there are 3 sets of 9 stairs [each]) were, in those days, again both perceptually and motorically enormous. I remember how proud I was to be able to "take" three of these steps in one stride and how tired I was by the time I arrived on the second floor. This summer the individual stairs seemed so shallow in height and slope that I* had *to take two with each step for otherwise I should have stumbled, and I reached the second floor without exertion and very quickly, so it seemed.*

Table A10.4. Reading

(1/0.5–4/56)

Reading my own handwriting is quite comfortable in 4 major orientations, though reading in the preexperimental orientation is still (again) preferred. During Stage 2, I could not read anything other than "normal" writing "normally" oriented. The order of difficulty in reading, from easiest to most difficult now *is:* (a) *Natural writing held right side up and read from left to right;* (b) *natural writing held geographically upside down and read from right to left;* (c) *carbon-copy-wrongly-placed* [*reversed*] *writing held right side up and read from right to left; and* (d) *most difficult, carbon-copy writing upside down and read from left to right (see Figure 9.4).*

Table A10.5. Telling Time

(1/0–4/56)

Trying to tell time causes hesitation: In fact, I now apply the self-same procedure which I applied when trying to tell time the first time I wore reversing prisms, namely, I check to see whether the numbers run clockwise or counterclockwise, whether the 7 comes before or after the 8, and so on. This method is slow but error-proof. Even 4 days later it takes several seconds to decide what time it is when my watch lies in odd positions relative to the posture of my head and body. The numbers on the face of the watch still look "different" from anything I have ever known.

Table A10.6. Visual Imagery

(1/2–2/28)

I have experienced no memories of any aspect of the up–down reversed world or of myself in it. This is true of visual imagery as well. In fact, I cannot conceive of what things were like unless I put my head between my knees (inversion) to get even an inkling of what the situation was like during the past 16 days.

B

Appendix: Apparatus and Time Course of the Prism Study

APPARATUS

Prisms

The two *reversing* prisms were prepared for joining by immersion in a bath of carbon tetrachloride to remove the tarlike protective coating on the silvering. The silvering of the hypotenuse face remained. The prisms were then washed in water and were ready to mount. No light passed through the plane where the two reversing prisms were joined because the protective copper plating prevented any light from penetrating the silvered surface. Hence, the reversing prism unit acted, functionally, as does a double-surfaced mirror held parallel to the ground plane, one surface facing skyward, the other, earthward.

Joining the two *nonreversing* prisms required, in addition, placing the prisms in a bath of 1:1 nitric acid to etch away the protective copper plating and finally, the silvering metal. Thus, light did pass through the joined hypotenuse faces of the nonreversing prisms because all protective plating as well as the silvering surface had been removed. The nonreversing prism unit acted, functionally, as does an Amici direct-vision prism, as a Kessler quadrilateral direct-vision prism, or as the rhomboidal form of a Kessler prism (Southall, 1964, pp. 497–499).

Both units were then mechanically mounted. The flatness of the hypotenuse faces precluded the need for any filler-type medium between the prisms to hold them together. Phenolic plastic was attached to the sides and joined along two longitudinal edges with 1.3-cm (1/2-in.) wide aluminum strips. Felt was used in all areas of prism contact. Holes were drilled into the phenolic plastic so that the prism could be screwed securely into the two metal bars along the right and left sides of the football helmet (see Figure 5.5). Further, an 8-mm deep, 22-mm wide (5/16-in.-×-14/16-in.) notch for the bridge of the nose was cut into the prism unit to bring the eyes as close to the glass as possible, thus maximizing the angular scope of the field of view (FV). This nose-groove was cut with a round "Remington" tungsten carbide hacksaw blade 1/8 in. thick. In the reversing prism unit, the notch was cut across the edge where the two hypotenuse faces of the two prisms were joined. Thus, when the reversing prism unit was mounted in the helmet and when the head was held in the primary position, the two jointed hypotenuse faces ran *parallel* to the ground. In the nonreversing prism unit, on the other hand, this notch was cut into the right-angle edge of one of the two prisms—where the two lateral faces of one of the prisms meet. Thus, when the nonreversing prism was mounted in the helmet and when the head was held in the primary position, the two jointed hypotenuse faces ran *perpendicular* to the ground. (Figure 5.5 also shows this second difference between the reversing and the normal-view unit.)

In both prism units, the observer looked through a geographically upper and lower sector. In the reversing prism unit, these two sectors were divided by a visible line of juncture, which joined the two hypotenuse faces. In the nonreversing unit, the two sectors were divided by the lateral edge of one of the nonreversing prisms. This visible line of juncture was 3 mm wide in both prism units and became readily unobtrusive.

Size of the Field of View and Point of Observation

Note that, as a general rule, the measured FV is greater when the observer maintains the eyes in the primary position than when he or she assumes extreme eye postures. This finding is counter-intuitive. An object just visible when the eyes are in the primary position will disappear from view when one tries to foveate it by an extreme eye movement excursion. Alternately, an object that is just out of the FV when an extreme eye posture is assumed will be represented in the array (and become visible) as soon as the primary eye position is assumed again.

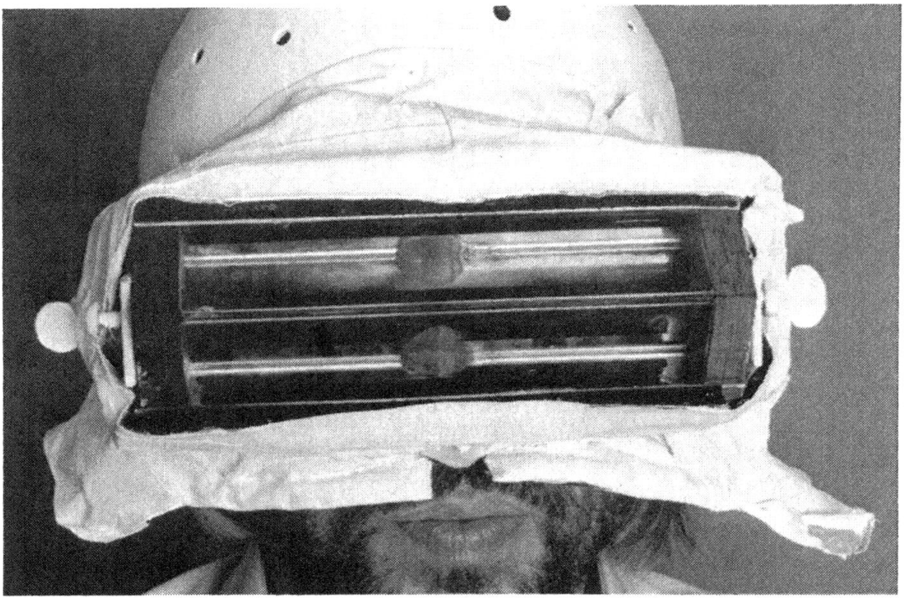

a

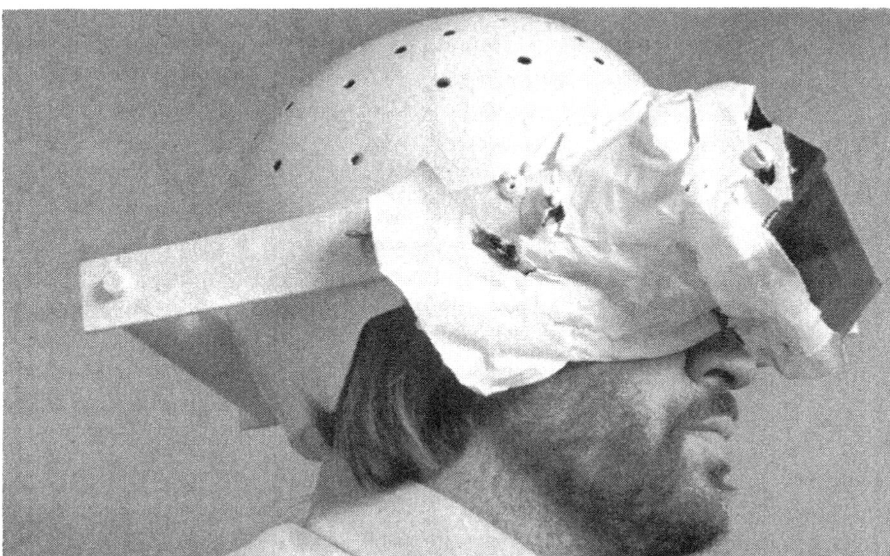

b

FIGURE B5.1. Helmet holding the prism units in place. Permanent, rear counterweight shown in *b*. Helmet reconstructed after wear and tear and studio-photographed following the Prism Study (2/79). The side flaps of the plastic hood are not as snug as during the study (cf. Figures 5.4 and 8.2b). The up–down reversing prisms of Stage 3 are shown.

The Helmet Holding the Prism Units

Figure B5.1 shows the helmet system during Stage 3. The helmet was a large (7 1/8 in.–7 1/4 in.) Spalding football helmet (Type 62–313). Many holes were drilled into it to provide ventilation and it was painted white to minimize absorption of light and heat-transmission to the head. Two steel bars (33 cm long × 3.7 cm wide [13 in. × 23/16 in.]) were screwed into each side of the helmet. These screws could be loosened or tightened at will to permit a snug fit, preventing movement of the helmet relative to the head during head movements. The two bars were permanently joined in the back of the helmet by a piece of pipe. This pipe served as an equalizing counterweight to the drag produced when either prism unit was inserted in the front. Once a prism unit was in place, the helmet system was dynamically balanced, no frontward or backward drag being produced. During Stages 1 and 5 of the study, I attached a pipe filled with lead to the front of the two bars. This front counterweight weighed the same as either prism unit (1.4 kg), and hence the helmet system remained both identical in weight (3.8 kg) and dynamically balanced throughout the experiment (see Figure B5.2).

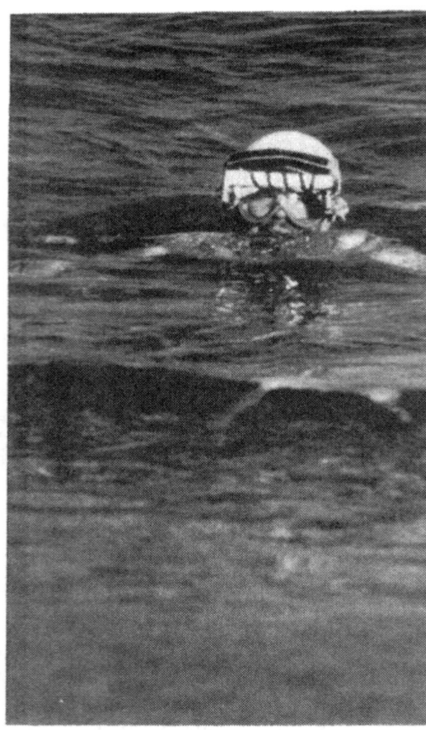

FIGURE B5.2. Adaptation to the increase in weight and size of the functional head during Stage 1. (With front counter weights used during Stages 1 and 5 in place.)

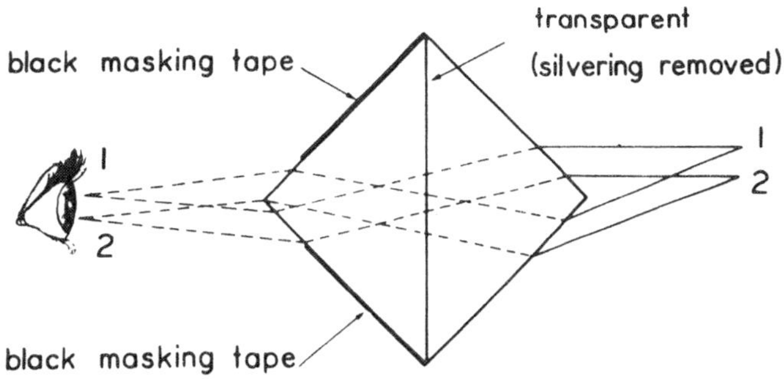

FIGURE B5.3. The path of light through the nonreversing prism unit (see Figure 5.5).

Geometrical Optics of Nonreversing Prisms

Figure B5.3 shows what happens to light when it passes through a pair of right-angle, isosceles glass prisms whose hypotenuse faces have been rotated 90° in the horizontal plane and from which the silvering has been removed (see also Figure 5.5).

Stray and Reflected Light

All light other than that coming through the prism units was very effectively prevented from reaching my eyes by an opaque, flexible hood made of thick plastic (as used for covering car seats). This plastic was painted white on the outside and black on the inside. On the upper side this hood was attached to the helmet. It was also attachable to the longitudinal side of either prism unit via a permanent, resealable adhesive. This hood itself was not in the visual field. On the underside (chinside), this hood also could be attached to either prism unit via a permanent adhesive. In this case, the hood covered the cheeks and part of the ears and closed tightly around the nose, leaving only the nostrils clear (see Figure B5.1 and 5.4). Each morning, before putting on the helmet, I cleaned the prisms with Spray-Kleen, an antifog and antistatic solution (made by the American Optical Company), which prevented them from "steaming up." I wore the backup system while cleaning the unit. During Stages 1 and 5, I wore clear plastic goggles, which were also cleaned with this solution.

Unless precaution is taken, there are two sources of light that can reach the eyes without being both properly transformed. First, some light is refracted through only the two lateral faces without ever reaching the silvered hypotenuse face to be reflected. When such light is reflected from normally oriented print, for example, the observer can read it per-

TABLE B5.1
Time Course of the Prism Study

Day of study	Stage of study	Day within stage	Sign in time (helmet, etc., on)	Sign out time (helmet, etc., off)	Relevant removal time: (e.g., of helmet for nap, shower). Observer's Eyes Closed (in minutes)	Total time with helmet system, small field, reversing or non-reversing prisms (in hours)	Mean number of waking hours for each stage
1	1	1	9:45 AM	9:00 PM	50	10.4	
2	1	2	7:30 AM	8:45 PM	75	12.0	
3	1	3	7:55 AM	10:15 PM	40	13.7	
4	1	4	8:00 AM	10:35 PM	20	14.25	
						50.3	12.6
5	2	1	8:30 AM	11:00 PM	00	14.5	
6	2	2	8:30 AM	10:00 PM	00	13.5	
7	2	3	8:00 AM	11:15 PM	00	15.25	
8	2	4	9:00 AM	11:25 PM	00	14.4	
9	2	5	9:15 AM	12:30 AM	00	15.25	
						73.0	14.6
10	3	1	8:45 AM	1:35 AM	240	12.8	
11	3	2	8:15 AM	1:30 AM	210	13.75	
12	3	3	8:30 AM	11:45 PM	00	15.25	
13	3	4	9:20 AM	12:30 AM	30	14.7	
14	3	5	[illegible]	[illegible]	00	[illegible]	

[illegible]	3	6	9:15 AM	11:30 PM	150	11.75	
16	3	7	9:30 AM	11:30 PM	00	14.0	
17	3	8	8:20 AM	11:00 PM	120	12.7	
18	3	9	9:30 AM	11:40 PM	00	14.2	
19	3	10	9:30 AM	11:25 PM	00	13.9	
20	3	11	8:15 AM	10:50 PM	00	14.6	
21	3	12	10:50 AM	11:00 PM	00	12.2	
22	3	13	8:55 AM	10:30 PM	00	13.6	
23	3	14	10:00 AM	12:30 AM	00	14.5	
24	3	15	9:10 AM	1:00 AM	00	15.8	
25	3	16	9:00 AM	11:15 AM	00	2.25	13.9
						211.2	(13.2)
25	4	1	11:15 AM	11:50 PM	00	12.6	
26	4	2	8:50 AM	1:00 AM	00	16.2	
27	4	3	9:35 AM	1:05 AM	00	15.5	
28	4	4	9:30 AM	12:45 AM	00	15.25	
29	4	5	8:30 AM	9:00 AM	00	00.5	14.9
						60.0	(12.0)
29	5	1	9:00 AM	1:00 AM	00	16.0	
30	5	2	9:30 AM	11:30 PM	00	14.0	
						30.0	15.0
31	6	1	8:00 AM	12:00 MID	00	16.0	
32	6	2	8:00 AM	12:00 MID	00	16.0	
33	6	3	9:00 AM	11:00 PM	00	14.0	
34	6	4	5:00 AM	11:00 PM	00	18.0	
						64.0	16.0

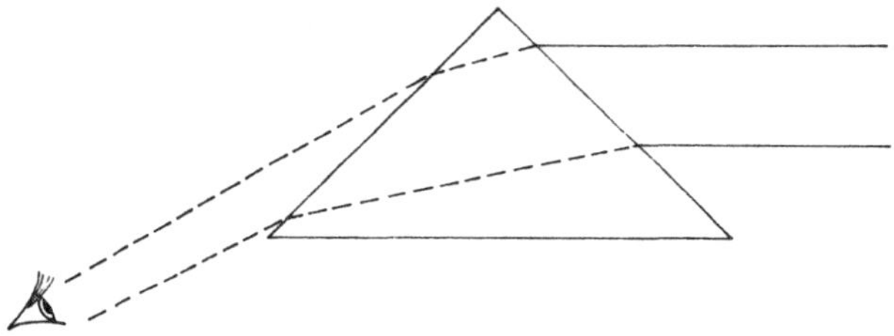

FIGURE B5.4. Pure refraction. Light entering the prism as shown is not up–down reversed by the prism. This light was prevented from reaching the eyes by the taping shown in Figure B5.3.

fectly well because no optical reversal has been effected. Figure B5.4 illustrates this case of pure refraction. Apparently, it occurs only at the extreme edges of the lateral faces (Southall, 1964, p. 122). Second, in addition to light being refracted through the lateral faces and reflected by the internal silvered hypotenuse faces, light is reflected from the external surfaces (lateral faces) of the prism on either side of the notch carved for the nose. Figure B5.5 shows this. These reflections are like the faint reflections sometimes seen in window-glass or "on" the surface of a calm body of water. In order to prevent either source of reflected light from entering the eyes, the two prism surfaces adjacent to the nose notch must be partially covered with two layers of black electrician's masking tape (see Figure B5.3). This was successfully accomplished by taping 38 mm of the two prism surfaces facing me. Thus, 11 mm of glass on either side of the nose notch remained visible. The size of the FV was not further restricted by this precaution because the two prism surfaces facing away from the observer determine the angular scope of light

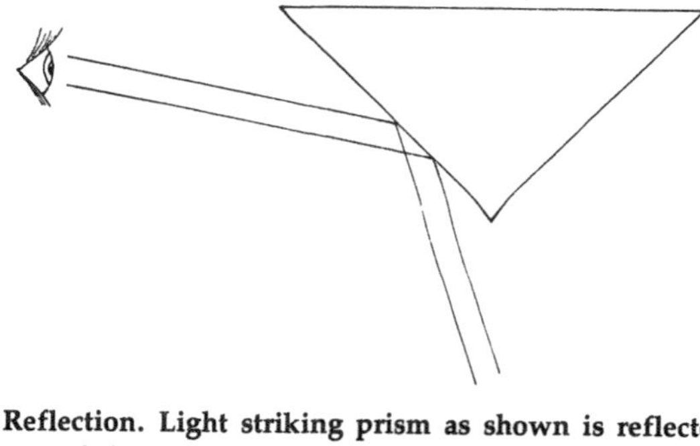

FIGURE B5.5. Reflection. Light striking prism as shown is reflected off its surface. Light-tight seal around the prism unit prevented this phenomenon (see Figure 5.4).

permitted to enter the prism unit and hence the eyes. All light undesirable from the standpoint of the experiment was thus eliminated. Both prism units were taped, although only the nonreversing unit is shown in Figure B5.3.

TIME COURSE

The duration of each stage of the Prism Study is shown in Table B5.1.

References

Agadzhanyan, N. A. *Medicine and space.* (NASA TT F-735). Washington, D.C.: National Aeronautics and Space Administration, 1973. (Originally published in Russian, 1971) (NTIS No. N73-18116).

Allen, S. R., Oswald, I., Lewis, S., & Tagney, J. The effects of distorted visual input on sleep. *Psychophysiology,* 1972, *9,* 498-504.

Alpern, M. Types of movement. In H. Davson (Ed.), *The eye* (Vol. 3), (2nd ed.). New York: Academic Press, 1969.

Ambler, R. K., & Guedry, F. E., Jr. Validity of a brief vestibular disorientation test in screening pilot trainees. *Aerospace Medicine,* 1966, *37,* 124-126.

Ardigò, R. Il fatto psicologico della percezione. *Opere Filosofiche* (3rd ed.). Padova, 1897 (?), *4,* Parte III, Ch. X, pp. 347-553.

Arora, H. L., & Sperry, R. W. Colour discrimination after optic nerve regeneration in the fish *Astromotus ocellatus. Developmental Biology,* 1963, *7,* 234-243.

Aubert, H. *Physiologie der Netzhaut.* Breslau: Morgenstern, 1865.

Baker, C. A. (Ed.). *Visual capabilities in the space environment.* New York: Pergamon Press, 1965.

Barnes, G. R. The role of the vestibulo-ocular reflex in visual target acquisition. *Journal of Physiology,* 1976, *258,* 65-66.

Bauer, J., & Held, R. Comparison of visually guided reaching in normal and deprived infant monkeys. *Journal of Experimental Psychology: Animal Behavior Processes,* 1975, *1,* 298-308.

Bauer, J., Woods, G., & Held, R. A device for rapid recording of positioning responses in two dimensions. *Behavioral Research Methods and Instrumentation,* 1969, *1,* 157-159.

Bender, M. B. The visual system: General considerations. In R. F. Naunton (Ed.), *The vestibular system.* New York: Academic Press, 1975.

Benson, A. J. Effect of diphenidol and prochlorperazine on semicircular canal function in man. *Aerospace Medicine,* 1969, *40,* 589-595.

Benson, A. J. & Brand, J. J. Some effects of 1-hyoscine hydrobromide on postrotatory sensation and nystagmus in man. *Quarterly Journal of Experimental Physiology,* 1968, *53,* 296-311.

Bergstedt, M. Vestibular problems in space travel. *Acta Oto-laryngologica,* 1966, supplement, *224,* 72-76.

Berkeley, G. *A new theory of vision.* London: J. M. Dent & Sons, 1969.

Berry, C. A., & Homick, G. L. Findings on American astronauts bearing on the issue of artificial gravity for future manned space vehicles. *Aerospace Medicine,* 1973, *44,* 163-168.

Bishop, H. E. *Innateness and learning in the visual perception of direction.* Unpublished doctoral dissertation, University of Chicago, 1959.

Bizzi, E., Kalil, R. E., Morasso, P., & Tagliasco, V. Central programming and peripheral feedback during eye-head co-ordination in monkeys. In J. Dichgans & E. Bizzi (Eds.), *Cerebral control of eye movements.* Basel: Karger, 1972.

Bizzi, E., Kalil, R. E., & Tagliasco, V. Eye-head coordination in monkeys: Evidence for centrally patterned organization. *Science,* 1971, *173,* 452-454.

Blum, G. S. A case study of hypnotically induced tubular vision. *The International Journal of Clinical and Experimental Hypnosis,* 1975, *23,* 111-119.

Boring, E. G. *A history of experimental psychology* (2nd ed.). New York: Appleton, Century, Crofts, 1950.

Bower, T. G. R. *Development in infancy.* San Francisco: Freeman, 1974.

Bower, T. G. R. *A primer of infant development.* San Francisco: Freeman, 1977.

Boynton, R. M. Summary and discussion. In A. Morris & E. P. Horne (Eds.), *Visual search.* Washingtin, D.C.: National Academy of Science, 1960.

Braine, L. G. A new slant on orientation perception. *American Psychologist,* 1978, *33,* 10-22.

Brand, J. J. A comparison of the effects of (-)-hyoscine and amylobarbitone sodium on measurements of post-rotational turning sensation and nystagmus. *Acta oto-laryngologica,* 1969, *68,* 427-434.

Brand, J. J., & Whittingham, P. Intramuscular hyoscine in control of motion sickness. *The Lancet,* 1970, *2,* 232-234.

Brecha, N., & Karten, H. J. Accessory optic projections upon oculomotor nuclei and vestibulocerebellum. *Science,* 1979, *203,* 913-916.

Brindley, G. S., Goodwin, G. M., Kolikowski, J. J., & Leighton, D. Stability of vision with a paralyzed eye. *Journal of Physiology,* 1976, *258,* 65-66.

Brindley, G. S., & Merton, P. A. The absence of position sense in the human eye. *Journal of Physiology,* 1960, *153,* 127-130.

Brown, G. G. Perception of depth with disoriented vision. *British Journal of Psychology,* 1928, *19,* 117-146.

Brown, J. L., (Ed.). *Sensory and perceptual problems related to space flight.* Washington, D.C.: National Academy of Sciences, 1961.

Brown, J. L. Visual elements in flight simulation. *Aviation, Space, and Environmental Medicine,* 1976, *47,* 913-924.

Brunswik, E. *The conceptual framework of psychology.* Chicago: University of Chicago Press, 1952.

Bursill, A. E. The restriction of peripheral vision during exposure to hot humid conditions. *Quarterly Journal of Experimental Psychology,* 1958, *10,* 114-129.

Carini, P. F. *Observation and description: An alternative methodology for the investigation of human phenomena.* Grand Forks, N.D.: University of North Dakota Press, 1975.

Carpenter, R. H. *Movements of the eyes.* London: Pion, 1977.

Carr, H. A. *An introduction to space perception.* New York: Longmans Green, 1935.

Chernik, D. A. Effect of REM sleep deprivation on learning and recall by humans. *Perceptual and Motor Skills,* 1972, *34,* 283–294.

Chkaidze, L. V. *Coordination of the voluntary movements of man in a zero gravitational field (under weightlessness)* (NASA TT F-578). (Aztec School of Languages, Inc. Maynard, Mass., Trans.). Washington: National Aeronautics and Space Administration, 1969. (Originally published in Russian, 1966.)

Clark, B. The vestibular system. *Annual Review of Psychology,* 1970, *21,* 273–306.

Clark, B., & Stewart, D. Vestibular and nonvestibular information in judgments of attitude and coriolis motion in a piloted flight simulator. *Aerospace Medicine,* 1967, *38,* 936–940.

Clark, B., & Stewart, D. Relationship between motion sickness experience and tests of the perception of rotation in pilots and nonpilots. *Aerospace Medicine,* 1973, *44,* 393–396.

Cohen, B. The vestibulo-ocular reflex arc. In H. H. Kornhuber (Ed.), *Handbook of Sensory Physiology* (Vol. VI/1). Berlin: Springer-Verlag, 1974.

Cohen, H. B. Some critical factors in prism-adaptation. *American Journal of Psychology,* 1966, *79,* 285–290.

Cohen, M. M. Continuous versus terminal feedback in prism aftereffects. *Perceptual and Motor Skills,* 1967, *24,* 295–302.

Cohen, M. M. Disorienting effects of aircraft catapult launchings: II. Visual and postural contributions. *Aviation, Space, and Environmental Medicine,* 1976, *47,* 39–41.

Cohen, M. M. Disorienting effects of aircraft catapult launchings: III. Cockpit displays and piloting performance. *Aviation, Space, and Environmental Medicine,* 1977, *48,* 797–804.

Cohen, W. Form recognition, spatial orientation, perception of movement in the uniform visual field. In A. Marris & E. Phorne (Eds.), *Visual search techniques.* Washington, D.C.: National Academy of Science National Research Council, 1960.

Collins, W. E. Vestibular responses from skaters. *Aerospace Medicine,* 1966, *37,* 1098.

Collins, W. E. Special effects of brief periods of visual fixation on nystagmus and sensations of turning. *Aerospace Medicine,* 1968, *39,* 257–266.

Collins, W. E. Habituation of vestibular responses with and without visual stimulation. In H. H. Kornhuber (Ed.), *Handbook of sensory physiology* (Vol. VI/2). Berlin: Springer-Verlag, 1974.

Collins, W. E., & Lentz, J. M. Some psychological correlates of motion sickness susceptibility. *Aviation, Space, and Environmental Medicine,* 1977, *48,* 587–594.

Coren, S. Adaptation to prismatic displacement as a function of the amount of available information. *Psychonomic Science,* 1966, *4,* 407–408.

Coren, S., & Festinger, L. An alternative view of the "Gibson normalization effect." *Perception and Psychophysics,* 1967, *2,* 621–626.

Craske, B., & Crawshaw, M. Prism adaptation while tracking and saccading. *Acta Psychologica,* 1979, *43,* 33–37.

Davies, P., & Melvill Jones, G. An adaptive neural model compatible with plastic changes induced in the human vestibulo-ocular reflex by prolonged optical reversal of vision. *Brain Research,* 1976, *103,* 546–550.

Da Vinci, L. *The notebooks of Leonardo Da Vinci* (E. MacCurdy, Ed. and trans.). New York: George Braziller, 1958.

Day, R. H., & Singer, G. Sensory adaptation and behavioral compensation with spatially transformed vision and hearing. *Psychological Bulletin,* 1967, *67,* 307–322.

Day, R. H., & Wade, N. J. Involvement of neck proprioceptive system in visual after-effect from prolonged head tilt. *Quarterly Journal of Experimental Psychology,* 1968, *20,* 290–293.

Dewan, E. M. The programming "P" hypothesis for REM sleep. In E. Hartmann (Ed.),

Sleep and dreaming (*International Psychiatry Clinics Series*, Vol. 7). Boston: Little Brown, 1970.

Dichgans, J. Spinal afferences to the oculomotor system: Physiological and clinical aspects. In G. Lennerstrand & P. Bach-y-Rita (Eds.), *Basic mechanisms of ocular motility*. Oxford: Pergamon Press, 1975.

Dichgans, J. The influence of peripheral vision on ambient ego-orientation. *Neurosciences Research Program Bulletin*, 1977, *15*, 376-385.

Dichgans, J., Held, R., Young, L., & Brandt, T. Moving visual scenes influence the apparent direction of gravity. *Science*, 1972, *178*, 1217-1219.

Ditchburn, R. W., & Ginsborg, B. L. Vision with a stabilized retinal image. *Nature* (London), 1952, *170*, 36-37.

Dix, M. R., & Hood, J. D. Observations upon the nervous mechanism of vestibular habituation. *Acta Otolaryngologica*, 1969, *67*, 310-318.

Dodge, R. Visual Perception during eye movement. *Psychological Review*, 1900, *7*, 454-465.

Dodge, R. Five types of eye movement in the horizontal meridian plane of the field of regard. *American Journal of Physiology*, 1903, *8*, 307-329.

Dodge, R. The illusion of clear vision during eye movement. *Psychological Bulletin*, 1905, *2*, 193-199.

Dodge, R. The latent time of compensatory eye-movements. *Journal of Experimental Psychology*, 1921, *4*, 247-269.

Dodge, R. Habituation to rotation. *Journal of Experimental Psychology*, 1923, *6*, 1-34. (a)

Dodge, R. Adequacy of reflex compensatory eye-movements including the effects of neural rivalry and competition. *Journal of Experimental Psychology*, 1923, *6*, 169-181. (b)

Dodwell, P. C. *Visual pattern recognition*. New York: Holt, 1970.

Dolezal, H. *Visual backward masking of blurred letters: Test of a luminance summation-contrast reduction and a contour rivalry hypothesis*. Unpublished master's thesis, State University of New York at Albany, 1968.

Dolezal, H. *Long-term perceptual and performatory adaptation to wearing up-down reversing prisms in the real world*. Unpublished manuscript, Cornell University, 1971.

Dolezal, H. In honor of Robert Brodie MacLeod: Psychological phenomenology face to face with the persistent problems of psychology. *Journal of the History of the Behavioral Sciences*, 1975, *11*, 223-234.

Dolezal, H. F. Long-term adaptation to up-down reversing the field of view: Complex changes afforded by optical invariants (Doctoral dissertation, Cornell University, 1976). *Dissertation Abstracts International*, 1977, *37*, 6364B-6365B. (University Microfilms No. 77-13,005)

Dolezal, H., & Held, R. *Two components of visually-induced tilt during rotary field motion*. Paper presented at the meeting of the Eastern Psychological Association, New York, April, 1975.

Dolezal, H., & Toleno, T. Introduction. In R. B. MacLeod, *The persistent problems of psychology* (M. Henle, & M. Wertheimer, Eds.). Pittsburgh: Duquesne University Press, 1975.

Donagan, A. Berkeley's theory of the immediate objects of vision. In P. K. Machamer & R. G. Turnbull (Eds.), *Studies in perception*. Columbus, Ohio: Ohio State University, 1978.

Dowd, P. J. Useful test in selecting motion-sick-prone individuals. *Space Life Sciences*, 1973, *4*, 391-401.

Duncker, K. Ueber induzierte Bewegung. *Psychologische Forschung*, 1929, *12*, 180-259.

Easton, R. D. Relation between optically induced and tracking-limb movement curvature in a visual capture phenomenon. *Perceptual and Motor Skills*, 1976, *43*, 363-369.

Easton, R. D., & Falzett, M. Finger pressure during tracking of curved contours: Implications for a visual dominance phenomenon. *Perception and Psychophysics*, 1978, *24*, 145-153.

Easton, R. D., & Moran, P. W. A quantitative confirmation of visual capture of curvature. *Journal of General Psychology*, 1978, *98*, 105-112.

Ebenholtz, S. The constancies in object orientation: An algorithm processing approach. In W. Epstein (Ed.), *Stability and constancy in visual perception: Mechanisms and processes*. New York: Wiley, 1977.

Ewert, P. H. A study of the effect of inverted retinal stimulation upon spatially coordinated behavior. *Genetic Psychology Monographs*, 1930, *7*, 177-363.

Ewert, P. H. Factors in space localization during inverted vision: I. Interference. *Psychological Review*, 1936, *43*, 522-546.

Ewert, P. H. Factors in space localization during inverted vision: II. An explanation of interference and adaptation. *Psychological Review*, 1937, *44*, 105-116.

Feinberg, I., & Evarts, E. V. Changing concepts of the function of sleep: Discovery of intense brain activity during sleep calls for revision of hypotheses as to its function. *Biological Psychiatry*, 1969, *1*, 331-348.

Festinger, L., Burnham, C. A., Ono, H., & Bamber, D. Efference and the conscious experience of perception. *Journal of Experimental Psychology Monograph*, 1967, *74*, (4, Whole No. 637).

Festinger, L., & Holtzman, J. D. Retinal image smear as a source of information about magnitude of eye movement. *Journal of Experimental Psychology: Human Perception and Performance*, 1978, *4*, 573-585.

Fieandt, K. von. Das phaenomenologische Problem von Licht und Schatten. *Acta Psychologica*, 1949, *6*, 337-357.

Fischer, M. H., & Kornmueller, A. E. Optokinetisch ausgeloeste Bewegungswahrnehmungen und optokinetischer Nystagmus. *Journal fuer Psychologie und Neurologie*, 1930, *41*, 273-308.

Flaherty, B. E. (Ed.). *Psychophysiological aspects of space flight*. New York: Columbia University Press, 1961.

Fleming, D. G., Vossius, G. W., Bowman, G., & Johnson, E. L. Adaptive properties of the eye-tracking system as revealed by moving-head and open-loop studies. *Annals of the New York Academy of Sciences*, 1969, *156*, 825-850.

Foley, J. P. An experimental investigation of the effect of prolonged inversion of the visual field in the rhesus monkey (macaca mulatta). *Journal of Genetic Psychology*, 1940, *56*, 21-51.

Ford, F. R., & Walsh, F. B. Clinical observations upon the importance of vestibular reflexes on ocular movements: Effects of section of one or both vestibular nerves. *Bulletin of the John Hopkins Hospital* (Baltimore), 1936, *58*, 80-88.

Franklin, S. S. The effect of modified correlation between eye movement and head movement on the perception of visual direction: An examination of Helmholtz's eye position hypothesis (Doctoral dissertation, University of Kansas, 1966). *Dissertation Abstracts*, 1967, *28*, 1123B-1124B. (University Microfilms No. 67-10, 803)

Freedman, S. J. On the mechanisms of perceptual compensation. In S. J. Freedman (Ed.), *The neuropsychology of spatially oriented behavior*. Homewood, Ill.: Dorsey, 1968.

Fukuda, T. Postural behavior and motion sickness. *Acta Otolaryngologica*, 1976, *81*, 237-241.

Gauthier, G. M., & Robinson, D. A. Adaptation of the human vestibulo-ocular reflex to magnifying lenses. *Brain Research*, 1975, *92*, 331-335.

Gernandt, B. E. Vestibular connections in the brainstem. In M. B. Bender (Ed.), *The oculomotor system*. New York: Harper & Row, 1964.

Giannitrapani, D. Changes in adaptation to prolonged perceptual distortion: A developmental study (Doctoral dissertation, Clark University, 1958). *Dissertation Abstracts*, 1959, *19*, 1835-1836. (University Microfilms No. 58-7084)

Gibson, E. J. *Principles of perceptual learning and development.* New York: Appleton, 1969.

Gibson, E. J., & Walk, R. D. The visual cliff. *Scientific American*, 1960, *202*(4), 64-71.

Gibson, J. J. Adaptation after-effect, and contrast in the perception of curved lines. *Journal of Experimental Psychology*, 1933, *16*, 1-31.

Gibson, J. J. *The perception of the visual world.* Boston: Houghton Mifflin, 1950.

Gibson, J. J. Visually controlled locomotion and visual orientation in animals. *British Journal of Psychology*, 1958, *49*, 182-194.

Gibson, J. J. Ecological optics. *Vision Research*, 1961, *1*, 253-262.

Gibson, J. J. *The senses considered as perceptual systems.* Boston: Houghton Mifflin, 1966.

Gibson, J. J. Invariant properties of changing stimulation as information for perception. In F. Klix (Ed.), *The organization of human information processing.* Berlin: Akademie-Verlag, 1967.

Gibson, J. J. What gives rise to the perception of motion? *Psychological Review*, 1968, *75*, 335-346.

Gibson, J. J. On theories for visual space perception: A reply to Johansson. *Scandinavian Journal of Psychology*, 1970, *2*, 75-79.

Gibson, J. J. Outline of a theory of direct visual perception. In J. R. Royce & W. W. Rozeboom (Eds.), *The psychology of knowing.* New York: Gordon & Breach, 1972.

Gibson, J. J. A note on ecological optics. In E. C. Carterette & M. P. Friedman (Eds.), *Handbook of perception* (Vol. I). New York: Academic Press, 1974.

Gibson, J. J. *The ecological approach to visual perception.* Boston: Houghton Mifflin, 1979.

Gibson, J. J., & Mowrer, O. H. Determinants of the perceived vertical and horizontal. *Psychological Review*, 1938, *45*, 300-323.

Gibson, J. J., & Waddell, E. Homogeneous retinal stimulation and visual perception. *American Journal of Psychology*, 1952, *65*, 263-270.

Gillingham, K. K., & McNaughton, G. B. Visual field contraction during G stress at 13deg., 45deg., and 65deg. seatback angles. *Aviation, Space, and Environmental Medicine*, 1977, *48*, 91-96.

Giurgea, C. E., Moeyersoons, F. E., & Evraerd, A. C. A GABA-related hypothesis on the mechanism of action of the antimotion sickness drugs. *Archives Internationales de Pharmaeodynamic et de Therapie*, 1967, *166*, 238-249.

Goldscheider, A. Untersuchungen ueber den Muskelsinn. I. Ueber die Bewegungsempfindung. In *Gesammelte Abhandlungen von A. Goldscheider* (Vol. II). Leipzig: Barth, 1898.

Goldstein, A. G. Recognition of inverted photographs of faces by children and adults. *Journal of Genetic Psychology*, 1975, *127*, 109-123.

Gonshor, A., & Melvill Jones, G. Vestibular habituation induced by mirror vision: An optimising process? *Proceedings of the Annual Scientific Meeting, Aerospace Medical Association*, Houston, 1971, 253-254.

Gonshor, A., & Melvill Jones, G. Changes of human vestibulo-ocular response induced by vision-reversal during head rotation. *Journal of Physiology*, 1973, *234*, 102P-103P.

Gonshor, A., & Melvill Jones, G. Short term adaptive changes in the human vestibulo-ocular reflex arc. *Journal of Physiology*, 1976, *256*, 361-379. (a)

Gonshor, A., & Melvill Jones, G. Extreme vestibulo-ocular adaptation induced by prolonged optical reversal of vision. *Journal of Physiology*, 1976, *256*, 381-414. (b)

Graham, C. H. Visual space perception. In C. H. Graham (Ed.), *Vision and visual perception.* New York: John Wiley & Sons, 1965.

Graybiel, A. Contributions of the space program to our knowledge of motion sickness. *Astronautica Acta*, 1972, *17*, 5-25.

Graybiel, A. Measurement of otolith function in man. In H. H. Kornhuber (Ed.), *Handbook of sensory physiology* (Vol. VI/2). Berlin: Springer-Verlag, 1974.

Graybiel, A., & Knepton, J. Sopite syndrome: A sometimes sole manifestation of motion sickness. *Aviation, Space, and Environmental Medicine,* 1976, *47,* 873–882.

Graybiel, A., Knepton, J., & Shaw, J. Prevention of experimental motion sickness by scopolamine absorbed through the skin. *Aviation, Space, and Environmental Medicine,* 1976, *47,* 1096–1100.

Graybiel, A., & Lackner, J. R. Comparison of susceptibility to motion sickness during rotation at 30 rpm in the earth-horizontal, 10 deg. head-up, and 10 deg. head-down positions. *Aviation, Space, and Environmental Medicine,* 1977, *48,* 7–11.

Graybiel, A., & Miller, E. F., II. A Z-axis recumbent rotating device for use in parabolic flight. *Aviation, Space, and Environmental Medicine,* 1976, *47,* 893.

Graybiel, A., Miller, E. F., and Homick, J. L. Experiment M-131, human vestibular function. *Proceedings of the Skylab Life Sciences Symposium, NASA Technical Memo,* JSC-09275, NASA TMX-S81S4, 1974, 169–220.

Graybiel, A., Wood, C. D., Knepton, J., Hoche, J. P., & Perkins, F. Human assay of antimotion sickness drugs. *Aviation, Space, and Environmental Medicine,* 1975, *46,* 1107–1118.

Green, J. A. Effectivity of antimotion sickness drugs during artificial gravity simulations. *Aerospace Medicine,* 1973, *44,* 1255–1260.

Greenberg, R., Horowitz, J., & Pearlman, C. The relation of dreaming to sensory motor adaptation. *Psychophysiology,* 1972, *9,* 145.

Greenberg, R., & Pearlman, C. Cutting the REM nerve: An approach to the adaptive role of REM sleep. *Perspectives in Biology and Medicine,* 1974, *17,* 513–521.

Greenberg, R., Pillard, R., & Pearlman, C. The effect of dream (Stage REM) deprivation on adaptation to stress. *Psychosomatic Medicine,* 1972, *34,* 257–262.

Gregory, R. L. Choosing a paradigm for perception. In E. Carterette & M. Friedman (Eds.), *Handbook of perception: Historical and philosophical roots of perception* (Vol. I). New York: Academic Press, 1974.

Gregory, R. L., & Wallace, J. G. Recovery from early blindness: A case study. *Experimental Psychology Society Monographs,* Cambridge, 1963, (No. 2).

Gresty, M., Trinder, E., & Leech, J. Perception of everyday visual environments during saccadic eye movements. *Aviation, Space, and Environmental Medicine,* 1976, *47,* 991–992.

Griffin, M. J. Levels of whole-body vibration affecting human vision. *Aviation, Space, and Environmental Medicine,* 1975, *46,* 1033–1040.

Grose, V. L. Deleterious effect on astronaut capability of vestibulo-ocular disturbance during spacecraft roll acceleration. *Aerospace Medicine,* 1967, *38,* 1138–1144.

Guedry, F. E. Psychophysiological studies of vestibular function. In W. D. Neff (Ed.), *Contributions to sensory physiology.* New York: Academic Press, 1965. (a)

Guedry, F. E. Habituation to complex vestibular stimulation in man: Transfer and retention of effects from twelve days of rotation at 10 rpm. *Perceptual and Motor Skills,* 1965, *21,* 459–481. (b)

Guedry, F. E. Relations between vestibular nystagmus and visual performance. *Aerospace Medicine,* 1968, *39,* 570–579.

Guedry, F. E. Psychophysics of vestibular sensation. In H. H. Kornhuber (Ed.), *Handbook of sensory physiology* (Vol. VI/2). Berlin: Springer-Verlag, 1974.

Gurovskiy, N. N., (Ed.). *Studies on the psychophysiology of the work of astronauts.* (NASA TT F-593). Washington, D.C.: National Aeronautics and Space Administration, 1970. (Originally published in Russian, 1967).

Gyr, S. W. Is a theory of direct visual perception adequate? *Psychological Bulletin,* 1972, *77,* 246–261.

Haber, R. N., & Hershenson, M. *The psychology of visual perception.* New York: Holt, 1973.

Hagen, M. A., Jones, R. K., & Reed, E. S. On a neglected variable in theories of pictoral perception: Truncation of the visual field. *Perception and Psychophysics*, 1978, *23*, 326–330.

Hallett, P. E., & Lightstone, A. D. Corrective saccades and visual inflow during the prior saccade. *Journal of the Optical Society of America*, 1973, *63*, 1311.

Hallett, P. E., & Lightstone, A. D. Saccadic eye movements towards stimuli triggered by prior saccades. *Vision Research*, 1976, *16*, 99–106.

Hanrahan, J. S., & Bushnell, D. *Space biology: The human factors in space flight*. New York: Basic Books, 1960.

Hardt, M. E., Held, R., & Steinbach, M. J. Adaptation to displaced vision: A change in the central control of sensorimotor coordination. *Journal of Experimental Psychology*, 1971, *89*, 229–239.

Harris, C. S. Adaptation to displaced vision: A proprioceptive change (Doctoral dissertation, Harvard University, 1963). (University Microfilms No. 68-8162) (a)

Harris, C. S. Adaptation to displaced vision: Visual, motor, or proprioceptive change? *Science*, 1963, *140*, 812–813. (b)

Harris, C. S. Adaptation to displaced vision: A proprioceptive change. *Dissertation Abstracts*, 1963, *24*, 2136–2137. (c)

Harris, C. S. Proprioceptive changes underlying adaptation to visual distortions. *American Psychologist*, 1964, *19*, 562. (Abstract)

Harris, C. S. Perceptual adaptation to inverted, reversed, and displaced vision. *Psychological Review*, 1965, *72*, 419–444.

Harris, C. S. *Through the looking glass: Adapting to an optically reversed world*. Paper presented at the Symposium on "Perceptual Change", American Association for the Advancement of Science, Washington, D.C., December, 1966.

Harris, C. S. Beware of the straight-ahead shift—a nonperceptual change in experiments on adaptation to displaced vision. *Perception*, 1974, *3*, 461–476.

Hay, J. C. Visual adaptation to an altered correlation between eye movement and head movement. *Science*, 1968, *160*, 429–430.

Hay, J. C. Does head-movement feedback calibrate the perceived direction of optical motions? *Perception & Psychophysics*, 1971, *10*, 286–288.

Hay, J. C. & Goldsmith, W. M. Space-time adaptation of visual position constancy. *Journal of Experimental Psychology*, 1973, *99*, 1–9.

Hay, J. C., & Pick, H. L., Jr. Gaze-contingent prism adaptation: Optical and motor factors. *Journal of Experimental Psychology*, 1966, *72*, 640–648.

Hay, J. C., Pick, H. L., Jr., & Ikeda, K. Visual capture produced by prism spectacles. *Psychonomic Science*, 1965, *2*, 215–216.

Hein, A., & Held, R. A neural model for labile sensorimotor coordinations. In E. E. Bernard & M. R. Kave (Eds.), *Biological prototypes and synthetic systems* (Vol. 1). New York: Plenum Press, 1962.

Held, R. Exposure-history as a factor in maintaining stability of perception and coordination. *Journal of Nervous and Mental Disease*, 1961, *132*, 26–32.

Held, R. Plasticity in sensorimotor systems. *Scientific American*, 1965, *213*(5), 84–94.

Held, R. Plasticity in sensorimotor coordination. In S. J. Freedman (Ed.), *The neuropsychology of spatially oriented behavior*. Homewood, Ill.: Dorsey Press, 1968. (a)

Held, R. Action contingent development in neonatal animals. In D. B. Kimble (Ed.), *Experience and capacity*. New York: New York Academy of Sciences, 1968. (b)

Held, R., & Bauer, J. A., Jr. Visually guided reaching in infant monkeys after restricted rearing. *Science*, 1967, *155*, 718–720.

Held, R., & Bauer, J. A., Jr. Development of sensorially-guided reaching in infant monkeys. *Brain Research*, 1974, *71*, 265–271.

Held, R., & Bossom, J. Neonatal deprivation and adult rearrangement: Complementary techniques for analyzing plastic sensory-motor coordinations. *Journal of Comparative and Physiological Psychology*, 1961, *54*, 33–37.

Held, R., Dichgans, J., & Bauer, J. Characteristics of moving visual scenes influencing spatial orientation. *Vision Research*, 1975, *15*, 357–365.

Held, R., & Freedman, S. Plasticity in human sensorimotor control. *Science*, 1963, *142*, 455–462.

Held, R., & Gottlieb, N. Technique for studying adaptation to disarranged hand–eye coordination. *Perceptual Motor Skills*, 1958, *8*, 83–86.

Held, R., & Hein, A. Adaptation of disarranged hand–eye coordination contingent upon reafferent stimulation. *Perceptual Motor Skills*, 1958, *8*, 87–90.

Held, R., & Hein, A. Movement-produced stimulation in the development of visually guided behavior. *Journal of Comparative and Physiological Psychology*, 1963, *56*, 872–876.

Held, R., & Mikaelian, H. Motor-sensory feedback versus need in adaptation to rearrangement, *Perceptual and Motor Skills*, 1964, *18*, 685–688.

Held, R., & Rekosh, J. Motor-sensory feedback and the geometry of visual space. *Science*, 1963, *141*, 722–723.

Helmholtz, H. von. *Handbuch der Physiologischen Optik* (Vol. 1) (1st ed.). Leipzig: Voss, 1867.

Helmholtz, H. von. *Handbuch der Physiologischen Optik* (Vol. 3) (3rd ed.). Leipzig: Voss, 1910.

Helmholtz, H. von. *Treatise on physiological optics* (Vols 1–3). (J. P. C. Southall, Ed.). New York: Dover Publications, 1962.

Hersen, M., & Barlow, D. *Single case experimental designs: Strategies for studying behavior change*. New York: Pergamon Press, 1976.

Hess, E. Space perception in the chick. *Scientific American*, 1956, *195*, 71–80.

Hochberg, J. In the minds eye. In R. N. Haber (Ed.), *Contemporary theory and research in visual perception*. New York: Holt, 1968.

Hochberg, J. Space and movement. In J. W. Kling & L. A. Riggs (Eds.), *Woodworth and Schlosberg's experimental psychology* (3rd ed.). New York: Holt, 1971.

Hochberg, J. *Perception* (2nd ed.). Englewood Cliffs, N.J.: Prentice-Hall, 1978.

Hochberg, J., & Brooks, V. Film cutting and visual momentum. In J. W. Senders, D. F. Fisher, & R. A. Monty (Eds.), *Eye movements and higher psychological functions*. Hillsdale, N.J.: Erlbaum, 1978.

Holst, E. von. Relations between the central nervous system and the peripheral organs. *British Journal of Animal Behavior*, 1954, 2, 89–94.

Holst, E. von, & Mittelstaedt, H. Das Reafferenzprinzip. *Naturwissenschaften*, 1950, *37*, 464–476.

Holway, A. H., & Boring, E. G. Determinants of apparent visual size with distance variant. *American Journal of Psychology*, 1941, *54*, 21–37.

Hornbostel, E. M. von. Die Einheit der Sinne. *Melos, Zeitschrift fuer Musik*, 1925, 4, 290–297. Translated as: The unity of the senses. *Psyche*, 1927, *7*, 83–89.

Howard, I. P. Displacing the optical array. In S. J. Freedman (Ed.), *The neuropsychology of spatially oriented behavior*. Homewood, Ill.: Dorsey Press, 1968.

Howard, I. P. The adaptability of the visual-motor system. In K. J. Connolly (Ed.), *Mechanisms of motor skill development*. London: Academic Press, 1970.

Howard, I. P. Perceptual learning and adaptation. *British Medical Bulletin*, 1971, *27*, 248–252.

Howard, I. P. Seeing space. *Transactions of the Opthalmological Societies of the United Kingdom*, 1973, *93*, 397–405.

Howard, I. P. Orientation and motion in space. In E. C. Carterette & M. P. Friedman (Eds.), *Handbook of perception* (Vol. III.). New York: Academic Press, 1974.

Howard, I. P. Effects of exposure to spatially distorted stimuli. In R. D. Walk and H. L. Pick (Eds.), *Perception and experience*. New York: Plenum, 1978.

Howard, I. P., Anstis, T., & Lucia, H. C. The relative lability of mobile and stationary components in a visual-motor adaptation task. *Quarterly Journal of Experimental Psychology*, 1974, *26*, 293–300.

Howard, I. P., Craske, B., & Templeton, W. B. Visuo-motor adaptation to discordant ex-afferent stimulation. *Journal of Experimental Psychology*, 1965, *70*, 189–191.

Howard, I. P., & Templeton, W. B. *Human spatial orientation*. London: Wiley, 1966.

Hubel, D. H., & Wiesel, T. N. Receptive fields of single neurons in the cat's striate cortex. *Journal of Physiology*, 1959, *148*, 574–591.

Hyslop, J. H. Upright vision. *Psychological Review*, 1897, *4*, 71–73. (a)

Hyslop, J. H. Upright vision. *Phychological Review*, 1897, *4*, 142–163. (b)

Itard, J. M. G. *The wild boy of Aveyron*. New York: Appleton, 1962.

James, W. *The principles of psychology*. New York: Dover, 1950. (Originally published, 1890).

Jenkins, J. G., & Dallenbach, K. M. Minor studies from the psychological laboratory of Cornell University. *American Journal of Psychology*, 1924, *35*, 605–612.

Johansson, G. Spatial constancy and motion in visual perception. In W. Epstein (Ed.), *Stability and constancy in visual perception: Mechanisms and processes*. New York: Wiley, 1977.

Johnson, W. H., & Jongkees, L. B. W. Motion Sickness. In H. H. Kornhuber (Ed.), *Handbook of sensory physiology* (Vol. VI/2). Berlin: Springer-Verlag, 1974.

Johnson, W. H., Money, K. E., & Graybiel, A. Airborne testing of three antimotion sickness preparations. *Aviation, Space, and Environmental Medicine*, 1976, *47*, 1214–1216.

Johnston, R. S., Dietlein, L. F., & Berry, C. A. (Eds.). *Biomedical results of Apollo* (NASA SP-368). Washington, D.C.: U.S. Government Printing Office, 1975.

Jung, R. Visual perception and neurophysiology. In R. Jung (Ed.), *Handbook of sensory physiology* (Vol. VII/3). Berlin: Springer-Verlag, 1973.

Kalil, R. E., & Freedman, S. J. Persistence of ocular rotation following compensation for displaced vision. *Perceptual and Motor Skills*, 1966, *22*, 135–139.

Kellogg, R. S. Vestibular influences on orientation in zero gravity, produced by parabolic flight. *Annals of the New York Academy of Sciences*, 1971, *188*, 217–223.

Kelso, J. A. S., & Frekany, G. A. Coding processes in preselected and constrained movements: Effect of vision. *Acta Psychologica*, 1978, *42*, 145–161.

Kinney, J. A. S., & Luria, S. M. Conflicting visual and tactual-kinesthetic stimulation. *Perception and Psychophysics*, 1970, *8*, 189–192.

Kinney, J. A. S., McKay, C. L., Luria, S. M., & Gratto, C. L. *The improvement of divers' compensation for underwater distortions* (NSMRL Report No. 633). U.S. Naval Submarine Medical Center, Groton, Conn., 1970.

Kobrick, J. L. Effects of hypoxia on peripheral visual response to dim stimuli. *Perceptual and Motor Skills*, 1975, *41*, 467–474.

Koehler, W., & Dinnerstein, D. Figural after-effects in kinaesthesis. In *Miscellanea Psychologia Albert Michotte*. Paris: Librarie Philosophique, 1947.

Koehler, W., & Wallach, H. Figural after-effects: An investigation of visual processes. *Proceedings of the American Philosophical Society*, 1944, *88*, 269–357.

Koffka, K. *Principles of gestalt psychology*. New York: Harcourt, 1935.

Kohler, I. *Ueber Aufbau und Wandlungen der Wahrnehmungswelt; Insbesondere Ueber "bedingte Empfindungen."* Vienna: Rohrer, 1951.

Kohler, I. Die Methode des Brillenversuchs in der Wahrnehmungspsychologie; mit Bemerkungen zur Lehre der Adaptation. *Zeitschrift fuer Experimentelle und Angewandte Psychologie,* 1956, *3,* 381–417.

Kohler, I. Experiments with goggles. *Scientific American,* 1962, *206*(5), 62–86.

Kohler, I. The formation and transformation of the perceptual world (H. Fiss, Trans.). *Psychological Issues,* 1964, *3,* 1-173. (Monograph)

Kohler, I. Die Zusammenarbeit der Sinne und das allgemeine Adaptationsproblem. In W. Metzger (Ed.), *Handbuch der Psychologie.* Goettingen: Verlag fuer Psychologie, 1966.

Kornheiser, A. S. Adaptation to laterally displaced vision: A review. *Psychological Bulletin,* 1976, *83,* 783–816.

Kornmueller, A. E. Eine experimentelle Anaesthesie der aeusseren Augenmuskeln am Menschen und ihre Auswirkungen. *Journal fuer Psychologie und Neurologie,* 1930, *41,* 354-366.

Kottenhoff, H. Situational and personal influences on space perception with experimental spectacles. *Acta Psychologica,* 1957, *13,* 79-97; 151-161.

Kottenhoff, H. *Was ist richtiges Sehen mit Umkehrbrillen und in welchem Sinne stellt sich das Sehen um?* Anton Hain, Germany: Meisnheim an Glan, 1961.

Kratochwill, T. R. *Single subject research: Strategies for evaluating change.* New York: Academic Press, 1978.

Lackner, J. R. A device for investigating adaptation to visual rearrangement. *Journal of Psychology,* 1973, *85,* 137-141.

Lackner, J. R. Adaptation to displaced vision: Role of proprioception. *Perceptual and Motor Skills,* 1974, *38,* 1251-1256.

Lackner, J. R. Influence of abnormal postural and sensory conditions on human sensorimotor localization. *Environmental Biology and Medicine,* 1976, *2,* 139-177.

Lackner, J. R. Adaptation to visual and proprioceptive rearrangement: Origin of the differential effectiveness of active and passive movements. *Perception and Psychophysics,* 1977, *21,* 55-59.

Lackner, J. R., & Graybiel, A. Elicitation of vestibular side effects by regional vibration of the head. *Aerospace Medicine,* 1974, *45,* 1267-1272.

Lackner, J. R., & Teixeira, R. A. Optokinetic motion sickness: Continuous head movements attenuate the visual induction of apparent self-rotation and symptoms of motion sickness. *Aviation, Space, and Environmental Medicine,* 1977, *48,* 248-253.

Lackner, J. R., & Zabkar, J. J. Proprioceptive information about target location suppresses autokinesis. *Vision Research,* 1977, *17,* 1225-1229.

Lee, D. N. The functions of vision. In H. L. Pick, Jr. & E. Saltzman (Eds.), *Modes of perceiving and processing information.* Hillsdale, N.J.: Lawrence Erlbaum, 1978.

Leibowitz, H. W., & Hennessy, R. T. The laser optometer and some implications for behavioral research. *American Psychologist,* 1975, *30,* 349-352.

Lentz, J. M. & Collins, W. E. Motion sickness susceptibility and related behavioral characteristics in men and women. *Aviation, Space, and Environmental Medicine,* 1977, *48,* 316-322.

Lenzi, G. L., Pompeiano, O., & Satoh, T. Transmission of labyrinthine volleys through the vestibular nuclei during sleep. *Archives Italiennes de Biologie,* 1969, *107,* 19–42.

Loftus, J. P. (Ed.). *Symposium on motion sickness with special reference to weightlessness* (AMRL-TDR-63-25). Wright-Patterson Air Force Base, Ohio: 6570th Aerospace Medical Research Laboratories, Aerospace Medical Division, June 1963.

Long, G. M., Ambler, R. K., & Guedry, F. E. Relationship between perceptual style and reactivity to motion. *Journal of Applied Psychology,* 1975, *60,* 599–605.

Luria, S. M. Stereoscopic and resolution acuity with various fields of view. *Science,* 1969, *164,* 452–453.

MacKay, D. M. Visual stability. *Investigative Ophthalmology,* 1972, *11,* 518-524.

MacKay, D. M. Visual stability and voluntary eye movements. In R. Jung (Ed.), *Handbook of sensory physiology* (Vol. VII/3). Berlin: Springer-Verlag, 1973.

MacLeod, R. B. Perceptual constancy and the problem of motivation. *Canadian Journal of Psychology,* 1949, *3,* 57-66.

MacLeod, R. B. Phenomenology. In D. L. Sills (Ed.), *International encyclopedia of the social sciences* (Vol. 12). New York: MacMillan, 1968.

MacLeod, R. B. Psychological phenomenology: A propaedeutic to a scientific psychology. In J. R. Royce (Ed.), *Toward unification in psychology.* Toronto: University of Toronto Press, 1970.

MacLeod, R. B. *The persistent problems of psychology* (M. Henle & M. Wertheimer, Eds.). Pittsburgh: Duquesne University Press, 1975.

Marks, L. E. *The unity of the senses.* New York: Academic Press, 1978.

Matin, L. Eye movements and perceived visual direction. In D. Jameson & L. M. Hurvich (Eds.), *Handbook of sensory physiology* (Vol. VII/4). Berlin: Springer-Verlag, 1972.

Matin, L. Saccades and extraretinal signal for visual direction. In R. A. Monty & J. W. Senders (Eds.), *Eye movements and psychological processes.* Hillsdale, N.J.: Lawrence Erlbaum, 1976.

Matin, L., Pearce, D., Matin, E., & Kibler, G. Visual perception of direction in the dark: Roles of local sign, eye movements, and ocular proprioception. *Vision Research,* 1966, *6,* 453-470.

McCarter, A., & Mikaelian, H. H. The role of acceleration information in prism adaptation. *Perception and Psychophysics,* 1978, *23,* 21-26.

McDonnell, P. M., & Abraham, W. Observations on a new illusion demonstrating touch dominance of vision. *Perceptual and Motor Skills,* 1978, *46,* 1240-1242.

McDonnell, P. M., & Duffett, J. Vision and touch: A reconsideration of conflict between the two senses. *Canadian Journal of Psychology,* 1972, *26,* 171-180.

McGinty, D. J., & Siegel, J. M. Neuronal activity patterns during rapid-eye movement sleep: Relation to waking patterns. In R. R. Drucker-Colin & J. L. McGaugh (Eds.), *Neurobiology of sleep and memory.* New York: Academic Press, 1977.

McGrath, M. J., & Cohen, D. B. REM sleep facilitation of adaptive waking behavior: A review of the literature. *Psychological Bulletin,* 1978, *85,* 24-57.

McLaughlin, S. C., Rifkin, K. I., & Webster, R. G. Oculomotor adaptation to wedge prisms with no part of the body seen. *Perception and Psychophysics,* 1966, *1,* 452-458.

McLaughlin, S. C., & Webster, R. C. Changes in straightahead eye position during adaptation to wedge prisms. *Perception & Psychophysics,* 1967, *2,* 37-44.

Medoff, J. A double-blind evaluation of the anti-emetic efficacy of benzquinamide, prochlorperazine and trimethobenzamide in office practice. *Current Therapeutic Research,* 1970, *12,* 706-710.

Melamed, L. E., Wallace, B., & Seyfried, B. Acceleration information for prism adaptation need not be reafferent: A comment on McCarter and Mikaelian (1978). *Perception and Psychophysics,* 1979, *25,* 70-72.

Melvill Jones, G. Origin, significance and amelioration of coriolis illusions from the semicircular canals: A non-mathematical appraisal. *Aerospace Medicine,* 1970, *41,* 483-490.

Melvill Jones, G. The vestibular system for eye movement control. In R. A. Monty & J. W. Senders (Eds.), *Eye movements and psychological processes.* Hillsdale, N.J.: Lawrence Erlbaum, 1976.

Melvill Jones, G., & Davies, P. Adaptation of cat vestibulo-ocular reflex to 200 days of optically reversed vision. *Brain Research,* 1976, *103,* 551-554.

Melvill Jones, G., & Gonshor, A. Extreme vestibular habituation to long-term reversal of vision during natural head movements. *Proceedings of the annual scientific meeting, Aerospace Medical Association,* Bal Harbour, Florida, May, 1972.

Melvill Jones, G., & Gonshor, A. Goal-directed flexibility in the vestibulo-ocular reflex arc. In G. Lennerstrand & P. Bach-y-Rita (Eds.), *Basic mechanisms of ocular motility and their clinical implications.* Oxford: Pergamon Press, 1975.

Merton, P. A. The accuracy of directing the eye and the hand in the dark. *Journal of Physiology,* 1961, *156,* 555-577.

Merton, P. A. Absence of conscious position sense in the human eye. In M. B. Bender (Ed.), *The oculomotor system.* New York: Harper and Row, 1964.

Metzger, W. Optische Untersuchungen am Ganzfeld. II. Zur Phaenomenologie des homogenen Ganzfelds. *Psychologische Forschung,* 1930, *13,* 6-29.

Miles, F. A., & Fuller, J. H. Adaptive plasticity in the vestibulo-ocular responses of the rhesus monkey. *Brain Research,* 1974, *80,* 512-516.

Miles, W. R. Movement interpretations of the silhouette of a revolving fan. *Amerian Journal of Psychology,* 1931, *43,* 392-405.

Miller, E. A. Interaction of vision and touch in conflict and nonconflict form perception tasks. *Journal of Experimental Psychology,* 1972, *96,* 114-123.

Miller, R. J., & Leibowitz, H. W. A signal detection analysis of hypnotically induced narrowing of the peripheral visual field. *Journal of Abnormal Psychology,* 1976, *85,* 445-454.

Money, K. E. Motion sickness. *Physiological Reviews,* 1970, *50,* 1-39.

Money, K. E., & Myles, W. S. Motion sickness and other vestibulo-gastric illnesses. In R. F. Naunton (Ed.), *The vestibular system.* New York: Academic Press, 1975.

Moruzzi, G. The functional significance of sleep with particular regard to the brain mechanisms underlying consciousness. In J. C. Eccles (Ed.), *Brain and conscious experience.* Berlin: Springer-Verlag, 1966.

Neisser, U. *Cognition and reality: Principles and implications of cognitive psychology.* San Francisco: Freeman, 1976.

Neisser, U. Perceiving, anticipating, and imagining. In C. W. Savage (Ed.), *Perception and cognition issues in the foundations of psychology* (Vol. IX). Minneapolis: University of Minnesota Press, 1978.

Ogle, K. N. Distortion of the images by prisms. *Journal of the Optical Society of America,* 1951, *41,* 1023-1028.

Ogle, K. N. Distortion of the image by ophthalmic prisms. *American Medical Association Archives of Ophthalmology,* 1952, *47,* 121-131.

Ogle, K. N. *Optics: An introduction for ophthalmologists* (2nd ed.). Springfield, Ill.: C. C. Thomas, 1968.

Osterhammel, P., Terkildsen, K., & Zilstorff, K. Vestibular habituation in ballet dancers. *Advances in Oto-Rhino-Laryngology,* 1970, *17,* 158-166.

Over, R. An experimentally induced conflict between vision and proprioception. *British Journal of Psychology,* 1966, *57,* 335-341.

Paap, K. R. Perceptual consequences of post-tetanic-potentiation: An alternative explanation for adaptation to wedge prisms (Doctoral dissertation, University of Wisconsin, 1975). *Dissertation Abstracts International,* 1976, *36,* 4737B. (University, Microfilms No. 75-28, 808)

Paap, K. R., & Ebenholtz, S. M. Concomitant direction and distance aftereffects of sustained convergence: A muscle potentiation explanation for eye-specific adaptation. *Perception and Psychophysics,* 1977, *21,* 307-314.

Parker, D. M. A psychophysiological test for motion-sickness susceptibility. *Journal of General Psychology,* 1971, *85,* 87-92.

Parker, D. M., Schaefer, J., & Cohen, E. The effect of past experience on motion sickness produced by visual stimuli. *Journal of General Psychology*, 1972, *87*, 65–68.

Peterson, J., & Peterson, J. K. Does practice with inverting lenses make vision normal? *Psychological Monographs*, 1938, *50*, (Whole No. 225).

Pfaltz, C. R. Vestibular habituation and central compensation. *Advances in Oto-Rhino-Laryngology*, 1977, *22*, 136–142.

Pfister, H. *Ueber das Verhalten der Huehner beim Tragen von Prismen*. Unpublished doctoral dissertation, University of Innsbruck, 1955.

Pick, H. L. Visual coding of nonvisual spatial information. In R. B. MacLeod & H. L. Pick (Eds.), *Perception: Essays in honor of James J. Gibson*, Ithaca, New York: Cornell University Press, 1974.

Pick, H. L., Jr., & Hay, J. C. Adaptation to prismatic distortion. *Psychonomic Science*, 1964, *1*, 199–200.

Pick, H. L., Jr., & Hay, J. C. A passive test of the Held reafference hypothesis. *Perceptual and Motor Skills*, 1965, *20*, 1070–1072.

Piercy, M., Poeck, K., & Held, R. The eighteenth international symposium of neuropsychology. Neuropsychologia, 1976, *14*, 265–268.

Pirie, N. W. (Ed.). *The biology of space travel*. London: The Institute of Biology, 1961.

Pitblado, C., & Mirabile, C. S., Jr. Relationship between visual orientation and susceptibility to motion sickness. *Perceptual and Motor Skills*, 1977, *44*, 267–273.

Polyak, S. L. *The retina*. Chicago: University of Chicago Press, 1941.

Polyak, S. L. *The vertebrate visual system*. Chicago: University of Chicago Press, 1957.

Pompeiano, O. Vestibular influences during sleep. In H. H. Kornhuber (Ed.), *Handbook of sensory physiology* (Vol. VI/1). Berlin: Springer-Verlag, 1974.

Posner, M. I., Nissen, M. J., & Klein, R. M. Visual dominance: An information-processing account of its origins and significance. *Psychological Review*, 1976, *83*, 157–171.

Potvin, A. R., Sadoff, M., & Billingham, J. Motion sickness and otolith sensitivity: A pilot study of habituation to linear acceleration. *Aviation, Space, and Environmental Medicine*, 1977, *48*, 1068–1075.

Prévost, F., De Koninck, J., Barry, W., & Broughton, R. Inversion of the visual field and REM sleep: Experimental reconciliation of the P hypothesis and scip hypothesis. *Sleep Research*, 1974, *3*, 89.

Prévost, F., De Koninck, J., & Proulx, G. Stage REM rapid eye movements following visual inversion: Further investigation and replication. *Sleep Research*, 1975, *4*, 57.

Raphan, T., & Cohen, B. Brainstem mechanisms for rapid and slow eye movements. *Annual Review of Physiology*, 1978, *40*, 527–552.

Rausch, E. *Struktur und Metrik figural-optischer Wahrnehmung*. Frankfurt: W. Kramer & Co., 1952.

Reason, J. T. Individual differences in motion sickness susceptibility: A further test of the 'receptivity' hypothesis. *British Journal of Psychology*, 1969, *60*, 321–328.

Redding, G. M. Visual adaptation to tilt and displacement: Same or different processes? *Perception and Psychophysics*, 1973, *14*, 193–200.

Redding, G. M. Decay of visual adaptation to tilt and displacement. *Perception and Psychophysics*, 1975, *17*, 203–208.

Redding, G. M. Additivity in adaptation to optical tilt. *Journal of Experimental Psychology: Human Perception and Performance*, 1978, *4*, 178–190.

Richards, W. Visual space perception. In E. C. Carterette & M. P. Friedman (Eds.), *Handbook of perception* (Vol. V). New York: Academic Press, 1975.

Rierdan, J. E., & Wapner, S. Adaptive changes in the relationship between visual and tactual-kinesthetic perception. *Psychonomic Science*, 1967, *7*, 61–62.

Riesen, A. H. Sensory deprivation: Facts in search of a theory. Studying perceptual development using the technique of sensory deprivation. *Journal of Nervous and Mental Disorders,* 1961, *132,* 21-25.

Rock, I. *The nature of perceptual adaptation.* New York: Basic Books, 1966.

Rock, I. *Orientation and form.* New York: Academic Press, 1973.

Rock, I. The perception of disoriented figures. *Scientific American,* 1974, *230*(1), 78-85.

Rock, I. *An introduction to perception.* New York: Macmillan, 1975.

Rock, I., Goldberg, J., & Mack, A. Immediate correction and adaptation based on viewing a prismatically displaced scene. *Perception and Psychophysics,* 1966, *1,* 351-354.

Rock, I., & Harris, C. S. Vision and touch. *Scientific American,* 1967, *216*(5), 96-104.

Rock, I., & Victor, J. Vision and touch: An experimentally created conflict between the two senses. *Science,* 1964, *143,* 594-596.

Ross, H. E. *Behavior and perception in strange environments.* New York: Basic Books, 1975.

Rossi, P. J. Adaptation and negative aftereffect to lateral optical displacement in newly hatched chicks. *Science,* 1968, *160,* 430-432.

Ryan, T. A., & Ryan, M. S. Geographical orientation. *American Journal of Psychology,* 1940, *53,* 204-215.

Ryback, R. S., Rudd, R. E., Matz, G. J., & Jennings, C. L. Motion sickness in USAF flying personnel. *Aerospace Medicine,* 1970, *41,* 672-677.

Sabra, A. I. Sensation and inference in Alhazen's theory of visual perception. In P. K. Machamer & R. G. Turnbull (Eds.), *Studies in perception.* Columbus: Ohio State University, 1978.

Sanderson, F. H., & Whiting, H. T. A. Dynamic visual acuity a possible factor in catching performance. *Journal of Motor Behavior,* 1978, *10,* 7-14.

Sandstroem, C. I. *Orientation in the present space.* Stockholm: Almquist & Wiksell, 1951.

Schiff, W., Caviness, J. A., & Gibson, J. J. Persistent fear responses in rhesus monkeys to the optical stimulus of "looming." *Science,* 1962, *136,* 982-983.

Schilder, P. *The image and appearance of the human body.* London: Kegan Paul, 1935.

Schlodtmann, W. Ein Beitrag zur Lehre von der optischen Lokalisation bei Blindgeborenen. *Archiv fuer Ophthalmologie,* 1902, *54,* 256-267.

Scholl, K. Vom Zielen und Zeigen. *Zeitschrift fuer die gesamte Neurologie und Psychiatrie,* 1925, *97,* 217-236.

Scholl, K. Das raeumliche Zusammenarbeiten von Auge und Hand. *Deutsche Zeitschrift fuer Nervenheilkunde,* 1926, *92,* 280-303.

Sedgwick, H. A. The visible horizon: A potential source of visual information for the perception of size and distance (Doctoral dissertation, Cornell University, 1973). *Dissertation Abstracts International,* 1973, *34,* 1301B-1302B. (University Microfilms No. 73-22, 530)

Sekuler, R. W., & Bauer, J., Jr. Adaptation to prismatic displacements: Hand position and target location. *Journal of Experimental Psychology,* 1966, *72,* 207-212.

Sells, S. B., & Berry, C. A. (Eds.). *Human factors in jet and space travel.* New York: The Ronald Press Company, 1961.

Senden, M. von. *Space and sight: The perception of space and shape in congenitally blind patients before and after operation* (P. Heath, Trans.). London: Methuen, 1960.

Shapiro, A. Dreaming and the physiology of sleep: A critical review of some empirical data and a proposal for a theoretical model of sleep and dreaming. *Experimental Neurology,* 1967, supplement, *4,* 56-81.

Shebilske, W. L. Visuomotor coordination in visual direction and position constancies. In W. Epstein (Ed.), *Stability and constancy in visual perception: Mechanisms and processes.* New York: Wiley, 1977.

Sherrington, C. S. *The integrative action of the nervous system.* Cambridge: Cambridge University Press, 1906.

Sherrington, C. S. Observations on the sensual role of the proprioceptive nerve-supply of the extrinsic ocular muscles. *Brain,* 1918, *41,* 332-343.

Shillinger, G. L., Baumgarten, R. J. von, & Baldrighi, G. The gravity reference response, the rotation sensation, and other illusory sensations experienced in aircraft and space flight. *Space Life Sciences,* 1973, 4, 368-390.

Siipola, E. M. Studies in mirror drawing. *Psychological Monographs,* 1935, *46,* 66-77.

Simons, J. C., Walk, D. E., & Sears, C. W. Motion performance of pressure-suited subjects under zero and lunar gravity conditions. *Aerospace Medicine,* 1965, *36,* 406-414.

Singer, G., & Day, R. H. Spatial adaptation and aftereffect with optically transformed vision: Effects of active and passive responding and the relationship between test and exposure responses. *Journal of Experimental Psychology,* 1966, *7,* 725-731.

Singer, G., & Day, R. H. Visual capture of haptically judged depth. *Perception and Psychophysics,* 1969, *5,* 315-316.

Sjöberg, A. Experimental studies of the eliciting mechanism of motion sickness. In *Fourth symposium on the role of the vestibular organs in space exploration* (NASA SP-187). Washington, D.C.: National Aeronautics and Space Administration, 1970.

Skavenski, A. A. The nature and role of extra retinal eye position information in visual localization. In R. A. Monty & J. W. Senders (Eds.), *Eye movements and psychological processes.* Hillsdale, N.J.: Lawrence Erlbaum, 1976.

Slotnick, R. S. Efference, eye movements and adaptation to curvature (Doctoral dissertation, Standford University, 1967). *Dissertation Abstracts,* 1967, *28,* 370B. (University Microfilms No. 67-7974)

Slotnick, R. S. Adaptation to curvature distortion. *Journal of Experimental Psychology,* 1969, *81,* 441-448.

Smiles, K. A., Hite, D., Hyams, V. J., & Junker, A. M. Effect of labyrinthectomy on the dynamic vestibulo-ocular counterroll reflex in the rhesus monkey. *Aviation, Space, and Environmental Medicine,* 1975, *46,* 1017-1022.

Smith, K. U. Cybernetic theory and analysis of learning. In E. A. Bilodeau (Ed.), *Acquisition of skill.* New York: Academic Press, 1966.

Snyder, F. W. Vibration and vision. In C. A. Baker (Ed.), *Visual capabilities in the space environment.* New York: Pergamon Press, 1965.

Snyder, F. W., & Pronko, N. H. *Vision with spatial inversion.* Wichita: University of Wichita Press, 1952.

Snyder, F. W., & Snyder, C. W. Vision with spatial inversion: A follow-up study. *Psychological Record,* 1957, *17,* 20-31.

Southall, J. P. C. *Mirrors, prisms and lenses* (3rd ed.). New York: Dover Publications, 1964.

Spector, M., (Ed.). *Dizziness and vertigo: Diagnosis and treatment.* New York: Grune and Stratton, 1974.

Sperry, R. W. Effect of 180 degree rotation of the retinal field on visuomotor coordination. *Journal of Experimental Zoology,* 1943, *92,* 263-279.

Sperry, R. W. Neural basis of the spontaneous optokinetic response produced by visual neural inversion. *Journal of Comparative and Physiological Psychology,* 1950, *43,* 482-489.

Spiegelberg, H. *The phenomenological movement: A historical introduction* (2nd ed.). The Hague: Martinus Nijhoff, 1965.

Stahle, J. (Ed.). *Vestibular function on earth and in space.* Oxford: Pergamon Press, 1968.

Starch, D. A demonstration of the trial and error method of learning. *Psychological Bulletin,* 1910, *7,* 20-23.

Steinman, R. M. Role of eye movements in maintaining a phenomenally clear and stable world. In R. A. Monty & J. W. Senders (Eds.), *Eye movements and psychological processes.* Hillsdale, N.J.: Lawrence Erlbaum, 1976.

Stelmach, G. E. (Ed.). *Motor control: Issues and trends.* New York: Academic Press, 1976.

Stevens, J. K., Emerson, R. C., Gerstein, G. L., Kallos, T., Neufeld, G. R., Nichols, C. W., & Rosenquist, A. C. Paralysis of the awake human: Visual perceptions. *Vision Research,* 1976, *16,* 93–98.

Stratton, G. M. Some preliminary experiments in vision without inversion of the retinal image. *Psychological Review,* 1896, *3,* 611–617.

Stratton, G. M. Upright vision and the retinal image. *Psychological Review,* 1897, *4,* 182–187. (a)

Stratton, G. M. Vision without inversion of the retinal image. *Psychological Review,* 1897, *4,* 341–360, 463–481. (b)

Stratton, G. M. The spatial harmony of touch and sight. *Mind,* 1899, *8,* 492–505.

Tastevin, J. En partant de l'experience d'Aristote. *L'Encephale,* 1937, *1,* 57–84, 140–158.

Taylor, J. G. *The behavioral basis of perception.* New Haven: Yale University Press, 1962.

Taylor, J. G. The prism illusion: A function of dislocated equivalence classes. *Perceptual and Motor Skills,* 1966, *22,* 219–232.

Templeton, W. B., Howard, I. P., & Lowman, A. E. Passively generated adaptation to prismatic distortion. *Perceptual and Motor Skills,* 1966, *22,* 140–142.

Teuber, H. L. Perception. In J. Field, H. W. Magoun, & V. E. Hall (Eds.), *Handbook of Physiology: Section 1. Neurophysiology* (Vol. 3). Washington, D.C.: American Physiological Society, 1960.

Teuber, H. L., Battersby, W. S., & Bender, M. B. *Visual field defects after penetrating missile wounds of the brain.* Cambridge, Mass.: Harvard University Press, 1960.

Thinès, G. *Phenomenology and the science of behavior.* London: George Allen and Unwin, 1977.

Thorpe, W. H. *Learning and instinct in animals* (2nd ed.). Cambridge, Mass.: Harvard University Press, 1963.

Thurner, F. *Studies of artificially disturbed sensory coordination in man* (AFOSR 67-1548). Innsbruck, Austria: Institut fuer Psychologie der Universitaet Innsbruck, 1967. (NTIS No. AD-655 128)

Trowbridge, C. C. On fundamental methods of orientation and imaginary maps. *Science,* 1913, *38,* 888–897.

Tschiassny, K. Perrotatory nystagmus in the ballet dancer, pigeon and blind person. *Annals of Otology,* 1957, *66,* 641.

Uhlarik, J. J. Role of cognitive factors on adaptation to prismatic displacement. *Journal of Experimental Psychology,* 1973, *98,* 223–232.

Volkmann, F. C., Schick, A. M. L., & Riggs, L. A. Time course of visual inhibition during voluntary saccades. *Journal of the Optical Society of America,* 1969, *58,* 562–569.

Walker, J. T., & Shea, K. S. A tactual size aftereffect contingent on hand position. *Journal of Experimental Psychology,* 1974, *103,* 668–674.

Wallace, B., Melamed, L. E., & Kaplan, C. Movement and illumination factors in adaptation to prismatic viewing. *Perception and Psychophysics,* 1973, *13,* 164–168.

Wallach, H. Informational discrepancy as a basis of perceptual adaptation. In S. J. Freedman (Ed.), *The neuropsychology of spatially oriented behavior.* Homewood, Ill.: Dorsey Press, 1968.

Wallach, H. *On perception.* New York: Quadrangle, 1976.

Wallach, H., & Canal, T. Two kinds of adaptation in the constancy of visual direction. *Perception and Psychophysics,* 1976, *19,* 445–449.

Wallach, H., & Floor, L. On the relation of adaptation to field displacement during head movements to the constancy of visual direction. *Perception & Psychophysics*, 1970, *8*, 95–98.

Wallach, H., & Frey, K. J. Adaptation in the constancy of visual direction measured by a one-trial method. *Perception & Psychophysics*, 1969, *5*, 249–252.

Wallach, H., & Frey, K. J. Adaptation in distance perception based on oculomotor cues. *Perception and Psychophysics*, 1972, *11*, 77–83.

Wallach, H., Frey, K. J., & Romney, G. Adaptation to field displacement during head movement unrelated to the constancy of visual direction. *Perception & Psychophysics*, 1969, *5*, 253–256.

Wallach, H., & Kravitz, J. H. The measurement of the constancy of visual direction and of its adaptation. *Psychonomic Science*, 1965, *2*, 217–218. (a)

Wallach, H., & Kravitz, J. H. Rapid adaptation in the constancy of visual direction with active and passive rotation. *Psychonomic Science*, 1965, *3*, 165–166. (b)

Wallach, H., & Kravitz, J. Adaptation in the constancy of visual direction tested by measuring the constancy of auditory direction. *Perception & Psychophysics*, 1968, *4*, 299–303.

Wallach, H., Kravitz, J. H., & Landauer, J. A passive condition for rapid adaptation to displaced visual direction. *American Journal of Psychology*, 1963, *76*, 568–578.

Walls, G. L. The problem of visual direction. *American Journal of Optometry & Archives of American Academy of Optometry*, 1951. (Monograph No. 117)

Warren, D. H., & Cleaves, W. T. Visual–proprioceptive interaction under large amounts of conflict. *Journal of Experimental Psychology*, 1971, *90*, 206–214.

Warren, D. H., & Platt, B. B. The subject: A neglected factor in recombination research. *Perception*, 1974, *3*, 421–438.

Warren, D. H., & Platt, B. B. Understanding prism adaptation: An individual differences approach. *Perception and Psychophysics*, 1975, *17*, 337–345.

Weinstein, S., Sersen, E. A., & Weinstein, D. S. An attempt to replicate a study of disarranged eye–hand coordination. *Perceptual and Motor Skills*, 1964, *18*, 629–632.

Welch, R. B. Adaptation to prism-displaced vision: The importance of target pointing. *Perception & Psychophysics*, 1969, *5*, 305–309.

Welch, R. B. Prism adaptation: The "target-pointing effect" as a function of exposure trials. *Perception and Psychophysics*, 1971, *9*, 102–104.

Welch, R. B. Research on adaptation to rearranged vision: 1966–1974. *Perception*, 1974, *3*, 367–392.

Welch, R. B. *Perceptual modification: Adapting to altered sensory environments*. New York: Academic Press, 1978.

Welch, R. B., Widawski, M. H., Harrington, J., & Warren, D. H. An examination of the relationship between visual capture and prism adaptation. *Perception and Psychophysics*, 1979, *25*, 126–132.

Wendt, G. R. The form of the vestibular eye-movement response in man. *Psychological Monographs*, 1936, *47*, 311–328.

Wendt, G. R. Vestibular functions. In S. S. Stevens (Ed.), *Handbook of experimental psychology*. New York: Wiley, 1951.

White, W. J., & Monty, R. A. Vision and unusual gravitational forces. In C. A. Baker (Ed.), *Visual capabilities in the space environment*. New York: Pergamon Press, 1965.

Whiteside, T. C. D. *The problems of vision in flight at high altitude*. London: Butterworths Scientific Publications, 1957.

Whitteridge, D. Central control of eye movements. In J. Field, H. W. Magoun, & V. E. Hall (Eds.), *Handbook of Physiology: Sec. 1. Neurophysiology* (Vol. II). Washington, D.C.: American Physiological Society, 1960.

Williams, I. D. Evidence for recognition and recall schemata. *Journal of Motor Behavior*, 1978, *10*, 45–52.

Witkin, H. A. Perception of body position and of the position of the visual field. *Psychological Monographs*, 1949, *63*(7, Whole No. 302).

Wohlwill, J. F. Perceptual learning. *Annual Review of Psychology*, 1966, *17*, 201-232.

Wood, C. D. Medications for vertigo and motion sickness. *American Journal of Nursing*, 1966, *66*, 1764-1767.

Wood, C. D., & Graybiel, A. A theory of motion sickness based on pharmacological reactions. *Clinical Pharmacology and Therapeutics*, 1970, *11*, 621-629.

Woodworth, R. S. Vision and localization during eye movements. *Psychological Bulletin*, 1906, *3*, 68-70.

Woodworth, R. S. *Experimental psychology*. New York: Holt, 1938.

Wooster, M. Certain factors in the development of a new spatial coordination. *Psychological Monographs*, 1923, *32*(4, Whole No. 146).

Wundt, W. Zur Theorie der raeumlichen Gesichtswahrnehmungen. *Philosophische Studien*, 1898, *14*, 11.

Yarbus, A. L. *Eye movements and vision*. New York: Plenum Press, 1967.

Yin, R. K. Looking at upside-down faces. *Journal of Experimental Psychology*, 1969, *81*, 141-145.

Yuganov, E. M., Gorshkov, A. I., Kasyan, I. I., Bryanov, I. I., Kolosov, I. A., Kopanev, V. I., Lebedev, V. I., Popov, N. I., & Solodovnic, F. A. Vestibular reactions of cosmonauts during the flight in the "Voskhod" spaceship. *Aerospace Medicine*, 1966, *37*, 691-694.

Zimmerman, J. T., Stoyva, J. M., & Metcalf, D. Distorted visual feedback and augmented REM sleep. *Psychophysiology*, 1970, *7*, 298.

Zimmerman, J. T., Stoyva, J. M., & Reite, M. L. Spatially rearranged vision and REM sleep: A lack of effect. *Biological Psychiatry*, 1978, *13*, 301-316.

Subject Index

R

S

W

www.ingramcontent.com/pod-product-compliance
Lightning Source LLC
LaVergne TN
LVHW011107300926
849160LV00008B/301
* 9 7 8 1 9 3 2 8 4 6 0 2 7 *